SUPERVISION, LEARNING AND ASSESSMENT IN **CLINICAL PRACTICE**

A Guide for Nurses, Midwives and Other Health Professionals

FOURTH EDITION

SUPERVISION, LEARNING AND ASSESSMENT IN CLINICAL PRACTICE

A Guide for Nurses, Midwives and Other Health Professionals

EDITED BY

Sue Woodward, PhD MSc PGCEA RN FRCN
Head of Clinical Education
Florence Nightingale Faculty of Nursing
    and Midwifery
King's College London
UK

Sam Bassett, DHC, MA, BSc(Hons), DipHe Mid, RGN, PGSHSCE, SFHEA
Lead Midwife for Education
Florence Nightingale Faculty of Nursing
    and Midwifery
King's College London
UK

FOREWORD BY

Ci Stuart, BAppSci MED RN RM MTD
City & Guilds Work Based Assessors' Awards
    D32 & D33
Formerly Senior Lecturer in Nursing and
    Midwifery, Faculty of Health and
Wellbeing
Sheffield Hallam University

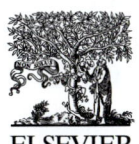

ELSEVIER

Notice

ISBN: 9780702077609

Printed in Poland

Last digit is the print number: 9 8 7 6 5 4 3 2 1

Content Strategist: Robert Edwards
Content Development Specialist: Robert Edwards
Project Manager: Kamatchi Madhavan
Design: Reid Margaret
Illustration Buyer: Narayanan Ramakrishnan
Marketing Manager: Tudin Belinda

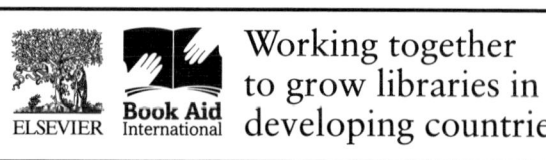

CONTENTS

LIST OF CONTRIBUTORS

Julie Bliss
Northwestern Michigan College

Chris Carter
Birmingham City University

Nigel Davies
University of East London

Michelle Ellis
City University of London

Jane Fish
Nurse

Yvonne Halpin
London South Bank University

Shaun Heath
University of Greenwich

Julie MacLaren
City University of London

Valerie Nangle
University of East London

Lynn Quinlivan
University of Hertfordshire

Jo Rixon
Bucks New University

Daniel Soto-Prieto
University of East London

Kathy Wilson
Middlesex University

The Purposes and Nature of Assessment and Clinical Assessment

Valerie Nangle and Nigel Davies

CHAPTER CONTENTS

INTRODUCTION

In this chapter, we consider the necessity for assessment in the health care professions together with the educational and professional purposes of assessment. Assessment will be explored in conjunction with the potential for short- and longer-term positive contributions for student learning. Mindful of the context of assessment being discussed throughout this book, this chapter will also look at the complexities involved with clinical assessment. The phrase 'complexities of clinical assessment' is used with intent on the assumption that, for many readers of this book, the nature of learning and assessing in the clinical setting will be close to their hearts as a direct result of significant and meaningful personal experiences of having been a learner and been assessed, and having worked and been an assessor, in that setting.

We have used the term 'assessment' in this chapter as a global term incorporating tests, assignments and examinations of coursework (whether oral or written), the judgement of performance during clinical practice and any other ways of measuring professional learning, competency and proficiency. Assessment of theory and clinical competence is central to any professional programme to ensure that health care practitioners are safe and competent as part of the obligation of public protection (Currer 2009). The term 'assessor' is used to encompass all clinical practitioners who support and assess students during practice, or lecturers from higher-education institutions (HEIs) who assess academic work and/or clinical practice. Sometimes as an assessor, you may be contributing to formative assessment through supervision and/or mentorship, whereas at other times, assessment will be summative with processes leading to grading and linked to progression and qualification awards. Formative assessment is considered more in Chapter 6 as part of the discussion about continuous assessment of practice.

THE NATURE OF ASSESSMENT

Assessment has an influence on all our lives in many and varying ways. Indeed, Rowntree (1987) points out that assessment is with us from the cradle to beyond the grave:

> Scarcely have we taken our first breath before we have a label fastened to our wrists, giving weight at, and method of, birth, and, somewhere, our first file (medical) has already been opened. And even in death we cannot escape the assessors – obituary-writers for the famous; just family, workmates and friends for the rest of us.
>
> **Rowntree (1987:xii)**

Consciously or subconsciously, we are assessing most of the time, be it at work, at home or at leisure. For students, this becomes all the more acute and consuming with discussion and attention to assessment not only taking place at university or on placement, but also a central feature of social life (Broadfoot 2012). As the results and consequences of "high stakes" assessment decisions can influence students confidence and career choices for the rest of their careers this is particularly important (Chimea et al 2020).

Passing judgement on people, on events, on ideas, on things and on values is part of the process of making sense of the world around us and where we stand in any given situation. Sometimes we judge to reassure ourselves – *I am glad I am not as selfish as she is* (and we might be rather lacking in self-awareness)! We are all assessors; even very young children are capable of making assessments. Ask a young child whether they like their new school, and, of course, the response will be either a yes or a no. The ability to respond implies that the child has activated the mental processes involving a mental review of perhaps the teachers, the other children, the events and the activities that they like or dislike and has applied more-or-less conscious criteria to what would constitute, for instance, a like or dislike of the teacher. In social settings and during social interactions, we may not be asked to justify our judgements and, indeed, may be most taken aback and even feel embarrassed if asked to do so. However, in educational and professional settings, such justification is frequently required because the process of assessment is overt, formalized and controlled. The criteria we use are often subject to scrutiny, and we are required to make our assessment decisions based on available evidence.

Much has been written about educational assessment because it is a legitimate concern of practitioners, learners, educators and those responsible for the development and accreditation of courses. Rightly or wrongly, assessment is assumed to be the nexus of learning. It might seem to be common sense, and, indeed, it is the 'custom and practice' today that students undertaking an educational programme should be assessed. It is easy to polarize to the position of unquestioning acceptance of the necessity for assessment because we have all been subject to some form of educational assessment ourselves, such as sitting through a timed, invigilated written examination or a multiple-choice paper, carrying out a practical procedure or enduring the agonies of an oral examination.

As a student of health care, you will have been observed, tested and questioned in both university and clinical settings, for example, while giving patient/client care, performing procedures in conjunction with care delivery and while giving individual and small group presentations. Consider Activity 1.1 and reflect on your own experiences of being assessed.

Activity 1.1   SWOT Analysis of Your Experience of Being Assessed

List the different ways in which you were assessed as part of your professional education.
- What were the strengths and weaknesses of each?
- What opportunities did the assessments give you for your future learning?
- Did you feel threatened by any of the assessment approaches?

The list of assessments you have experienced is undoubtably long. You may recall that, on your 'good' days, after completion of a span of duty, you left the clinical area feeling glad to have been on duty because you had had a positive and productive day where you had learnt from feedback from your assessors. Conversely, you may also remember 'bad' days when you may have cried and contemplated discontinuing your course! Staff might have been too busy to help and supervise what you were doing, you perhaps made errors, and staff and patients did not comment favourably about your contribution or work. This may have left you feeling emotionally and physically drained and demoralized, and you possibly perceived that your time had been wasted because you had not learnt on those types of days. Assessment can lead us to experience extremes of emotions and often provoke anxiety, something we consider later in the chapter in the section on resilience.

Learning and assessment in clinical practice continues to be seen as hit-and-miss affairs, with students' evaluations showing a range of positive and negative experiences, even in similar or the same environments. Clinical placements provide the realistic context for students in the health professions to develop the knowledge, skills, attitudes and values of a registered practitioner and enables integration of theory and practice while under supervision. Effective clinical placements are essential to the success of nursing and health professions educational programs (Henderson et al 2012; Stayt & Merriman 2013).

The quality of assessment in clinical practice is dependent on the clinical environment, the engagement, the dedication and motivation of the student to learn and, importantly, the clinical supervisor, clinical assessor or mentor. You may wish to consider Activity 1.2 at this point before moving on to the next section, which will consider why assessment is necessary.

Activity 1.2   Your Role Models

Think about someone who was an inspirational mentor or role model for you during your professional education.
- What key qualities did they have that you would now like to emulate to be a successful practice supervisor or mentor?
- Did you think about different people and different qualities for the different roles of mentor, supervisor and assessor?

THE PURPOSES OF ASSESSMENT

The nursing, midwifery and medical professions have required their trainees to be examined since the 19th century, with certificates being awarded on successful completion of study. Legislation starting with *The Midwives Act* in 1902, and subsequently during the 20th century for other professions, has led to a statutory requirement for professional registration based on not only completion of an education programme but also candidates being able to successfully pass examinations or other forms of assessment.

Eraut states that the major purpose of assessment is: 'to provide guidance and feedback to those involved in caring or learning activities or who influence the contexts in which they take place; and that assessment plays an important role in professional accountability and … in organizational or policy accountability for contextual factors. To this, it is useful to add that assessment is used to inform "high-stakes" decisions which have a major impact on the lives of clients or learners'. (Eraut 2003:177).

Professionally, then, nurses, midwives and allied health professionals have experienced assessment as part of the process to achieving professional registration and are likely to have internalized this value as part of the norm. However, to accept the necessity for assessment unthinkingly denies a complex debate concerning the purposes of assessments, the effects of assessment on learners both as individuals and as wider members of a peer group, and its impact on the curriculum and overall approaches to teaching and learning (Broadfoot 2012). Critically reviewing 'why' we assess may make us consider more carefully whether our assessments are fair, valid, reasonable and just. Both the Nursing and Midwifery Council (NMC) and the Health and Care Professions Council (HCPC) set out their expectations for assessment in their respective standards (Health and Care Professions Council 2017b; Nursing and Midwifery Council 2018c). As regulators, their primary function is protection of the public, but they also acknowledge that assessment occurs as part of practitioner preparation programmes for other reasons too. The following sections concentrate on what we see as the four main reasons commonly advanced for assessment in professional health care education:
- Selection for entry into the profession;
- For quality control and to ensure public protection obligations;
- As a form of motivation for students;
- To support teaching and learning.

Assessment for Entry Into the Profession
Application and Student Selection
Assessment for entry into a profession starts at the point of application for entry onto the professional course. Candidates are typically screened against two broad criteria:
- Academic qualifications and potential;
- Personal qualities and health care values associated with care and compassion.

Different professions will have different baseline levels of academic qualifications, with minimum requirements being set as professional standards. However, entry to some HEIs may require higher qualifications. In the UK, for nursing and midwifery, the NMC specify base-level entry for programmes leading to Registered Nurse or Registered Midwife which include English and mathematics at level 2 (General Certificate of Secondary Education [GCSE] pass equivalent) or for nursing associate programmes for this to be achieved as part of the course. Additionally, other higher qualifications are required, but with applications from candidates from increasingly diverse backgrounds, there are a variety of acceptable qualifications for entry, which now complement typical secondary school–level qualifications. These include entry based on completion of Access to Higher Education courses and other vocation qualifications, such as Business and Technology Education Council (BTEC) and National Vocational Qualification (NVQ) qualifications. The range of acceptable qualifications is now great, but most university admissions departments can provide advice on the equivalence of qualifications gained both in the UK and overseas. General information about routes into nursing can be found online as part of information sponsored by Health Education England (see https://www. hee.nhs.uk/our-work/capitalnurse/workstreams/routes-nursing) or by looking specifically at individual university websites.

A similar situation exists for Allied Health Professions, with entry-level qualifications being part determined by the programme requirements and by popularity and demand for places on some courses. There is wide variation in academic entry requirements across the 16 professions regulated by the HCPC. What is common across all professions is that this academic element of assessment for entry to the professions is judged against external criteria, based on assessment of potential students' prior learning.

In contrast, the other elements of assessment for entry to the education programme will be completed, in most cases, at the education institution to whom the student has applied. Generally, assessment processes involve a collaborative approach between universities and their practice partners, and, indeed, for nursing, this is a requirement for course approval. Different approaches have been used over the years for this stage of assessment, with debates about the efficacy and efficiency of traditional interviews. Following criticisms about standards of fundamental care associated with various failings or scandals in health care between 2005 and 2010 (Hutchison 2015), new procedures were introduced widely referred to as 'Values Based Recruitment' (Health Education England 2016) to ensure potential students espouse values of care and compassion in accordance with those expressed in the National Health Service (NHS) Constitution (Department of Health 2015). Practice-based staff are often asked to participate in this stage of the student assessment process and find attending student interviews interesting and developmental. If you are asked to participate, you may find it helpful to read further information about values-based recruitment (Health Education England 2016) or about the use and background to multiple mini-interviews that have been widely adopted for student recruitment across the health professions (Gale et al 2016; Morgan & Bendall 2016; Callwood et al 2018).

One of the assumptions implicit in this selection procedure is that only those who are deemed capable of successfully completing the programme are accepted and offered a place in the course. Disappointingly, the correlation between fulfilment of selection criteria and successful completion of education is low. Levels of discontinuation from preregistration health care practitioner courses have been a source of concern for some time, with estimates that this is currently between 15% and 25% (Health Education England 2018; Buchan et al 2019). Table 1.1 illustrates the

TABLE 1.1   Attrition Rates for Preregistration Nursing, Midwifery and Therapeutic Radiography Students in the UK: 2009–2015

Subject/Cohort	2009–10	2010–11	2011–12	2012–13	2013–14	2014–15	Trend	Average Attrition	% Change in Expected Attrition 2009–10 to 2014–15
Midwifery	15.0%	15.8%	14.2%	15.9%	12.1%	11.5%		13.6%	−23%
Nursing – adult	17.5%	16.4%	15.6%	13.6%	10.9%	9.6%		14.0%	−45%
Nursing – childern	14.4%	15.5%	14.0%	13.1%	11.0%	9.9%		13.0%	−31%
Nursing – learning disability	16.9%	17.2%	19.2%	15.2%	14.8%	18.3%		16.9%	8%
Nursing – mental health	19.2%	16.3%	14.4%	13.4%	12.0%	12.9%		14.7%	−33%
Radiography – therapeutic	35.1%	28.3%	21.5%	19.7%	17.0%	15.1%		22.8%	−57%
Total	**17.5%**	**16.4%**	**15.3%**	**13.6%**	**11.3%**	**10.5%**		**14.1%**	**−40%**

Source: HEE analysis of HESA student records, 2009–10 to 2016–17. *HEE,* Health Education England; *HESA,* Higher Education Statistics Agency.
From Table 3 page 29 from HEE RePAIR report (Health Education England 2018).

change for nursing, midwifery and therapeutic radiography students between 2010 and 2015 and suggests the situation may be improving in some fields of practice; however, caution is suggested because the impact of changes to student funding in nursing (the move away from funded bursaries to self-funded student loans) is not yet known. Exact rates are often difficult to find and are influenced by the varying inclusion and exclusion criteria. Health Education England's RePAIR (Reducing Pre-registration Attrition and Improving Retention) report noted the difficulty and used observed expected attrition rather than pure attrition, as reported by the Health Foundation (Buchan et al 2019), so that reasons such as students taking longer to complete courses were considered. A similar picture can be seen in many of the allied health professions, for example, as shown in therapeutic radiography (Health Education England 2018), occupational therapy (Ilott & Murphy 1999) and midwifery (Buchan et al 2019).

Internationally, the scale of the problem is difficult to quantify from the literature because of differences in definition and because of incomplete and noncomparable data. Results from the United States report even higher levels of attrition, with rates reported to be 50% for students enrolled in baccalaureate nursing programs and 47% for students enrolled in associate degree nursing programs (Newton & Moore 2009; Harris, Rosenberg, & O'Rourke 2013). Merkley (2016) reviews the literature from the United States and suggests similar reasons for attrition to the UK. With the change to student nurse financing since 2017, parallels with the United States may become more pertinent, especially as Health Education England (2018) already identified finances as one of the main factors cited by student nurses for discontinuation before the funding changes.

Hence, attrition rates are concerning, and factors contributing to attrition are complex with multiple reasons cited for attrition (Table 1.2), many enduring over time and related to the clinical learning environment, not just academic failure. Pertinent here, where we are considering selection for entry to health professional courses, is that the reasons for attrition casts some doubt over the assumption that those who perform best in current selection assessments are those who will complete the course or become the most capable as a result of further educational investment. You should therefore be mindful of the assessment approaches used for selection and also perhaps consider factors such as maturity, personality and motivation together with family support and the culture of the clinical settings. Readers are directed to discussions of these issues by Deary, Watson and Hogston (2003), Vergel et al (2018) and Buchan et al (2019).

Approaches and the nature of assessment right from this early stage are critical. Of the candidates we reject, we

TABLE 1.2	Reasons for Discontinuation of Nursing and Health Profession Programme over Four Decades	
Author	**Year**	**Reasons**
Health Education England (2018)	2018	• Financial pressures • Student confidence • Poor clinical supervision • Culture in clinical settings
Merkley (2016) (Review)	2016	• Multiple factors • Precourse preparation • Outside/family support • Lack of confidence in ability/competence
Waters (2010)	2010	• Financial pressures • Academic failure • Wrong career choice
Urwin et al (2010)	2009	• Academic failure • Wrong career choice • Personal problems • Financial pressures • Dissatisfaction with the course and clinical placements
White, Williams and Green (1999)	1999	• Academic failure • Personal problems • Wrong career choice
Braithwaite, Elzubeir & Stark (1994)	1994	• Academic failure • Disciplinary proceedings • Personal problems • Disillusionment
Lindop (1987)	1987	• Unsatisfactory performance • Not suited to nursing • Personality disorders

will never know how many would have become the sensitive and caring nurse, midwife or allied health professional with their potential may never realized. The academic high flyer may not be the better practitioner if she/he does not possess the right values such as compassion and empathy.

Ensuring Students are Fit to Qualify

The primary purpose of statutory regulation is to protect the public, with regulation of health professionals now well established. This has evolved since the first requirements for medical practitioners in the 19th century. Regulation by bodies such as the NMC or the HCPC is overseen in the UK by the Professional Standards Authority, who ensure that the statutes or laws relating to a range of health and social care practitioners, from acupuncturists to yoga therapists, are properly regulated (Professional Standards Authority 2019). The NMC regulates the practice of nurses, midwives and now nursing associates (Nursing and Midwifery Council 2019d), whereas the HCPC currently regulates 16 professions (Health and Care Professions Council 2018b). A feature of statutory regulation is that Parliament grants a profession the right to self-regulation. This means that a profession is given the right to maintain professional discipline, standards of conduct and entry into the profession.

The standards of conduct, performance and ethics of the NMC (Nursing and Midwifery Council 2018f) and the HCPC (Health and Care Professions Council 2016) are concerned with maintaining a standard of practice so that high-quality care is provided to the recipients of health care at all times. One subsidiary but important feature of this is to set the standards for education and training, which include how potential practitioners (i.e., students) will be assessed for entry to the profession. The NMC reviewed its nursing education standards in 2018 (Nursing and Midwifery Council 2018c, 2018d, 2018e) and has launched new midwifery standards in 2020 (Nursing and Midwifery Council 2019a). The HCPC published its most recent standards for education in 2017 (Health and Care Professions Council 2017b) and updated standards of proficiency for all professions regulated by the HCPC came into effect on 1st September 2023. The primary aim of the standards is to ensure public protection for anyone who receives care from someone who has a 'license' to practice. The public has a fundamental right to expect competence from the qualified professional in health care, and protection against unsafe, unscrupulous or incompetent practice. The recent updates followed criticisms, rightly or wrongly, mainly of nursing (Reeves, Ross & Harris 2014), but of other health professionals too, following national outrage about failings in care. A review of education was commissioned by Health Education England and led by an independent chair, Lord Willis, to look at the 'future shape of caring' professional education (Health Education England 2015).

The educational and professional outcome of preregistration education is a competent practitioner who is fit to practise. Both the NMC and the HCPC make it clear that fitness to practise is a registrant's suitability to be on the register without restrictions. This means that, before being admitted to the professional registers, there must be evidence that the student is able to uphold the standards of conduct, performance and ethics expected of registrants set out in the respective professional's codes of practice. It is incumbent upon practitioners to facilitate the learning and development of students so that evidence of fitness to practise is generated and provided through assessment processes. This evidence needs to be valid and reliable to

provide the objective data upon which assessment decisions of fitness to practise can then be made.

There is long-standing debate concerning the interpretation of competence in clinical practice (Yanhua & Watson 2011; Garside & Nhemachena 2013). Complications arise because of reported difficulties concerning the validity and reliability of competence assessment tools (Cassidy et al 2012), and reasons for this are wide-ranging (Jervis & Tilki 2011; Brown & Crookes 2016). Competence assessment is widely used in undergraduate preregistration nursing programmes to determine student achievement and eligibility for professional registration (O'Driscoll, Allan & Smith 2010; Cant, McKenna & Cooper 2013). Other studies reported assessors' lack of skills, knowledge and confidence to assess and report underperformance to take the necessary remedial action (Dudek, Marks & Regehr 2005; Cleland et al 2008; Luhanga, Yonge & Myrick 2008) and to make assessment decisions using expectations of an 'idealized student' (Burden, Topping & O'Halloran 2018). Equally, assessors are often also placed under stress and intimidation from students to pass them automatically (Hunt et al 2016).

Some of these issues could be alleviated if a standard and consistent rating scale was applied during assessments, as suggested by Bondy (1983). These concepts have been incorporated widely into specific student clinical assessment documentation. Table 1.3 shows how Bondy suggested that students could be graded at different levels based on the standards and quality of their practice and the level of assistance or supervision required. The narrative descriptors in the table help assessors to be more consistent in the grade they apply to either individual aspects of care or overall performance. Bondy's principles have been applied to the nursing practice assessment document (PAD) originally used in London and now used widely throughout the UK (see later) (Fish & Wilson 2018).

If the purpose of assessing students for entry into the profession is to be achieved with validity, there needs to be a more careful examination of how preregistration health care education, including the assessment of clinical practice, can be managed better, so that when students qualify, they can meet service needs and requirements – that is, they are 'fit for practice' and 'fit for purpose' (Benton 2011). Within this framework, more concerted efforts are required to make valid and reliable assessments of students' clinical practice.

Assessment as a Form of Quality Control

Closely related to the purpose of assessing for entry into the profession is this second overall purpose of assessment. In industry such as manufacturing, quality control of production enables those items below the required standard to

TABLE 1.3 Assessment – Evaluation of Clinical Performance Scale

Scale Label	No	Standard of Procedure	Quality of Performance	Level of Assistance Required
Independent	5	• Safe • Accurate • Achieved intended outcome • Behaviour is appropriate to context	• Proficient • Confident • Expedient	• No supporting cues required
Supervised	4	• Safe • Accurate • Achieved intended outcome • Behaviour is appropriate to context	• Proficient • Confident • Reasonably expedient	• Requires occasional supportive cues
Assisted	3	• Safe • Accurate • Achieved most objectives for intended outcome • Behaviour generally appropriate to context	• Proficient throughout most of performance when assisted	• Required frequent verbal and occasional physical directives in addition to supportive cues
Marginal	2	• Safe only with guidance • Not completely accurate • Incomplete achievement of intended outcome	• Unskilled • Inefficient	• Required continuous verbal and frequent physical directive cues
Dependent	1	• Unsafe • Unable to demonstrate behaviour • Lack of insight into behaviour appropriate to context	• Unskilled • Unable to demonstrate behaviour/procedure	• Required continuous verbal and continuous physical directive cues
X	0	Not observed		

From Bondy KN. Criterion-referenced definitions for rating scales in clinical evaluation. *J Nurs Ed*, 1983;22(9):376–382.

be rejected. The aim of this purpose of assessment is to identify those students and practitioners who have not achieved or maintained the required educational standards and therefore ensure those who are not competent are not on the professional register. For this to happen, there are recognised governance processes related to both preregistration students and existing professionals.

Preregistration Students

Among other roles, assessors need to be the 'gatekeepers' of their profession to achieve the quality control function of assessment. A crucial question to ask is: How adequately, or how well, is this gatekeeping role being performed? Again, the answer is that this purpose of assessment is not always fully realized because gatekeeping can be inadequate with 'failure to fail'. This complex problem is not new and appears to be a continuing challenge for assessors of students on preregistration professional courses (Dudek, Marks & Regehr 2005; Scholes & Albarran 2005; Luhanga, Yonge & Myrick 2008; Chambers et al 2019; Hughes, Mitchell & Johnston 2016; Cassidy, Coffey & Murphy 2017;

Timmins et al 2017). References are made to assessors giving students the benefit of the doubt in marginal situations instead of awarding a fail when it was clearly warranted. The points of fitness to practise and fitness for practice will be developed in Chapter 3 and issues of failure to fail in Chapter 7.

To determine whether preregistration students have achieved the threshold standards or competence, assessors must make the crucial pass/fail assessment decision. HEIs must make decisions of impairment of fitness to practise. These vital decisions protect the public from unsafe, incompetent or unscrupulous practitioners. This is crucial for quality control, and, as one of the purposes of assessment, it also serves to safeguard the standards of the profession.

In relation to undergraduate health professions students, this function of assessment is often over and above what HEIs recognise as the purpose of assessment for other students. Often collectively referred to as professional and statutory board requirements, these take into account specific requirements of bodies such as the NMC (Nursing and Midwifery Council 2018c) or HCPC (Health and Care Professions Council 2017a) and also other obligations, for example, apprenticeship standards (Institute for Apprenticeships and Technical Education 2019).

Qualified Professionals

The quality control purpose of assessment for registered professionals falls into two categories: professional conduct and education and training. Over the last few decades, this has received increasing recognition, with formal standards and renewal requirements now set. Many of these require practitioners to self-assess or provide confirmatory review or assessment of their peers. This is therefore an important aspect of assessment related to professional regulation.

The NMC and HCPC maintain registers of practitioners who have met the standards for entry to the professions. This is central to their roles in protecting the public. Being on the NMC and HCPC registers demonstrates to the public that practitioners have accepted the responsibilities and accountability that go along with registration and that they will abide by the professional standards set by the NMC and the HCPC. This is done through professional self-regulation. Professional self-regulation means that, in exercising professional accountability, professional knowledge, judgement and skill are used to interpret and apply professional standards in practice. Although the NMC and the HCPC administer the system of professional self-regulation, it is through its practitioners who are accountable for their own practice that professional standards are maintained in the workplace.

The professional standards for conduct of the NMC and the HCPC (Health and Care Professions Council 2016; Nursing and Midwifery Council 2018f) are the basis of the regulatory framework. Practitioners are required to monitor and maintain not only their own professional standards but also those of their colleagues. In exercising individual professional responsibility and accountability, the standards require practitioners to report to an appropriate person or authority any circumstances that may put patients and clients at risk. Practitioners must act without delay if they believe anyone's practice may be putting patients or clients at risk and that there should be transparency if errors occur, with service users and their families being consulted and kept fully informed. This duty of candour has been endorsed by the professions (Professional Standards Authority 2013; Nursing and Midwifery Council and General Medical Council, 2015) and guardians also appointed to encourage freedom to speak up (Care Quality Commission 2019).

The guidance provided by these publications reinforces the quality control purpose of assessment of practitioners, which, in turn, supports the primary mandate of the NMC

and the HCPC; to safeguard the health and well-being of the general public. In 2017 to 2018, the NMC received 5509 new concerns (0.8% of registrants) against its registrants for their fitness to practise (Nursing and Midwifery Council 2018a), and the HCPC received 2259 allegations (0.64% of registrants) (Health and Care Professions Council 2018a). The allegations of fitness to practise against these practitioners indicate that the quality control purpose of assessment of practitioners is necessary.

The importance of continuing professional development (CPD) is recognized to ensure professionals demonstrate that their professional knowledge and competence are maintained and continue to be developed. Practitioners must undertake and record their CPD to renew their registration. Nurses and midwives must have undertaken 35 hours of CPD relevant to their scope of practice in the previous 3-year period (Nursing and Midwifery Council 2019b), whereas the HCPC has a flexible approach but requires a declaration that CPD is relevant to current and future practice, contributes to practice and service delivery, and benefits service users (Health and Care Professions Council 2018c).

The standards set by the professions, together with guidance from the NHS – for example, the NHS Knowledge and Skills Framework (NHS – Employers 2018) and good organisational people (human resource) processes, including annual performance reviews or appraisals–provide a more consistent structure for postregistration development and CPD of health care professionals. This has facilitated the process of defining criteria for demonstrating continuing levels of competence throughout a professional career and has thus made the quality control of practice more consistent.

Assessment for the Motivation of Students

Assessments serve as a powerful motivating force for students–were it not for the carrot of success or stick of failure created by summative assessments, many students, it is claimed, would lack any real incentive to work. With motivation, assessment is used to encourage the student to learn. From this standpoint, assessments are seen as a form of positive help to students. Assessments can be used as an instrument of coercion, as a means of getting students to do something they might not otherwise do. The line between coercion and encouragement is hard to draw and may well be related to students' understanding, or lack of understanding, of the longer-term goals. One key aim of nursing or health professions' programmes is to prepare practitioners who are safe and competent. Of necessity, then, students are assessed for their achievement of statutory standards of proficiency. How else can we measure such learning? Failure to pass these standards of proficiency results in them being discontinued from the course. You may wish to decide whether assessments in this instance are used to coerce or encourage the student.

It is important not to take too simplistic a view of motivation and assessment because motivation is a complex concept. A high level of motivation is not a sufficient condition but is a necessary one for learning. Motivation on its own is not sufficient for achievement, but it is a necessary precursor for success. Conversely, negative motivational influences, such as fear of failure, feelings of helplessness, lack of confidence, and feeling that one's fate is largely controlled by external factors rather than by one's self, almost certainly have effects that restrict a student's achievements.

The responses of individual students to educational experiences and tasks are complex functions of their abilities and personalities, their past educational experiences, their current attitudes, self-perception and motivational states, together with the nature of their current experiences and tasks. Assessment is also important in defining the attitude students take towards their work, their sense of ownership and control of their own learning, the strategies they employ in learning and their confidence and self-esteem – all of which impact profoundly on the quality of learning achieved. The significant effects of assessment on motivation for learning and their implications for assessment in health care education are discussed later.

It is also important to consider the type of assessment and what the purpose is. Overall assessment can be classified in four ways. Table 1.4 summarizes the different types, the reasons for and the functions of assessment, and provides some health care examples. From this, you can see that the reason for the assessment will influence student motivation and that different types of assessment will motivate students at different stages of their programme in different ways. For example, a new first-year student may find it motivational to undertake a diagnostic assessment that tests their mathematical ability and is related to medication administration, as they will perceive this will help them learn in the future, whereas a final-year student may be motivated to complete a similar drugs test, not for its future learning potential but because it is viewed as a gatekeeping exercise related to job-seeking opportunities where the motivation is not about learning but about gaining employment.

Student Self-Efficacy

Self-efficacy refers to students' perceptions of their capability to perform certain tasks. Perceptions of self-efficacy have a strong influence on effort and persistence with difficult tasks, or after experiences of failure: under such circumstances, students high in self-efficacy usually redouble their efforts, whereas students low in self-efficacy tend to make minimal efforts or avoid such tasks. Self-efficacy can be developed if repeated success is experienced. Conversely, repeated failures lead to lowered self-efficacy. Success at tasks perceived to be difficult or challenging is more influential than success on easier tasks.

Self-efficacy is best enhanced if longer-term goals are supported by a carefully sequenced series of subgoals with clear criteria that students find attainable. In addition, standards must be clearly specified. The setting of clear and attainable goals has significant implications for strategies used by clinical assessors in relation to the level and type of work that is aimed at individual students. These important points are discussed further in Chapters 6 and 7.

Intrinsic Motivation and Continuing Motivation

Intrinsic motivation to learn (defined as a self-sustaining desire to learn) and continuing motivation (defined as a tendency to return to and continue working on tasks away

TABLE 1.4	**Typical Types, Reasons and Functions of Assessment**		
Type	**Reason**	**Function**	**Health Care Student Example**
Diagnostic	Assessment for learning	To determine previous knowledge to help focus and plan learning	Numeracy or literacy test at commencement of course
Formative	Assessment as learning	To support student learning to enhance progress through feedback	Student reflective account as part of a midway placement review
Summative	Assessment of learning	To evaluate or grade achievement at the end of a module or placement	Objective structured clinical examination to assess patient assessment skills
Certificate evaluation	Confirmation of learning	To confirm competency at completion of a task or course	Basic life support or other statutory or mandatory training

from the instructional context in which they were initially confronted) are highly related concepts. Both, in turn, are closely related to interest in the material that is being studied. Where students initially lack intrinsic motivation in a subject area, a carefully planned programme of positive educational experiences accompanied by extrinsic motivation can lead to the development of interest in the area and thus to intrinsic motivation. On the other hand, where students are initially intrinsically motivated, attempting to stimulate learning through extrinsic motivation usually leads to decreased intrinsic motivation, especially on challenging tasks.

These findings have obvious implications for teachers and assessors when designing learning experiences for students. Crooks' (1988) classic statement that effective education requires the fusing of 'skill and will' reminds us that we need to consider carefully which assessment strategies we use so we can help our students develop and/or maintain intrinsic and continuing motivation.

This aspect of learning and assessment is explored in Chapter 6.

Assessment Anxiety

The fact that clinical experience is overwhelming and stressful for many students is well documented (see, for example, James & Chapman 2009–2010; Lincoln et al 2004; Deary et al 2003; Phillips et al 2000; Smith 1992; Williams 1993; Kleehammer et al 1990; Parkes 1985). These authors also reported that anxiety can contribute to decreased learning. To be subject to assessment in the face of this negative emotion can only compound the situation. Crooks (1988) found that the debilitating effects for high-anxiety students are greater when the student perceives good performance to be particularly important, when the test is expected to be difficult and when the testing conditions are particularly intrusive (e.g., rigid timing). Although extrapolations must be made with caution, it seems possible to draw parallels between these findings and the circumstances faced by health care students during clinical practice. The performance of students in the clinical setting must meet the required standards within the timeframe of the clinical placement. The achievement of some aspects of care can be difficult, such as being able to perform cardiopulmonary resuscitation, communicating with the very ill/dying client/patient and managing the care of a group of clients/patients. For some students, experiences of assessment may then be rather dispiriting and demotivating.

Assessment to Support Teaching and Learning

Assessment helps to make understanding and knowledge, as Hattie (2012) described it, 'more visible'. Adopting strategies that encourage assessment for learning helps students understand what good practice and excellence look like and how they can develop their own work to reach that level. This is equally true in the classroom and clinical setting. Feedback, particularly about their own work, has a positive effect on student achievement.

Health care students appreciate feedback and benefit from it, but it is not always done well (Fitzgerald, Gibson & Gunn 2010; Walsh 2014). Students look to, and indeed expect and welcome, constructive feedback from their teachers and assessors (Neary 2001; Embo et al 2010) and also from their peers (Rohatinsky, Harding & Carriere 2017; Vandal et al 2018) and look to friends and family for support (Royal College of Nursing 2008). Students' skills of self-assessment and motivation for self-directed learning improved when feedback on practice-based learning was linked to constructive feedback on performance (Embo et al 2010).

For feedback of this nature to be effective, assessment needs to be used as a diagnostic aid to learning throughout the course so that it becomes an integral part of the educational process, continually providing both feedback and 'feed forward' (Ferrell & Gray 2013) for both students and assessors. This formative element of the assessment process will then have a positive impact on learning, particularly if it focuses on helping the student to achieve short-term goals and provides specific and detailed feedback on progress. Some aspects, which we typically have come to expect of assessment, like the award of marks and grades, may be unhelpful. In summary, being awarded just a mark or a pass or a fail does not indicate to the student how well or badly they may have performed in aspects of the assessment exercise. Such grades are meted out by the teacher at the end of a term or a course. Students may therefore not know how to improve future performance. Generally, such feedback can only begin to be useful only when it includes narrative or verbal comments. Feedback is explored further in Chapter 7.

Insofar as assessment evidence reveals the quality and quantity of learning, the assessor may be able to identify what has been taught well and what has not been so well explained and therefore may have confused the issue for the student, what further experiences are required and so on. In the clinical setting, such information will further enable the assessor to plan those clinical experiences and teaching sessions the student will require to achieve learning outcomes. The use of the formative assessment process is explored in Chapter 6, where the process of the continuous assessment of clinical practice is discussed.

Assessment practices have an impact on student learning, and the approaches used influence how students go about studying and learning. Students' approaches to learning tasks can be categorized into two broad categories: deep or surface approaches. Deep approaches involve an active search for meaning to understand material for oneself. The content is interacted with vigorously and critically. Organizing principles are used to integrate ideas. Surface approaches, in contrast, rely primarily on attempts to memorize course material, treating the material as if different facts and topics were unrelated. Snelgrove (2004) found that most student nurses were taking a surface approach. Those students exhibiting deep approaches to learning correlated positively and significantly with overall higher assessment scores.

Assessment strategies should encourage deep learning, higher-order thinking and self-monitoring, alongside the acquisition of knowledge, from the earliest stages of professional education to develop the practitioner who is fit for practice (HCPC 2007; NMC 2018b). Higher-order learning is retained longer and encourages the development of intrinsic motivation and positive attitudes to continued learning. The health care professions can only stand to benefit given the professions' aim of developing and fostering the attitude of lifelong learning in its practitioners to strive constantly to improve standards and quality of client/patient care (Department of Health 2015; HCPC 2010; NMC 2008b).

Complexities Faced by Students

When using assessment to support learning, remember that students individually face a variety of issues and challenges to their learning. These might include:

- Difficulties with learning, such as dyslexia or dyscalculia (Ridley 2011);
- English not being their first language (Olson 2012);
- Responsibilities associated with family roles as a parent or as a carer;
- Issues associated with being a mature student. This may include coping with return to study, negotiating roles in the classroom with younger peers, false expectations in practice of greater skills or knowledge and loss and grief for former status and role;
- A culture of consumer expectations in fee-paying students where the nature of practice-based assessments are not fully appreciated and are perceived as unpaid work and where mentors are expected to pass students (Hunt et al 2016).

Good preparation of students at the start of their programme can often alleviate many of these issues either by ensuring students receive appropriate specialist support or they gain good insights into what is required as part of the socialisation to becoming a health care professional.

Look at Activity 1.3 and consider what your development needs as an assessor are.

Activity 1.3   Your Learning Needs as an Assessor

Considering your own development, what gaps do you recognize in your preparation to become a good practice supervisor or mentor?

Think about:

- What development opportunities are there within your workplace?
- Whether you have access to online resources

Access any practice learning resources or training packages available to you (e.g., from the university your students attend) or on the Pan-London Practice Learning Group's webpage and consider if any are relevant for your development.

Web link: https://plplg.uk/e-learning-resources/

ASSESSMENT IN CLINICAL PRACTICE

The Nature of Clinical Assessment

You may be able to recall your experiences of being assessed when you were a student. Some of these memories may, no doubt, be rather vivid! Not only were you required to sit written tests and be subjected to oral and practical examinations, but also you were assessed while you were working. In the classroom, your teacher gave you feedback on your test papers and assignments. In the clinical area, your assessor gave you feedback, thus implying that some form of assessment of your practice had taken place. At a personal level, you were either pleased or dissatisfied with your performance – you had therefore assessed yourself. Colleagues may have indicated to you how they thought you were doing on a surgical ward – they had assessed you. Patients gave you feedback on the care you had given them – you were subject to yet further assessment!

All in all, you may have frequently felt quite overwhelmed because you knew that what you said or did or the way you behaved, or even the way you dressed, was under scrutiny. If we reflect on our experiences of being assessed as a health care student, some of us may even begin to say that we experienced assessment as though we had experienced a phenomenon. What is the nature of this phenomenon? Pause for a moment to reconsider Activity 1.1.

In most instances feedback you received about your performance and abilities or otherwise was probably based on another person's inferences and estimations of your actions and behaviours. In other words, you had been judged by someone else. Assessment in education occurs whenever one person is conscious of obtaining and interpreting information about the knowledge, understanding, abilities and attitudes of another person.

Assessors of health care students make judgements about, for example, how students are integrating into the clinical team, how they are developing as practitioners, what they are learning and what they have accomplished. Assessments may reveal the positive changes in the student's knowledge, understanding, abilities and attitudes as a result of supervision and guidance, together with the practical experiences and other influences and effects of the clinical setting on the student. The nature of clinical practice, and the clinical milieu itself, places multiple demands on the skills of the practitioner as mentor, assessor and teacher. The dynamic clinical setting is ever changing and unstructured. It provides a range of clients whose conditions are varied and changeable. Learning experiences for students are therefore not consistent. Each of these situations has to be dealt with in a different way. Real people in the real world of practice do not see things in a uniform way. Our own values will also influence the interpretations we make of situations. The subjectivity of the clinical world will inevitably mean that assessments we make are likely to be influenced by our own personal and professional experiences and perceptions of the situation.

The diversity of context and the differing demands of each context also mean that the student's knowledge, understanding, abilities and attitudes can be assessed only within those contexts that the student has encountered. While we are observing, we cannot be sure that we have picked up every aspect of performance; there may have been some aspect of care or nuance that has been missed, or the interpretation of ability to perform or otherwise may have been made based on our personal biases for, or against, the student. During clinical placements then, finding out about a student's abilities to perform is done mainly through informal processes and as opportunities arise. Because assessments are likely to be based on short allocations or placements, there is a need to question how well we truly know the student. Knowledge of the student's achievements is, of course, important when assessment decisions are made, be they formative or summative.

As the student works alongside us, we hope that they are learning through observation of our practices. Throughout the student's placement, their learning is facilitated through instruction, guidance and supervision as they participate in care delivery. While they are adjusting to clients, staff and other personnel and also learning to perform care, students are being assessed and given feedback on their performance. This means that while the student is learning, they are being assessed. Working in the demanding clinical setting may prevent practitioners from carrying out their roles of mentor and assessor as effectively as they would wish to. At the grassroots level, the first responsibility of health care practitioners is to care for clients.

BOX 1.1   Guidelines for Assessment in Clinical Practice

The following are links to assessment in clinical practice guidelines for different health care professions. The list is not exhaustive but, as a starting point, will help guide you to a range of resources:

Nursing and Midwifery
- Nursing and Midwifery Council (2019c) https://www.nmc.org.uk/supporting-information-on-standards-for-student-supervision-and-assessment/
- Pan London Practice Learning Group (Fish & Wilson 2018): https://plplg.uk
- Midwifery practice learning: http://www.mentoringat-mdx.co.uk/practice-learning-midwifery/

Allied Health Professions
- Health and Care Professions: https://www.hcpc-uk.org/standards/standards-relevant-to-education-and-training/set/
- Practice education guidance for all Health and Care professions: https://www.sor.org/system/files/section/201809/hcp_practice_education_guidance.pdf
- National Association of Educators in: http://naep-uk.org/about/

Consequently, even the extremely important activity of teaching and assessing students comes second to this.

Although students are supernumerary–that is, not part of the employed workforce–it is important that they experience the realities of health care delivery and therefore work alongside mentors and supervisors. However, as Allan et al (2011) reported, students were left unsupervised and often with an allocated workload. There were also instances when students were not directly supervised or allocated to work alongside supervisors and mentors. It is therefore difficult to ensure that students are learning what they should to achieve professional competence. Strategies to facilitate more effective learning and assessment are made in Chapters 7 and 9. Links to some guidelines for assessment in clinical practice are listed in Box 1.1.

The Complexities of Clinical Assessment

From this discussion, the nature of clinical assessment is complex. There is much in the literature that says the assessment of students in clinical practice is a continuing challenge (Cleland et al 2008; Fitzgerald, Gibson & Gunn 2010; Duffy 2013) with a variety of issues suggested including:
- Assessment is often based on the potentially biased and subjective human observation of practice;

- Students are subject to multiple assessments, giving a sense of overassessment;
- Students experience multiple placements, many of a short duration, with interaction with many different professionals and client groups;
- There is unpredictability in the learning opportunities because of the dynamic and diverse nature of clinical environments, with variation for students within and across placements;
- The requirements of the HCPC and NMC (Health and Care Professions Council 2017b; Nursing and Midwifery Council 2018b) for students to achieve mandatory standards of proficiency;
- Difficulties of achieving uniformity, consistency and fairness – this is considered in greater detail in Chapters 4 and 5;
- Pressures on clinical environments to accommodate large numbers of students, meaning even the most committed practitioners are hard-pressed to support students with mentor overload (Hurley & Snowden 2008; Hallin & Danielson 2009);
- Failure to fail has been identified as an increasing concern in both nursing and allied health programmes (Chambers et al 2019; Hughes, Mitchell & Johnston 2016);
- Concerns about a continuing theory-practice gap (Asokan 2012; Monaghan 2015) in health care professional education accentuated by divisions between university and practice teaching;
- Assessment is often based on learning assumed to have taken place before allocation to the placement–that is, in the university–yet Eraut's (2003) work has shown that this is cognitively difficult and learning needs to be contextual;
- Clinical assessors often do not have a good knowledge of what actually has been taught in the classroom;
- Accurate feedback on professional values and behaviours has been seen to frequently not be given (Fitzgerald, Gibson & Gunn 2010; Miller 2010).

Now look at Activity 1.4 and reflect on your role as an assessor.

Activity 1.4   Your Experience as an Assessor

Thinking about your experiences up to now of assessing students:
- Recall a specific situation where you gave positive feedback to a student. How did you feel?
- Now consider a situation where you gave a student feedback that they found challenging. How did you feel?
- How have these experiences influenced or changed your practice as an assessor for future students?

Approaches to Improve Clinical Assessment

Increasing awareness about the different purposes of assessment, together with the desires to address many of the complexities of clinical assessment discussed, have led to measures to improve the assessment process in clinical settings. Much of this work has led to initiatives that aim to provide greater consistency for students and standardization of documentation for clinical assessors.

Practice Assessment Documentation

In nursing, an initiative to develop a Pan-London PAD (Baillie et al 2016) has now spread across much of the UK. The aim was to develop a PAD that would rigorously assess student nurses reflecting the changing health and social care policies and environments where students are placed. To this end, a unified PAD to meet the NMC standards (Nursing and Midwifery Council 2018b) was first validated in 2012 and updated in 2019 (Fish & Wilson 2018), following extensive engagement and consultation with academics, practice partners, students and service users. The pan-London PAD has been used by over 10,000 students in London in over 40 NHS trusts and other independent and voluntary sector health care providers under the auspices of 12 universities. It is also now being used in other parts of the UK.

The document is underpinned by Benner's (1984) model of skill development, together with Bondy's (1983) scale for a standardized rating of nursing practice (see the section earlier in this chapter) and the concepts underpinning situated learning (Evans 2012) and the social dimensions of learning originally espoused by Wenger (Morley 2016). The approach recognizes the work and emotional dimensions of clinical practice learning.

The benefits of this PAD approach (Fish & Wilson 2018) are summarized as follows:
- A unified document across London with universal support from health care provider organizations;
- The document structure facilitates rigorous assessment of students;
- There is explicit assessment of professional values;
- The inclusion of patient or service user feedback;
- Practice assessors with students from multiple universities and different fields do not have to become familiar with multiple documents;
- Supervisor or mentor time can be focussed on individual student support and assessment;
- Greater constituency around the concept of competence;
- Improves the quality of assessment with improved reliability of assessment.

Team-Based Approaches

Demand for more clinical placements as universities increase their intakes of nursing and health care students to address workforce shortages and increasing population health needs has led to debate about alternative ways to the traditional one-to-one student/mentor or student/practice educator relationship (Hurley & Snowden 2008). In parallel, the NMC's standards for student supervision and assessment (Nursing and Midwifery Council 2018d) require a separation, with different people undertaking the practice supervisor and practice assessor roles. Alternative models have, therefore, been suggested to enhance practice learning (Royal College of Nursing 2015).

One suggestion is for a new clinical supervision model, such as the Collaborative Learning in Practice (CLiP) project (Lobo, Arthur & Lattimer 2014). This approach advocates student peer support, for example, with third-year students mentoring junior students with oversight from a designated qualified nurse as the practice supervisor. This approach reinforces the development of the leadership and supervision role in the student nurse with a greater coaching, rather than mentoring role, from the overseeing registered nurse (Huggins 2016; Clarke, Williamson & Kane 2018).

Another initiative is the Health Education England–sponsored Strengthening Team-based Education in Practice (STEP) project led by Middlesex University that works to support the whole practice-based team in understanding ways to promote student learning and provide them with key resources to do so (Morley, Wilson & McDermott 2017).

What is clear from these initiatives is that the direction of change in student supervision is from a model based on teaching to one based on coaching and away from a one-to-one mentor/mentee system to a team approach to support students. This is also taking place against a backdrop of a diverse range of students following different entry routes and different university and work-based programmes, such as apprenticeships with greater interprofessional supervision of health care students. What is not yet clear in the literature is the effect these initiatives will have on the assessment of students. Will an assessor working at arm's-length from the student be able to effectively assess students? Will students' feel these assessments are fair and just? Alternatively, do they offer an opportunity to tackle many of the challenges presented earlier in this chapter and help provide greater rigour, help eliminate bias and ensure fitness to practise?

Considering these changes, look at Activity 1.5.

Activity 1.5   Comparing Assessment Resources Interprofessionally

First search online for resources related to assessment in clinical practice that are relevant to your own profession. Some suggested links are given in Box 1.1.

- Consider current professional guidance and think about how this is either the same as, or different from, when you were a student.
- Have a look at guidance for other professions. What are the similarities and differences in approach?
- Think about interprofessional education opportunities in your workplace and how you can contribute to student assessment across the health care professions.

CONCLUSION

Four broad categories of purpose for assessment in health care professional education have been outlined. These are not entirely without overlap and continue to generate debate about what works and what is effective. Assessors of learners in the health care professions need to consider carefully the learning that must be achieved and balance this against the needs of the learner, as an individual, and the wider responsibilities for ensuring safe patient care. At times, these may conflict, adding to the challenge and complexity of student assessment in clinical practice. Reflecting and developing a clear personal philosophy of what is important for students to learn in clinical practice is key to determining attitudes and approaches to the assessment. This, in turn, influences our use of and approach to assessment systems, tools and procedures. As we examine the nature of clinical assessment further throughout this book, it is important to begin to analyse the reasons underpinning our attitudes toward learning and assessment in clinical practice and to question who is responsible and accountable. These issues will be examined in the next chapter.

KEY POINTS FOR REFLECTION

1. To accept the necessity for assessment unthinkingly denies a complex debate around the purposes of assessments. It may also make us overlook the effects of the assessment on the learner as an individual and its impact on the curriculum, teaching and learning. Critically reviewing 'why' we assess may make us consider

more carefully whether our assessments are reasonable and just. Four key purposes of assessment in professional education put forward are:

a. To regulate entry into the profession through:
   - Selection for training where only those who we perceive fulfil our selection criteria are admitted. These are those who are supposed to be the best and who will complete the course successfully. Noncompletion and discontinuation rates tell us that our stringent selection criteria may not be so valid and reliable.
   - Assessment of preregistration students so that they achieve fitness for practice. Concern about the competence (and by implication, the fitness for practice) of newly qualified nurses and midwives has a long history. Recent failings in health care provision–where nursing, rightly or wrongly (Reeves, Ross & Harris 2014), was criticized–have continued this debate and led to a review of education and recommendations to raise standards (Health Education England 2015) and to both the Nursing and Midwifery Council (2018b) and the Health and Care Professions Council (2017a) updating their standards for education.

b. To use assessment as a quality control mechanism for the profession through:
   - Assessment of students in training so that only those who are safe and competent are registered. There is overwhelming evidence that there is a failure to fail marginal students, and therefore, there are practitioners on professional registers who are not safe and competent.
   - The quality control purpose of assessment for qualified professionals serves to maintain the standards of the profession through the regulation of the education, training and the continuing fitness to practise of its registrants. Regulations are in place for the reporting of fitness to practise and to ensure the CPD of practitioners.

c. To motivate students:
   - Assessments can encourage or discourage students to learn. They define the attitude students take towards their work, their sense of ownership and control of their own learning, the strategies they employ in learning and their confidence and self-esteem, all of which impact profoundly on the quality of learning achieved.

d. To support teaching and learning:
   - Feedback is vital for learning. Feedback needs to become an integral part of the educational process, continually providing both feedback and feedforward (Ferrell & Gray 2013) for both students and assessors so that strengths and weaknesses in student learning and teaching by the practitioner can be identified. Specific and detailed feedback is required to enable students to progress.

2. Teaching and assessing activities in clinical areas are frequently left to chance. As assessments of competence are frequently based on 'snapshots' of practice, the validity and reliability of assessment decisions are questionable. Reliability is compromised further by the subjective nature of clinical assessments.

3. The dynamic nature of clinical practice militates against consistency of experience and learning. This is likely to lead to variations in fitness to practise at the point of registration.

REFERENCES

Allan HT, Smith P, O'Driscoll M. Experiences of supernumerary status and the hidden curriculum in nursing: a new twist in the theory-practice gap? *J Clin Nurs*, 2011;20(5–6):847–855.

Asokan GV. Evidence-based practice curriculum in allied health professions for teaching-research-practice nexus. *J Evid-Based Med*, 2012;5(4):226–231.

Baillie L. Fish J, Barclay J, et al. Assessing nursing students in practice: a mixed method evaluation of a unified assessment document, in HEA Health and Social Care conference, Glasgow; 2016. Available: https://www.researchgate.net/publication/308077744_Enter_titleAssessing_nursing_students_in_practice_a_mixed_method_evaluation_of_a_unified_assessment_document. Accessed: 13 March 2020

Benner P. *From Novice to Expert: Excellence and Power in Clinical Nursing Practice.* Addison-Wesley, Menlo Park, CA;1984.

Benton D. Nurses fit for purpose, award and practice? *Int Nurs Rev*, 2011;58(3):276–276.

Bondy KN. Criterion-referenced definitions for rating scales in clinical evaluation. *J Nurs Educ*, 1983;22(9):376–382.

Braithwaite DN, Elzubeir M, Stark S. Project 2000 student wastage: a case study. *Nurs Educ Today*, 1994;14(1):15–21.

Broadfoot, P. (2012) Assessment, Schools and Society. 2nd ed. Routlege, Abingdon, UK.

Brown RA, Crookes PA. What level of competency do experienced nurses expect from a newly graduated registered nurse? Results of an Australian modified Delphi study. *BMC Nurs*, 2016;15(1):45.

Buchan J, Charlesworth A, Gershlick B, et al. A critical moment: NHS staffing trends, retention and attrition. London:2019. Available: https://www.health.org.uk/sites/default/files/upload/publications/2019/A%20Critical%20Moment_1.pdf (Accessed: 13 March 2020)

Burden S, Topping AE, O'Halloran C. Mentor judgements and decision-making in the assessment of student nurse competence in practice: a mixed-methods study. *J Advanc Nur*, 2018;74(5):1078–1089.

Callwood A, Jeevaratnam K, Kotronoulas G, et al. Personal domains assessed in multiple mini interviews (MMIs) for healthcare student selection: a narrative synthesis systematic review. *Nurs Educ Today*, 2018;64:56–64.

Cant R, McKenna L, Cooper S. Assessing preregistration nursing students' clinical competence: a systematic review of objective measures'. *Int J Nurs Prac*, 2013;19(2):163–176.

Care Quality Commission. National Guardian's Office: 2019. Available: https://www.cqc.org.uk/national-guardians-office/content/national-guardians-office. Accessed: 1 July 2019.

Cassidy I, Butler MP, Quillinan B, et al. Preceptors' views of assessing nursing students using a competency based approach. *Nurs Edus Prac*, 2012;12(6):346–351.

Cassidy S, Coffey M, Murphy F. "Seeking authorization": a grounded theory exploration of mentors' experiences of assessing nursing students on the borderline of achievement of competence in clinical practice. *J Ad Nurs*, 2017;73(9):2167–2178.

Chambers M, Hickey G, Borghini G, et al. Preparation for practice: the role of the HCPC's standards of education and training in ensuring that newly qualified professionals are fit to practise. London:2019. Available: https://www.hcpc-uk.org/globalassets/resources/reports/preparation-for-practice.pdf. Accessed: 13 March 2020.

Chimea T, Kanji Z, Schmitz S. Assessment of clinical competence in competency-based education. *Can J Dent Hyg*. 2020;54(2):83–91.

Clarke D, Williamson GR, Kane A. Could students' experiences of clinical placements be enhanced by implementing a Collaborative Learning in Practice (CliP) model? *Nurs Edus Prac*, 2018;33:A3–A5.

Cleland JA, Knight LV, Rees CE, et al. Is it me or is it them? Factors that influence the passing of underperforming students. *Med Edus*, 2008;42(8):800–809.

Currer C. Assessing student social workers' professional suitability: comparing university procedures in England. *Br J Soc Work*, 2009;39(8):1481–1498.

Deary IJ, Watson R, Hogston R. A longitudinal cohort study of burnout and attrition in nursing students. *J Adv Nurs*, 2003;43(1):71–81.

Department of Health. The NHS Constitution. London:2015. Available: https://assets.publishing.service.gov.uk/government/uploads/system/uploads/attachment_data/file/480482/NHS_Constitution_WEB.pdf. Accessed: 13 March 2020.

Dudek NL, Marks MB, Regehr G. Failure to fail: the perspectives of clinical supervisors. *Acad Med*, 2005;80(Suppl):S84–S87.

Duffy K. Providing constructive feedback to students during mentoring. *Nurs Stan*, 2013;27(31):50–56.

Embo MPC et al. Assessment and feedback to facilitate self-directed learning in clinical practice of Midwifery students. *Med Teach*, 2010;32(7):e263–e269.

Eraut M. Assessment in a wider context'. *Learn Health Soc Care*, 2003;2(4):77–180.

Evans K. Introduction: working to learn in clinical practice. In: Cook V, Daly C, Newman M, Work-Based Learning in Clinical Settings, Insights From Socio-Cultural Perspectives. Radcliffe Publishing, London:2012.

Ferrell G, Gray L. Feedback and feed forward. Using technology to support students' progression over time. 2013. Available: https://www.jisc.ac.uk/guides/feedback-and-feed-forward. Accessed: 16 July 2019.

Fish J, Wilson K. Developing a second pan London practice assessment document for preregistration Nursing in London. In: 29th International Networking for Healthcare Education Conference. Churchill College, Cambridge, 4–6 September 2018. Available: https://www.heacademy.ac.uk/system/files/downloads/Strands 2A-2I_1.pdf.

Fitzgerald M, Gibson F, Gunn K. Contemporary issues relating to assessment of pre-registration nursing students in practice. *Nurs Educ Prac*, 2010;10(3):158–163.

Gale J, Ooms A, Gran R, et al. Student nurse selection and predictability of academic success: the Multiple Mini Interview project. *Nurs Edus Today*, 2016;40(May):123–127.

Garside JR, Nhemachena JZZ. A concept analysis of competence and its transition in nursing. *Nurs Edus Today*, 2013;33(5):541–545.

Hallin K, Danielson E. Being a personal preceptor for nursing students: Registered Nurses' experiences before and after introduction of a preceptor model. *J Adv Nurs*, 2009;65(1):161–174.

Harris RC, Rosenberg L, O'Rourke ME. Addressing the challenges of nursing student attrition. *J Nurs Educ*, 2013;53(1):31–37.

Hattie J. Visible Learning for Teachers: Maximising Impact on Learning. Routlege, Abingdon, UK:2012.

Health and Care Professions Council. *Standards of Conduct, Performance and Ethics.* London:2016. Available at: https://www.hcpc-uk.org/standards/standards-of-conduct-performance-and-ethics/ (Accessed: 13 March 2020)

Health and Care Professions Council. Standards of education and training. London.2017a. Available: https://www.hcpc-uk.org/globalassets/resources/standards/standards-of-education-and-training.pdf. Accessed: 13 March 2020.

Health and Care Professions Council. Fitness to Practice Report 2017. London:2017b.

Health and Care Professions Council. HCPC–what we do. 2018b. Available: https://www.hcpc-uk.org/about-us/what-we-do/. Accessed: 25 June 2019.

Health and Care Professions Council. Standards of Continuing Professional Development. London:2018c. Available: https://www.hcpc-uk.org/standards/standards-of-continuing-professional-development/. Accessed: 1 July 2019.

Health Education England. Raising the Bar: Shape of Caring: A Review of the Future Education and Training of Registered Nurses and Care Assistants (Chair: Lord Willis). London:2015.

Health Education England. Values Based Recruitment Framework. London:2016.

Health Education England. RePAIR (Reducing Pre-registration Attrition and Improving Retention Report. London:2018.

Henderson A, Cooke M, Creedy DK, et al. Nursing students' perceptions of learning in practice environments: a review'. *Nurs Edus Today*, 2012;32(3):299–302.

Huggins D. Enhancing nursing students' education by coaching mentors. *Nurs Manag*, 2016,23(1).30 32.

Hughes LJ, Mitchell M, Johnston ANB. "Failure to fail" in nursing – a catch phrase or a real issue? A systematic integrative literature review. *Nurs Educ Prac*, 2016;20:54–63.

Hunt LA McGee P, Gutteridge R, et al. Manipulating mentors' assessment decisions: do underperforming student nurses use coercive strategies to influence mentors' practical assessment decisions? *Nurs Educ Prac*, 2016;20(Sept):154–162.

Hurley C, Snowden S. Mentoring in times of change. *Nurs Crit Care*, 2008;13(5):269–275.

Hutchison JS. Scandals in health-care: their impact on health policy and nursing. *Nurs Inq*, 2015;23:32–41.

Ilott I, Murphy R. Success and Failure in Professional Education: Assessing the Evidence. Whurr, London:1999.

Institute for Apprenticeships and Technical Education. Apprenticeship Standards. 2019. Available: https://www.institutefor apprenticeships.org/apprenticeship-standards/. Accessed: 1 July 2019.

Jervis A, Tilki M. Why are nurse mentors failing to student nurses who do not meet clinical performance standards? *Br J Nurs*, 2011;20(9):582–587.

Lindop E. Factors associated with student and pupil nurse wastage. *J Adv Nurs*, 1987;12(6):751–756.

Lobo C, Arthur A, Lattimer V. Collaborative Learning in Practice (CLiP) for Pre-registration Nursing Students. 2014. Available: https://www.charleneloboconsulting.com/wp-content/uploads/CLiP-Paper-final-version-Sept-14.pdf. Accessed: 13 March 2020.

Luhanga F, Yonge OJ, Myrick F. Failure to assign failing grades. *Int J Nurs Educ Schola*, 2008;5(1):article 8.

Merkley B. Student nurse attrition: a half century of research. *J Nurs Educ Prac*, 2016;6(3):71–75.

Miller C. Improving and enhancing performance in the affective domain of nursing students: insights from the literature for clinical educators. *Contemp Nurse*, 2010;35(1):2–17.

Monaghan T. A critical analysis of the literature and theoretical perspectives on theory–practice gap amongst newly qualified nurses within the United Kingdom. *Nurs Educ Today*, 2015;35(8):e1–e7.

Morgan J, Bendall A. Candidate evaluation of the Multiple Mini-interview (MMI) as a selection tool for physiotherapy undergraduate students, Presented at: Welsh Board of the Chartered Society of Physiotherapy Conference, Cardiff, UK, 28 June 2016. 2016. Available: http://orca.cf.ac.uk/92281/2/CSP Wales MMI Candidate Evaluation.pdf. Accessed: 13 March 2020.

Morley D. Applying Wenger's communities of practice theory to placement learning. *Nurs Educ Today*, 2016;39:161–162.

Morley DA, Wilson K, McDermott J. Changing the practice learning landscape. *Nurs Educ Prac*, 2017;27:169–171.

Neary M. Responsive assessment: assessing student nurses' clinical competence. *Nurs Educ Today*, 2001;21(1):3–17.

Newton SE, Moore G. Use of Aptitude to understand bachelor of science in nursing student attrition and readiness for the National Council Licensure Examination-registered nurse. *J Prof Nurs*, 2009;25(5):273–278

NHS Employers. Simplified Knowledge and Skills Framework (KSF). 2018. Available. https://www.nhsemployers.org/SimplifiedKSF. Accessed: 1 July 2019.

Nursing and Midwifery Council and General Medical Council. Openness and honesty when things go wrong: the professional duty of candour (joint statement). London:2015.

Nursing and Midwifery Council. Annual Fitness to Practice Report. London:2018a.

Nursing and Midwifery Council. Future nurse: standards of proficiency for registered nurses. London:2018b.

Nursing and Midwifery Council. Realising professionalism: standards for education and training Part 1: standards framework for nursing and midwifery education. London:2018c.

Nursing and Midwifery Council. Realising professionalism: standards for education and training Part 2: standards for student supervision and assessment. London:2018d.

Nursing and Midwifery Council. Realising professionalism: standards for education and training Part 3: standards for pre-registration nursing programmes. London:2018e.

Nursing and Midwifery Council. The Code: Professional standards of practice and behaviour for nurses, midwives and nursing associates (updated). London:2018f. Available: https://www.nmc.org.uk/standards/code/.

Nursing and Midwifery Council. Future midwife. 2019a. Available: https://www.nmc.org.uk/standards/midwifery/education. Accessed: 25 June 2019.

Nursing and Midwifery Council. Revalidation: continuing professional development. 2019b. Available: http://revalidation. nmc.org.uk/what-you-need-to-do/continuing-professional-development/index.html. Accessed: 1 July 2019.

Nursing and Midwifery Council. Supporting information on standards for student supervision and assessment. 2019c. Available: https://www.nmc.org.uk/supporting-information-on-standards-for-student-supervision-and-assessment. Accessed: 15 July 2019.

Nursing and Midwifery Council. What we do. 2019d. Available: https://www.nmc.org.uk/about-us/our-role. Accessed: 25 June 2019.

O'Driscoll MF, Allan HT, Smith PA. Still looking for leadership – who is responsible for student nurses' learning in practice? *Nurs Educ Today*, 2010;30(3):212–217.

Olson MA. English-as-a-Second Language (ESL) nursing student success: a critical review of the literature. *J Cult Divers*, 2012;19(1):26–32.

Professional Standards Authority. Candour, disclosure and openness. London:2013.

Professional Standards Authority. What we do. 2019. Available: https://www.professionalstandards.org.uk/what-we-do. Accessed: 25 June 2019.

Reeves S, Ross F, Harris R. Fostering a 'common culture'? Responses to the Francis Inquiry demonstrate the need for an interprofessional response. *J Interpro Care*, 2014;28(5):387–389.

Ridley C. The experiences of nursing students with dyslexia. *Nurs Stan*, 2011;25(24):35–41.

Rohatinsky N, Harding K, Carriere T. Nursing student peer mentorship: a review of the literature. *Ment Tut Partner Learn*, 2017;25(1):61–77.

Rowntree D. Assessing Students: How Shall We Know Them? 2nd ed. London: Kogan Page:1987.

Royal College of Nursing, Nursing our future: an RCN study into the challenges facing today's nursing students in Wales. London:2008. Available: https://www.rcn.org.uk/-/media/royal-college-of-nursing/documents/publications/2009/november/pub-003309.pdf. Accessed: 13 March 2020.

Royal College of Nursing, RCN Mentorship Project 2015: From today's support in practice to tomorrow's vision for excellence. London:2015. Available: https://www.rcn.org.uk/professional-development/publications/pub-005455. Accessed: 13 March 2020.

Scholes J, Albarran J. Failure to fail: facing the consequences of inaction. *BACCN Nurs Crit Care*, 2005;10(3):113–115.

Snelgrove SR. Approaches to learning of student nurses. *Nurs Educ Today*, 2004;24(8):605–614.

Stayt LC, Merriman C. A descriptive survey investigating pre-registration student nurses' perceptions of clinical skill development in clinical placements. *Nurs Educ Today*, 2013;33(4):425–430.

Timmins F, Cassidy, S., Nugent, O., et al. Reluctance to fail nursing students in practice-implications for nurse managers'. *J Nurs Man*, 2017;25(7):489–490.

Urwin S, Stanley R, Jones M, et al. Understanding student nurse attrition: learning from the literature'. *Nurs Educ Today*, 2010;30(2):202–207.

Vandal N, Leung K, Sanzone L, et al. Exploring the student peer mentor's experience in a nursing peer mentorship program'. *J Nurs Educ*, 2018;57(7):422–425.

Vergel J, Quintero GA, Isaza-Restrepo A, et al. The influence of different curriculum designs on students' dropout rate: a case study'. *Med Educ Online*, 2018;23(1):1432963.

Walsh D. The Nurse Mentor's Handbook: Supporting Students in Clinical Practice: Supporting Students in Clinical Practice. 2nd ed McGraw-Hill, Maidenhead, UK:2014.

Waters A. The question for universities: how can they win the war on attrition? *Nurs Stan*, 2010;24(24):12–15.

White J, Williams RW, Green BF. Discontinuation, leaving reasons and course evaluation comments of students on the common foundation programme. *Nurs Educ Today*, 1999;19(2):142–150.

Yanhua C, Watson R. A review of clinical competence assessment in nursing. *Nurs Educ Today*, 2011;31(8):832–836.

Responsibility and Accountability Surrounding Clinical Assessment

CHAPTER CONTENTS

INTRODUCTION

For busy nursing and midwifery practitioners, having the additional role of educating and assessing students can be seen as adding to role strain (Han et al 2013; Allan et al 2011; Dolan 2003). As appropriate, the demands of clinical practice take priority, and as such, tasks are often viewed as add-on activities attended to only when time permits. Not surprisingly, practitioners in this unenviable position frequently report feeling frustrated and unhappy that their role in the supervision and support of students cannot be made more of a priority (Wisdom 2011; Vinales 2015). As a result, what students learn can be left to chance, with decisions about performance sometimes made without any real concrete evidence of the student's confidence and competence (Gainsbury 2010; Lawson [unpublished report] 2010, Cassidy 2017). However, such decisions are not without legal and ethical ramifications.

This chapter will explore issues of responsibility and accountability surrounding assessment in preregistration health care education and professional practice. It begins with a discussion of the meanings and implications of the concepts of responsibility and accountability in professional practice and continues with an exploration of two key questions surrounding the assessment of clinical practice:

- What are health professionals responsible and accountable for?
- Who are health professionals responsible and accountable to?

ACCOUNTABILITY AND PROFESSIONALISM

As professions such as nursing and midwifery, regulated by the Nursing and Midwifery Council (NMC) and other health care professions regulated by the Health and Care Professions Council (HCPC) strive for professional status and self-regulation, the term 'accountability' has assumed increasing importance and is now considered as an integral part of health care practice in the UK (Allen & Dennis 2010; Ormerod 1993; Emerton 1992; RCN 2019). Society places a high value on the health care professions. The confidence and trust in which health care professionals are held are measures of the special relationship with the vulnerable patients and clients in their care, with health care professionals required to consider and observe, often simultaneously, ethical, psychological, ethnic and human rights aspects in their day-to-day work. As a result, not surprisingly, accountability remains high on the agenda of both the NMC and the HCPC.

In the UK, both the NMC and HCPC came into being in 2002. The HCPC was established under the Health Professions Order 2001 in February 2002 (HCPC 2001; SI 2002 No. 254), and the NMC was established under the Nurses and Midwives Order 2001 in April 2002 (NMC 2001; SI 2002 No. 253). The primary mandate of both is to safeguard the health and well-being of the general public by keeping a register of all their registrants and ensuring they are fit to practice. In addition, they also set the standards for the education, training and conduct of those on the register. However, note that they do not work in isolation but rather in collaboration with others, including statutory and professional bodies, education providers, employers and education commissioners.

In 2002, the NMC published its first code of professional conduct, now known as The Code: Professional Standards of Practice and Behaviour for Nurses, Midwives and Nursing Associates (NMC 2018a). Likewise, the HCPC published Standards of Conduct, Performance and Ethics for its registrants in 2003 when their register opened that year, with the latest edition published in 2016 (HCPC 2016). Although safeguarding standards and principles of practice for patients and clients remain core to both publications, they are also intended to assist individual practitioners by an expression of the components of acceptable professional practice and related ethical considerations. As a result, they set out the responsibilities and accountability of the registered practitioner, and, facilitating the basis of the regulatory framework, they stress the personal accountability of each practitioner for their own practice, making it clear that this may not be delegated or transferred to another person. They also expressly require that the interests of patients and clients should take precedence over all other considerations.

Accountability becomes strikingly real when set in the context of clinical situations where professional knowledge and competence are exercised, caring for the diverse range of patients and clients. It is evident that professional accountability in the health care professions is a complex matter, which, as Caulfield (2005) proposed, can be viewed as being derived from four pillars: professional, ethical, lawful and employment/contractual.

ACCOUNTABILITY AND RESPONSIBILITY

There are many questions that can be asked about accountability in general. You may wish to carry out Activity 2.1 before progressing, with an exploration of the concept of accountability.

> ### Activity 2.1
>
> What is meant by accountability? What is the relationship between responsibility and accountability?

However, it is not possible within the realms of this chapter to enter into an extensive philosophical discussion of the concepts of accountability and responsibility. As such, discussion is therefore limited to aspects relevant to the educational role of practitioners.

Responsibility is linked inextricably with accountability. However, the focus of responsibility is on the task at hand and not on accounting for it (Cornock 2011). We talk of a 'responsible person' as one who accepts and executes an undertaking so long as it is within their capabilities (RCN 2019). To be responsible implies being answerable to either another or oneself for an act; it implies a moral accountability for one's actions as long as the individual is capable of rational conduct and fulfilling obligations for vested trust (Brykczynska 2003). Bergman (1981) goes on to state that although responsibility is only a part of accountability, it is a key component. Cornock (2011) suggests that accountability is a higher-level activity than responsibility because the person is not only responsible for an action undertaken but is also required to give an account, reason or explanation for the action, either right or wrong.

In the case of nurses and midwives who assess the clinical practice of preregistration students in the UK, the NMC states that they are accountable for confirming that students have met, or not met, the NMC standards in practice (NMC 2018b). However, before one can be accountable, several preconditions must be present, as shown in the model used by Bergman (2003:55) (Fig. 2.1). The basic precondition is that individuals need to have the ability (knowledge, skills, values) to decide and act on a specific issue to be able to act autonomously. The individual must then be given, or take, the responsibility to carry out that action as well as the autonomy to carry out the action

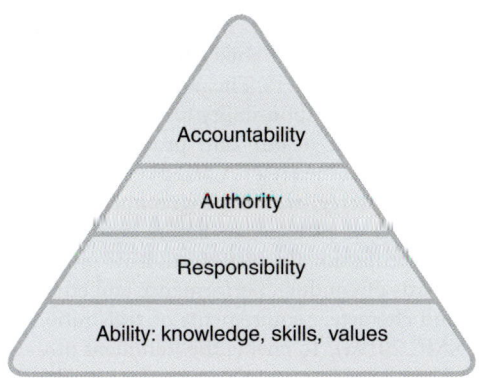

Fig. 2.1 Model of the preconditions leading to accountability. (From Bergman R. Accountability – definition and dimensions. *Int Nurs Rev,* 1981;28(2):53–59. With permission.)

(Cornock 2011). The link between accountability and autonomy here is key because without the autonomy to make decisions freely about the form of action to be taken, a practitioner is unable to be accountable. For example, in the situation where a health professional is instructed to undertake an action as well as the way it should be undertaken, then the health professional is not, in fact, accountable but responsible.

Champion (1991) describes two forms of autonomy: personal and structural. Personal autonomy refers to the expertise, knowledge and skills related to the defined area of work, the understanding of personal limits of competence and the willingness to take responsibility, whereas structural autonomy is the authority to act given by the organisation. It can thus be expected that an accountable person does not undertake an action merely because someone in authority says to do so. Instead, the accountable person examines a situation, explores the various options available, demonstrates a knowledgeable understanding of the possible consequences of options and decides for action which can be justified from a knowledge base (Marks-Maran 2003; Cornock 2011).

Professional accountability involves accepting responsibility for professional decisions. Stated more simply, practitioners are 'entrusted with, answerable for, take the credit and blame for and can be judged within legal and moral boundaries' (Castledine 1991). The Royal College of Nursing (RCN) (2023) suggests that to be accountable, practitioners must:

- have the ability to perform the activity or intervention
- accept responsibility for doing the activity
- have the authority to perform the activity, through delegation and the policies and protocols of the organisation.

In view of the substantial clinical role of practitioners, the HCPC Standards of Conduct, Performance and Ethics (HCPC 2016) appropriately focus on professional accountability to patients and clients. Generally, such practitioners are in little doubt about their professional accountability towards their patients and clients. However, professional accountability for nursing and midwifery education did not receive the same attention and interest (Marks-Maran 2003; Harding & Greig 1994) until the publication of the NMC Standards to Support Learning and Assessment in Practice (NMC 2008). It was then that accountability for student learning and assessment in clinical practice started to receive due attention.

There can be few health care practitioners who are not in some way involved in the training and supervision of others, and such roles frequently form part of the contract of employment.

NMC registrants who support preregistration nursing or midwifery students and make summative assessment decisions were traditionally termed as mentors and sign-off mentors, and within this model, students were expected to work at least 40% of their time with a mentor and be signed off as proficient by a sign-off mentor at the end of their programme. However, in 2018, the NMC published their Standards for Student Supervision and Assessment, and these have been in effect since 28 January 2019 (NMC 2018b). Within these, the NMC introduced three roles to the supervision and assessment of students: practice supervisors, who must be registered with a professional regulator such as the NMC, General Medical Council (GMC) or HCPC, who support and supervise nursing and midwifery students in practice; practice assessors, registrants with appropriate equivalent experience for the student's field of practice (for midwifery, this has to be a midwife) who are responsible for the assessment and confirmation of the achievement of proficiencies and programme outcomes; and academic assessors, registrants usually from an approved academic institute, with appropriate equivalent experience for the student's field of practice who, in partnership with the practice assessor, are responsible for collating and confirming the achievement of proficiencies and programme outcomes. The overall aim stated by the NMC for this change was to give approved education institutions and practice learning partners more flexibility to develop creative approaches to education while still being accountable for the local delivery and management of approved programmes in line with NMC standards (NMC 2018b).

In the case of registrants on the HCPC register, practice educators must also have relevant knowledge, skills and experience to support safe and effective learning and be on the relevant part of the HCPC register (HCPC 2018a). However, akin to the NMC, they also recognize that in some circumstances, there may be other appropriate practice educators whose backgrounds do not match the specific profession that the student is studying but whose knowledge, skills and experience mean that they are well suited to support and develop learners in a particular area. For example, occupational therapists may supervise physiotherapy students in areas such as hand therapy, and nurses may supervise radiographers in aseptic techniques (HCPC 2017). In such circumstances, the HCPC acknowledges that 'other arrangements are appropriate' and could include professionals registered with a different regulator. Although the Standards of Education and Training of the HCPC (HCPC 2018a) state that practice educators involved in formative and summative assessment 'must undertake regular training which is appropriate to their, role, learner's needs and the delivery of the learning outcomes of the programme', they don't specify any precise standards to guide this practice.

The requirements for training, supervision and support of preregistration health care students, and the concomitant assessment of learning, mean that such roles are now often integral to practitioners' day-to-day practice. Dimond (1994:272) says that 'for the most part this is unlikely to give rise to many legal issues'. However, an awareness of the potential pitfalls and problems associated with these roles may prevent grief from arising. The rest of the chapter therefore examines accountability issues surrounding the assessment of clinical practice, providing an exploration of the moral and legal obligations that practice educators have to fulfil. The rights of learners and why they have legal means of redress will also be explained.

Because of the differences in terminology used by the NMC and the HCPC for the educational role of registrants to preregistration students in clinical practice, all health care practitioners who support and supervise preregistration students and conduct their summative assessments during clinical practice are referred to as 'practice educators' in the rest of this book.

ACCOUNTABILITY FOR THE ASSESSMENT OF CLINICAL PRACTICE

Before going on to explore this section, consider the questions posed in Activity 2.2.

Activity 2.2

What are practice educators responsible and accountable **for**?
Who are practice educators responsible and accountable **to**?

Almost 25 years ago, in its document *Making a Difference* (Department of Health 1999:24), the government made it clear that the National Health Service (NHS)

needed practitioners who are fit for purpose, with excellent skills, the knowledge and ability to provide the best care possible in a modern NHS. The point made was that every practitioner shares responsibility to support and teach the next generation of health care professionals. Both the NMC (2018b) and the HCPC (2018b) expect that students who complete preregistration programmes must have met their standards of proficiency. Before entry to the NMC and HCPC professional registers, students must also meet the standards of conduct, performance and ethics and the health and character requirements of registration (HCPC 2016; NMC 2019a). To enable the fulfilment of these professional requirements, practice educators need to be cognizant of their responsibility and accountability for the supervision and assessment of clinical practice.

The following section examines what the practice educator is responsible and accountable for when supervising and assessing learners.

RESPONSIBILITY AND ACCOUNTABILITY FOR WHAT?

For nurses and midwives, direct reference is made to professional accountability for the support and supervision of learners in the NMC Code: Professional Standards of Practice and Behaviour for Nurses, Midwives and Nursing Associates (NMC 2018a). The Standards state:

> You must support students' and colleagues' learning to help them develop their professional competence and confidence.

In regard to accountability, both standards, the NMC Code (2018a) and HCPC Standards of Conduct, Performance and Ethics (2016), make it clear that no one else can answer for you, and it will be no defence to say that you were acting on someone else's orders. The NMC states:

> The professional commitment to work within one's competence is a key underpinning principle of the Code.

The HCPC also states:

> You must keep within your scope of practice by only practicing in the areas you have appropriate knowledge, skills and experience for.

Both sets of standards also make it clear that, if you delegate work to someone, your responsibility and accountability is to make sure that the person who does the work is able to carry out your instructions safely and effectively and that proper supervision and support are provided. The NMC further states that nurses and midwives must also confirm that the outcome of any delegated tasks meets required standards.

When these requirements for professional practice are applied to assessment, it can be seen that the practitioner has professional responsibility and accountability to fulfil in her/his role as a practice educator. It is suggested here that the practice educator can be answerable for standards of personal professional practice, with its inevitable impact on learning, and the following aspects of supervision and assessment:

- standards of personal professional practice
- standards of care delivery by learners
- what is taught, learned and assessed
- standards of teaching and assessing
- professional judgements about student performance.

PERSONAL PROFESSIONAL STANDARDS OF PRACTICE

As discussed in Chapter 1, one of the purposes of assessment in preregistration health care education is as a form of quality control for the outcome of the educational process. The educational and professional outcome is a professional who can apply their knowledge, understanding and skills to perform to the standards required in employment. As such, this professional must have met the standards of proficiency required (NMC 2018b; HCPC 2023), and before entry to both professional registers, students must also meet the standards of conduct, performance and ethics, as well as the health and character requirements of registration.

The full realization of this outcome is dependent on the successful achievement of both theoretical and clinical learning and professional development measured by assessment. As such, assessment is an integral part of professional health care programmes. The processes of clinical teaching, learning and assessment are complex. The committed input of practice educators is required to plan and implement these processes if learning outcomes are to be achieved successfully. I would suggest that this commitment starts with the individual practitioner's competence and standard of practice. Eraut et al (1995) state that, if aspects of clinicians' practice are ill-defined, lack quality or make insufficient use of scientific knowledge, the next generation of practitioners will suffer.

Much of the learning that takes place in professional education does so in the practice setting. Role modelling is an important (Fowler 2008; Pollard 2008; Spouse 1998; Wood 1987), and an almost inevitable, learning strategy in this environment. Within social learning theory, Bandura (1977) suggests that, in role modelling, one person sets a pattern of behaviour that is then copied by another. Learning takes place constantly from observing role models deliver care – these practices are subsequently emulated (Charters 2000). Jack et al's (2017) study of role modelling illustrated that students highly valued exposure to positive role models in the clinical setting, seeing them as both beneficial to learning and inspirational to the type of nurse they aspired to become. Conversely, exposure to negative role models led to adverse effects on learning, poor practice and disillusionment with the profession. As stated succinctly by McAllister et al (2009:205), 'students are a product of their schooling'. It is therefore important for the practice educator to adhere to high standards of professional practice so that students learn this high standard of care and are assessed against these professional practices. A high standard of care from students cannot be expected if this is not role modelled. Without modelling high standards of practice, one aspect of professional and moral accountability will not be fulfilled.

Nicklin and Kenworthy (2000:72) say that 'assessment inevitably takes place in a role-relationship'. The usual relationship that exists between a student and a practice educator is hierarchical in nature. Neary (2000) pointed out that many practice educators take for granted their position of power in the assessment relationship. Her study in 1996 (in Neary 2000) showed the extent to which this 'taken-for-granted' power imbalance became explicit at early stages of the relationship when practice educators quickly confirmed their expertise and established the subordination of their students. In a review of the literature on how practice educators influence practice, Armstrong (2010) found that a student's actual experience is one of control and coercion. Students felt powerless in challenging practice owing to their lack of status and the fear of jeopardizing their clinical assessment and securing a job.

Within this hierarchical situation, one assumption made of the practitioner as practice educator is that they possess the requisite professional qualities and can recognize these in the learner (Harding & Greig 1994). This assumption is, of course, open to debate. Hepworth (1991:46) expressed her disagreement when she said that: 'the assessor of a student's clinical nursing skills can only assess the student in the light of her [sic] own perceptions of the nursing situation, and her own nursing expertise'.

Our assessments, then, are likely to be based on our own standards of practice and perceptions of the situation. Therefore, as practitioners who are also practice educators, there is the responsibility for maintaining competent practice so that assessments are made against these standards. Furthermore, in exercising professional accountability, the NMC (2018a) and the HCPC (2016) require their practitioners on the professional registers to maintain and improve professional knowledge and competence. One point arising from debates on competence is the requirement for the practitioner to keep up to date to claim that practice is competent (Hager & Gonczi 1995; McGaghie 1991). Notwithstanding professional requirements, the bottom line in the argument for keeping up to date must be the legal requirement that professional health care practitioners can exercise contemporary professional practices because the law expects current practice to be the accepted practice (Dimond 2019; Young 2009). There is an expectation that practitioners will employ evidence-based practice, and, generally speaking, judges will take a dim view of practitioners who fail to follow the latest clinical guidelines (Young 2009). The duty of care to patients requires practitioners to keep their knowledge and practice up to date (Griffith & Tengnah 2016).

Young (1994) states that the legal implication of omitting certain information, or of giving wrong information, is potential negligence on the part of the instructor. This potential exists whenever a failure in instruction jeopardizes the safety of the learner being instructed, or of the patient in her care. I would also suggest that, unless a practice educator is also a competent practitioner, training requirements may not be fulfilled owing to the inability to teach what constitutes competent practice. The practice educator thus has a legal duty, as well as moral and professional accountability to fulfil, in terms of keeping up to date and maintaining competent practice. If it could be established that a patient/client suffered harm as a consequence of negligent instruction (e.g. incorrect information to a student), the patient/client could instigate legal action against the instructor.

STANDARDS OF CARE DELIVERY BY LEARNERS

The practice educator has a dual responsibility: to the patient/client and to the student. A major aspect of the concept of professional negligence in clinical practice is that practice educators have a 'specific duty or responsibility to foresee or anticipate the possible adverse outcomes of their actions' (Gunby 2008:414). This applies to both client care and supervision of students. Practice educators must meet a standard of care with respect to the patient/client and a standard of conduct with respect to the student. Practice educators must ensure that students have the necessary clinical experiences and supervision to develop professional competencies in such a way that the patient/client is not harmed in any way while the student is giving the care. The NMC (2018a) and the HCPC (2016) state that patient safety must always take precedence above all else. The NMC Code: Professional Standards of Practice and Behaviour for Nurses, Midwives and Nursing Associates (2018a) and HCPC Standards of Conduct, Performance and Ethics (HCPC 2016) make sure that practitioners put the interests of patients, clients and the public before their own interests and those of professional colleagues, that is, accountability to the patient is always more important than to the student.

The Bolam test (see later discussion) applies to delegation (Dimond 2019). In the eyes of the law, the student's performance must be equal to that of a registered practitioner. The law is quite clear that a lack of experience or knowledge is never an excuse for incompetent care (Griffith & Tengnah 2016; Young 1994). Students of health care are thus required to provide care equivalent to that of the registered practitioner. One judge (in Young 1994:56) adopted the following view:

> The law requires the trainee or learner to be judged by the same standard as his more experienced colleagues. If it did not, inexperience would frequently be urged as a defence to an action for professional negligence.

Another judge linked the expected standard of care to that of the post rather than to the status of the person performing the care, saying:

> To my mind the notion of a duty tailored to the actor, rather than to the act which he elects to perform, has no place in the law of tort.

Therefore, in a highly specialized clinical setting, the standard must be 'not just that of the averagely competent and well-informed [nurse] but of such a person who fills a post in a unit offering a highly specialized service' (Wilsher v Essex AHA 1988, in Young 1994).

For students to deliver care to a standard equivalent to that of a registered practitioner, that care to be given must be within the student's capabilities. So far as the NMC (2018a) and HCPC (2016) are concerned, it is the registered practitioner working with the student who is professionally responsible for the consequences of the actions and omissions of that student. A preregistration student, or any other unqualified staff, who is not on the professional register cannot be called to account for their actions or omissions because registered practitioners are accountable for care given, whether directly or through delegation. It is the personal and professional responsibility of the practitioner who delegates an activity to make sure that the person carrying out the activity is trained and competent and has the necessary experience to undertake the activity safely (Dimond 2019). The delegating professional must also make sure that the appropriate level of supervision is provided. The provision of appropriate levels of supervision are developed in Chapter 7.

A number of cases of qualified staff were reported to the then UK Central Council for Nursing, Midwifery and Health Visiting (UKCC 1996) for inappropriate delegation of responsibilities. One case, which was closed by the Preliminary Proceedings Committee (PPC) of the UKCC, concerned the delegation, by a nurse to a care assistant, of the task of administering an insulin injection. The case was reported on the basis that such administration by a care assistant was prima facie wrong. The issue considered by the PPC was not that the care assistant could not give the injection, but whether the person to whom the responsibility was being delegated was competent to carry out the task. The UKCC concluded that the issue was about supervision, the appropriateness of the delegation and the instruction of unqualified staff, and not about the rigid demarcation of work into tasks to be done by one group or another.

It is therefore important to know when and to whom it is safe to delegate. To delegate safely and to avoid negligent delegation, the practitioner must be satisfied that the person performing the delegated task is competent to carry it out (Dimond 2019; Young 1994). Making the following two checks may help you to decide when it is safe to delegate. Assess:

- The extent of the person's knowledge and understanding of the task. This requires skilful questioning of the person. This point is developed in Chapter 4.
- How skilful the person is in the task delegated. This may require observation and close supervision of the person initially. It is important to provide ongoing supervision. The amount and extent of the supervision will vary from person to person. However, Wood (1987) holds that students must be under strict supervision at all times. This point on supervision of students will be developed in Chapter 6 when management of the continuous assessment process is discussed.

The learning and assessment programme for the student must therefore be planned so that the patient/client is protected from harm while the student is enabled to develop and achieve the professional standards of proficiency required.

The NMC (2018c) has issued detailed guidance on delegation that is available on its website. The guidance considers the principles of delegation by nurses and midwives, the responsibility and accountability of the practitioner who delegates and the documentation required.

WHAT IS TAUGHT, LEARNED AND ASSESSED

The practice educator has the responsibility for ensuring that the learning environment is conducive to learning. A wide range of high-quality learning opportunities should be arranged and provided to enable the student to achieve learning outcomes and competencies. The Nursing and Midwifery Order 2001 (NMC 2001) and the Health Professions Order 2001 (HCPC 2001) require the NMC and HCPC to determine the standard, kind and content of training to be undertaken with a view to registration. The standards of proficiency and standards of education required for all preregistration health care education regulated by the NMC and the HCPC are set out in the text of the legislation for regulation in the Registration Rules (NMC 2004) and Standards of Education and Training under Article 15(1) – (9) of the Health Professions Order, 2001, respectively.

Preregistration nursing and midwifery programmes in the UK now require students to achieve national NMC standards of proficiency (NMC 2018d). In the case of professions regulated by the HCPC, in addition to standards all professionals must meet to become registered, each profession has defined its own standards of proficiency that apply to their scope of practice with varied dates of implementation (HCPC 2023).

It is a requirement that preregistration programmes must be designed to enable students to apply knowledge, understanding and skills when performing to the standards required in employment and to provide the care that patients/clients require, safely and competently, to assume, on registration, the responsibilities and accountability necessary for public protection. Both the NMC and HCPC make it clear that these standards of proficiency are achieved under the direction of the practice educator. In accepting the roles of practice educator as defined by the NMC and the HCPC (NMC 2018b; HCPC 2018a,), the practitioner is responsible for ensuring that teaching and learning activities, including clinical experiences, assist the student in achieving these standards of proficiency. This requires practitioners to have a sound knowledge and understanding of the learning outcomes to be achieved and expectations of professional conduct and assessment procedures, including the implications of, and any action to be taken in the case of, failure to progress. This will enable the practice educator to identify and plan appropriate teaching and learning activities and clinical experiences.

As in any practice discipline, it is not enough just to have 'knowledge of' – one also needs to know what to do with that knowledge. This leads into the next 'what for' aspect of accountability of the practice educator: namely, that of facilitating and measuring that learning.

STANDARDS OF TEACHING AND ASSESSING

The student is entitled to the best instruction available (Young 1994; Wood 1987). Failure to instruct properly could be construed as a negligent act (Dimond 2019, Goclowski 1985). The standard of teaching and learning that an academic institution is expected to provide is generally stated in the educational institution's student charter. Service providers for patient/client care enter into contracts with higher-education institutions to provide clinical experience for students. Within such contracts is an agreement to provide a standard of teaching and learning in the clinical setting commensurate with that set by the educational institution. To achieve the required standards of the teaching and assessment of clinical practice, practice educators need to attain and maintain competent practice in these roles (HCPC 2016; NMC 2018b). It is recognized that clinical staff exercise a major influence on the quality of preregistration programmes (Allan et al 2011; Eraut et al 1995). They do much of the teaching, supervision and assessment of students, and because it is likely that this will continue, it is imperative that they are capable of fulfilling these roles. Activities that practice educators are expected to provide will include planning learning opportunities for and with students to enable them to achieve their individual learning needs, facilitating and supporting the learning process, assessing learning and providing feedback to students on their performance (NMC 2018b; Neary 2000; Eraut et al 1995). To support these educational processes in the clinical setting, higher-education institutions include a policy for the management of the assessment of clinical practice in its curriculum document. Generally, the practice educator is required to carry out an initial interview with the student to negotiate and formulate a learning contract/plan to facilitate the achievement of learning outcomes and standards of proficiency. Subsequently, an intermediate interview should take place halfway through the placement to review the student's progress and achievement, and formal feedback should be given and documented. A final interview allows the practice educator to make a summative assessment of whether the student has achieved the learning outcomes of the placement.

Practice educators must be aware of, and be careful that, any policy regulating the assessment of practice is followed, as any deviation from such regulations could give rise to students appealing against any unfavourable assessment decision on the grounds of not having received the supervision, guidance and support to which they are entitled. Cases of students suing nursing institutions in the courts using the above grounds as educational malpractice are well documented in the North American literature (see, for example, Johnson 2012; Goudreau & Chasens 2002; Graveley & Stanley 1993; Goclowski 1985; Spink 1983). Courts have recognized that, by virtue of their training, practice educators are uniquely qualified to observe and judge all aspects of their students' performance. Court decisions ruling in favour of the student have been on the basis of practice educators not following established guidelines for the supervision of the student.

Practice educators require adequate preparation to enable them to manage the educational activities to support learning and assessment. Subsequently, regular updates are important to keep abreast of developments and/or changes in the curriculum, the assessment process and new local and national policies influencing health care education. In the case of nurses and midwives and registrants with the HCPC, the NMC and HCPC require practice educators to update regularly (HCPC 2018a; NMC 2018b). The practices of supervision and assessing can be enhanced if these 'update' sessions are also used as opportunities to discuss assessment problems and how these had been dealt with by individuals.

However, unfortunately, the perineal debate about the expertise of practice educators remains, with research highlighting factors such as emotions, insufficient competence and insufficient support both in the working environment and from the university (Duffy 2004; Hughes et al 2016; Bachmann et al 2019). Whereas practice educators are personally accountable for their practice of the supervision and assessment of students (HCPC 2016; NMC 2018b), service providers and higher-education institutions have joint responsibility for ensuring that training, support and updating opportunities are provided for practitioners to develop their role as practice educator (HCPC 2018a; NMC 2018b).

PROFESSIONAL JUDGEMENTS ABOUT STUDENT PERFORMANCE

By virtue of their role, practice educators have the right to make, and are indeed vested with the onerous responsibility and accountability for making, professional judgements about the performance of students (HCPC 2018a; NMC 2018b). These professional judgements require the practice educator to make and report on two important professional decisions: first, they are reporting on the degree to which a student has met the programme learning outcomes and standard; second, they are reporting on the ability of the student to provide professionally competent and safe care to the public. Practice educators to students on NMC-approved programmes leading to registration, or a qualification that is recordable on the register, are **accountable** to the NMC for their assessment decisions about fitness to practise of students to enter the register and whether they have the necessary knowledge, skills and competence to take on the role of registered nurse, midwife or specialist community public health nurse (NMC 2018b). Although the HCPC does not make a direct reference to accountability for summative assessment decisions, it may be inferred from the Standards of Conduct, Performance and Ethics (HCPC 2016) that HCPC registrants who are practice educators are also accountable, thus:

'As a registrant, you are personally responsible for the way you behave. You will need to use your judgement so that you make informed and reasonable decisions and meet the standards. You must always be prepared to justify your decisions and actions' (p. 4).

It is important for the practice educator to remember that professional judgements not only assess the student's current competence but also provide a prediction of the student's potential ability to practise as a professional nurse or midwife, physiotherapist, or social worker and so on. Therefore, the conclusion about a student's performance should attempt to elicit reliability and predictive validity. These important criteria of sound assessments are discussed in Chapter 5.

Literature on the assessment of clinical practice abounds with discussions about the subjective nature of this process. Ashworth and Morrison (1991:260) stated that:

> … assessing involves the perception of evidence about performance by an assessor, and the arrival at a decision concerning the level of performance of the person being assessed. Here there is enormous, unavoidable scope for subjectivity especially when the competencies being assessed are relatively intangible ones.

Assessments about a student's performance frequently reflect the practice educator's personal perception of what performance constitutes professional practice. Such an assessment is based on both objective and subjective criteria. There is, therefore, a danger that some decisions about student performance may be biased and unfair. Practice educators should be aware that many factors, some of which they are unaware of, can interfere with fair and equitable professional judgements, resulting in the student being treated unfairly.

As noted earlier, students have the right to expect that they will be notified of any deficiencies in their performance. The practice educator is behaving unfairly and unethically if the student is not informed about unsatisfactory performance (Orchard 1994). Furthermore, practice educators who fail to evaluate a student's unsatisfactory performance accurately, either through reluctance to expose the student to the experience of failure or through a fear of potential redress by the student, are guilty of misleading the student, potentially jeopardizing patient/client care and placing the higher-education institution in a difficult situation. It is much fairer to students to inform them of unsatisfactory performance as soon as such performance is identified. Informing students of deficiencies in a caring and constructive way allows students the opportunity to improve their performance; not to inform them denies them this opportunity and right (Killam et al 2010; Johnson 2012).

Practice educators have a moral responsibility to fail incompetent students (Gopee 2008; Beaumont 2004; Ilott & Murphy 1999). Beaumont's call came after Duffy (2004) reported that practice educators were 'failing to fail' nursing students. Being 'kind' to students by not failing them is not in the best interest of the student, especially when there is a delay to fail until late into the programme, such as in the final year. Having to inform family and friends that one will now not be able to graduate owing to failure, after having been on the programme for 2 years, can do untold damage to the self-esteem of that student, not to mention the accrual of student loans to be repaid. Failing to fail students is also not in the best interest of the profession for obvious reasons. An awareness of those factors that contribute to failure to fail may be a first step to understanding why difficulties are experienced when dealing with a failing student, and may assist the practice educator in not passing a student when a fail is clearly warranted. It is suggested here that the responsibility for seeking assistance and/or support to make valid summative assessment decisions rests with the individual practice educator. The issues of the unsafe student and 'failure to fail' will be explored further in Chapter 7.

I have put forward what I see are the main aspects that practice educators are responsible and accountable for when they supervise and assess learners. The next section examines the 'to whom?' aspects.

RESPONSIBILITY AND ACCOUNTABILITY TO WHOM?

As discussed earlier, one position that the RCN takes in relationship to professional accountability is that it comprises ethical, societal and public duty and protective elements for patients and clients. These elements of professional accountability may also be applied to the supervision and assessment of learners. With professional registration, each practitioner is vested with personal autonomy. A contract of employment gives the structural autonomy for the authority to act in the best interests of patients and clients. This contract frequently also requires the practitioner to take on the role of practice educator; this gives the practice educator the authority to act in the best interests of the learner.

Based on the context of accountability, and extrapolating from the work of mainstream education, practice educators responsible for the supervision and assessment of clinical practice can be seen to assume the three aspects of educational accountability described by Becher et al (1981):

- professional accountability: responsibility to self, colleagues and the profession
- contractual accountability: accountability to the employer or someone in authority
- moral accountability: answerability to students.

Teachers are accountable for their professional conduct, such as the selection and implementation of appropriate forms of practice. Contractually, they are under an obligation to report to, and be partly directed by, a specific person or group of persons. A teacher in mainstream education is contractually accountable to the head teacher. Moral accountability is of special importance in education because it pervades the teacher–pupil relationship. These aspects of accountability will now be used to examine the to whom aspects of responsibility and accountability when supervising and assessing the clinical practice of students. Before you proceed, you may wish to try Activity 2.3.

Activity 2.3

Make a list of the individuals and bodies that you consider you are responsible for and accountable to when you supervise and assess students. Why do you think you are responsible for and accountable to them?

These individuals and bodies are listed in Fig. 2.2. In acknowledgement of professional responsibility and accountability required of the practitioner by the NMC and HCPC, the most important individual would be the patient/client.

Each of the previously mentioned individuals and bodies shown in Fig. 2.2 will now be considered in an examination of why you might be responsible and accountable to them. This will be developed in four sections, namely, that of responsibility and accountability to:

- the patient/client
- the student
- the trust/employing authority and the higher-education institution
- yourself, colleagues and your profession.

THE PATIENT/CLIENT

The practitioner on the NMC or HCPC professional register has both a legal and a professional duty of care to patients and clients. In law, the courts could find a registered practitioner negligent if a person suffers harm because the practitioner has failed to provide proper care to that person. Professionally, the NMC's and HCPC's Fitness to Practice Committee can find a registered practitioner guilty of misconduct and remove the practitioner from the register if there has been failure to provide adequate care

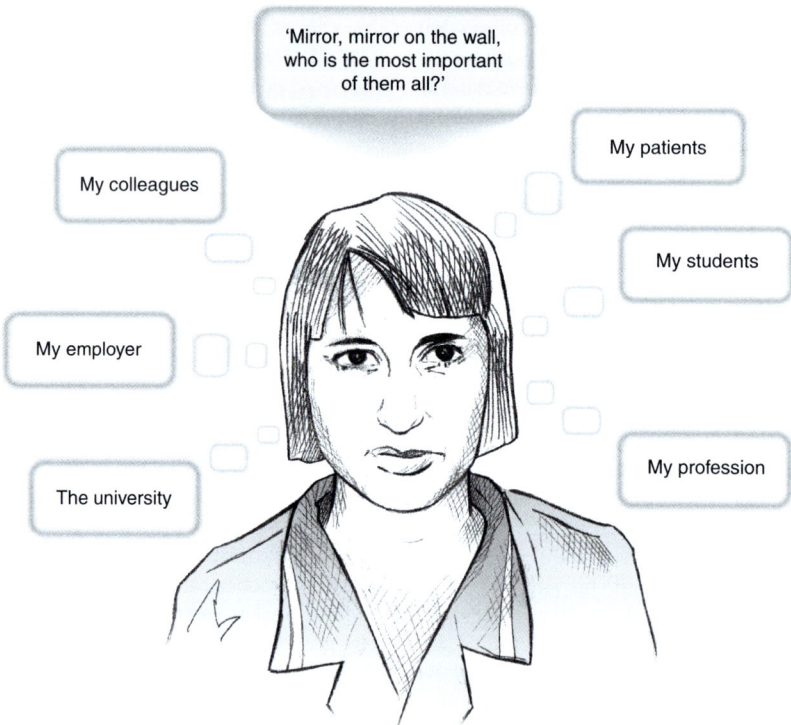

Fig. 2.2 Juggling responsibilities?

for patients/clients (HCPC Tribunal Service 2019; NMC 2019b). The practitioner's accountability and duty of care to the patient/client when supervising students has been discussed at some length in the previous section (see responsibility and accountability for standards of care delivery by learners). It will be reiterated here that the preregistration student cannot be called to account by the NMC or HCPC for any actions and omissions. It is the registered practitioner with whom the student is working who is professionally responsible and accountable for the consequences of the student's actions and omissions. In law, the practitioner could also be found to be negligent for the actions and omissions of the student (Goudreau & Chasens 2002). These authors reported the case of a patient in North America who was injured while under the care of a medical student who had been left to make inappropriate decisions. The courts determined that the supervisor was negligent in his duty because of lack of adequate supervision of the student.

When making arrangements for students to care for patients and clients, the wishes of patients and clients should be respected at all times. Under the NHS Constitution for England, patients/clients have the right to choose whether or not to take part in medical research or student training (Department of Health & Social Care 2015). This right should be made clear to them when they are first given information about care they will receive from students. Their rights as patients or clients supersede at all times the student's rights to knowledge and experience (NMC 2018a; HCPC 2016).

THE STUDENT

Students have rights; practice educators need to respect these while maintaining professional standards and expectations of their performance at the same time. Students also have obligations and responsibilities to fulfil. It is important for the practice educator to recognize what these rights, obligations and responsibilities are so that the student may be assisted in the most appropriate ways to succeed during clinical practice. The practice educator also needs to recognize that there are legal, professional and moral obligations towards students under supervision.

STUDENT RIGHTS, OBLIGATIONS, RESPONSIBILITIES AND ACCOUNTABILITY

Student Rights

Higher-education institutions have the right to set academic standards for students. They have the responsibility to communicate those standards to students. Institutions have written policies that govern student progression, grading and discipline. In line with CMA (Competition and Markets Authority) consumer law obligation (CMA 2015), all higher-education providers now have to give an overview of these in advance to all prospective students, with detailed policies then made available to students through the use of a student/programme handbook (Johnson 2012). Policies made within a programme of study regarding progression, grading and dismissal of students must be in line with the institution's policies. Any student who has enrolled in a course has implicitly agreed to abide by the policies of the course and those of the higher-education institution. Within assessment regulations (Johnson 2012), students have the following rights:

- to know the professional conduct and competencies that are expected of them to pass the clinical placement successfully;
- to receive timely feedback about their performance and conduct, and the opportunity and support to correct unsatisfactory performance and conduct;
- to be made aware that their performance is not meeting the criteria that have been set for satisfactory performance before being failed;
- to work under the supervision of a qualified practitioner who has been appropriately trained to be a practice educator.

Within any scheme of the continuous assessment of practice, there must be formalized meetings between the student and the practice educator to guide student learning, which will also enable these rights to be met. Assessment regulations relating to the continuous assessment of practice generally require practice educators to conduct a minimum of three documented formal interviews with student nurses and student midwives. Failure to do so could give rise to grounds for student appeal against an unfavourable assessment decision.

All higher-education institutions have established policies for hearing student grievances and appeals. These policies exist to protect students' rights and to provide student recourse to appeal assessment decisions previously made (Johnson 2012). The grievance and student appeal process provides the opportunity for the original assessment decision to be reassessed. Generally, the assessment grade and/or summative assessment decision cannot be altered, but it is likely to be declared null and void if those educational processes that were in place to support student learning and progression had been violated.

Student Obligations and Responsibility

As stated, any student who has enrolled in a course has agreed to abide by the policies of the course and those of the higher-education institution. Higher-education institutions generally have regulations governing the progress and discipline of students. Practice educators have the responsibility of assisting higher-education institutions to uphold these regulations. These regulations serve to safeguard standards of training and conduct. Failure to fulfil and/or comply with these regulations could result in the student being dismissed from the course. Students are thus directly accountable to their higher-education institution. I have known students to be disciplined by the higher-education institution for falsifying their practice educators' signatures in the assessment of practice records. This misconduct has resulted in those students being dismissed from their course.

Several responsibilities are conferred on the student. Higher-education institutions can expect students:

- to fulfil regulations governing the progress of students
- not to behave in ways that can be alleged as misconduct.

Additionally, nursing and midwifery students need to abide by the guidance set out in the NMC document The Code: Professional Standards of practice and behaviour for nurses, midwives and nursing associates (NMC 2018a). Students studying for a profession regulated by the HCPC need to abide by the guidance set out in the HCPC document Guidance on Conduct and Ethics for Students (HCPC 2016).

The NMC (2018a) and HCPC (2016) and higher-education institutions make it clear to students that they must always work under the supervision of a registered practitioner. Furthermore, students should not participate in any procedure for which they have not been fully prepared or in which they are not adequately supervised (NMC 2018a; HCPC 2016). Students must learn when to ask for help and not to allow themselves to be placed in situations where practice becomes unsafe. Working in collaboration with their practice educator, students must learn to appraise for themselves whether they are personally willing to take any risks that may be involved in any caregiving situations (Goudreau & Chasens 2002). In general, students should be allowed to practise only to the level of competence consistent with course requirements. When it becomes unclear whether engagement in an aspect of care delivery could be beyond the student's usual scope of practice, it becomes incumbent upon the student, and the practice educator, to seek guidance from the educational institution.

Student Accountability

The student can also be called to account by the law for the consequences of actions or omissions as a preregistration student (NMC 2018a; HCPC 2016). The student must behave in a reasonable way (Castledine 2000), but what is reasonable? The case of Bolam v Friern Hospital Management Committee produced the Bolam test of what is reasonable (Dimond 2019; UKCC 1996). The test derives from a case heard in 1957 where a psychiatric patient was given electroconvulsive therapy without any relaxant drugs or restraint. He suffered several fractures and claimed compensation. The judge, in deciding how to determine the standard that should have been followed, said:

> When you get a situation that involved the use of some special skill or competence, then the test as to whether there has been negligence or not is the standard of the ordinary skilled man exercising and professing to have that special skill. A man need not possess the highest expert skill; it is well established that it is sufficient if he exercises the ordinary skill of an ordinary competent man exercising that particular art.

> He is not guilty of negligence if he has acted in accordance with a practice accepted as proper by a responsible body of medical men skilled in that particular art.
> **Dimond (1994:115).**

Although the case concerned a doctor, the Bolam test can be used to examine the actions of any professional person. Thus the negligence of a professional (e.g. a nurse) is to be determined by the standard of the ordinary skilled nurse exercising and professing to have the skills of a nurse.

The case of Wilsher versus Essex AHA (1986, in Dimond 2019:66, 419) sets the standard of reasonable care to be expected of students and junior staff. The case involved a premature baby in the special care baby unit who required oxygen therapy. The junior doctor inadvertently inserted the catheter to monitor blood levels of oxygen into a vein rather than an artery. He had asked the senior registrar to check the position of the catheter following the procedure. The registrar failed to see the mistake. This resulted in incorrect oxygen levels being monitored with the consequent administration of too much oxygen. The outcome was that the baby developed near blindness resulting from incurable damage to the retina. The Bolam test was applied. The court ruled that the standard of care required was that of the ordinary skilled person, but that standard was to be determined in the context of the particular posts in the unit rather than according to the general rank or status of the post holder. The duty ought to be tailored to the act performed rather than to the doctor himself. Therefore, inexperience is no defence to an action for negligence. The judges held that the junior doctor had not been negligent and had upheld the relevant standard of care by consulting his superior. Because students have to practise under supervision (direct or indirect) at all times, they can be held liable for what they chose to do or failed to do under their own volition and will be judged according to the standards expected of a student.

GOOD HEALTH AND GOOD CHARACTER

The requirement for good health and good character to enter the professional registers and renewing registration are laid down in legislation. The Nursing and Midwifery Order (the Order; NMC 2001) and the Health Professions Order 2001 state that these regulatory bodies must prescribe the requirements to be met as to the evidence of good health and good character to satisfy the NMC and HCPC registrars that an applicant is capable of safe and effective practice without supervision; that is, the registrant is fit to practise. The requirement for evidence of good health and good character was introduced into the Order to enhance protection of the public, following a number of high-profile cases involving the health and character of doctors and nurses; see, for example, the cases that involved the nurse, Beverly Allitt (Clothier 1994), the doctor, Harold Shipman (Baker 2001) and more recently the neonatal nurse Lucy Letby.

For the purposes of the NMC's and HCPC's legislation, the term 'good health' is a relative concept. The NMC (2019a) defines good health as the capability of 'safe and effective practice without supervision. It does not mean the absence of any disability or health condition. Many disabled people and those with health conditions are able to practise with or without adjustments to support their practice'. A registrant may have a disability, such as impaired hearing, or a health condition, such as depression, epilepsy, diabetes or heart disease, and yet be perfectly capable of safe and effective practice. However, there are some conditions that would be likely to affect a practitioner's ability to practise safely and effectively, such as alcoholism or other substance misuse. In 2018 to 2019, the NMC (NMC 2019c) reviewed 1990 cases by means of a full investigation, 661 of which resulted in a hearing or meeting. Of these, 25% of practitioners were struck off the register, 35% suspended, 15% given conditions of practice, 8% a caution, 3% case not proven and 14% fitness to practice not impaired. In 2017 to 2018, Health Committee panels of the HCPC considered 432 cases, 414 relating to conduct and competence, 17 relating to physical and/or mental health and 1 to fraudulent entry. Of these, 51% resulted in a sanction that prevented them from practice, 12% restricted practice, 12% a caution entry on the register and 24% of cases were considered not well founded or resulted in no further action (HCPC 2018c).

Good character is central to the Standards of Conduct, Performance and Ethics in that practitioners must be honest and trustworthy. The NMC (2019a) states that 'good character is based on an individual's conduct, behaviour and attitude. It also takes into account any convictions, cautions and pending charges that are likely to be incompatible with professional registration. A person's character must be sufficiently good for them to be capable of safe and effective practice without supervision'. Both the NMC and HCPC state that an important determinant of good character is the individual's commitment to compliance with the Standards of Conduct, Performance and Ethics (HCPC 2017a; NMC 2019a, 2019b). Examples of the nature of the allegations made in cases considered by panels of the Conduct and Competence Committee during this time included dishonesty (e.g. falsifying records, fraud or a false claim of sick leave), breach of professional boundaries with service users (e.g. verbal/physical/sexual abuse of a patient or inappropriate relationships with patients), attending work under the influence of alcohol, convictions and/or theft of drugs (NMC 2019c; HCPC 2018c).

Before being admitted to a preregistration health programme, good health will normally be checked and assessed by a local occupational health department. This includes the completion of a health questionnaire. Additionally, students are required to declare their good health annually during the programme. Good character will normally be assessed by taking up character references from reliable referees. Programme providers are also required by the NMC and HCPC to carry out an enhanced criminal conviction check through the Disclosure and Barring Service or equivalent (Disclosure Scotland, Access Northern Ireland) and request confirmation that the person is not barred from working with children or vulnerable adults.

Students are required to maintain good health and good character throughout the educational programme. Students must inform the programme provider immediately if they have any charges, convictions or cautions during the programme.

Programme providers are required by the NMC and HCPC to set up processes to monitor good health and good character throughout the programme to deal with any new issues that arise. A local fitness to practise process and panel must be in place to consider any health or character issues to ensure that public protection is maintained. Concerns include those relating to a student's health, behaviour or attitude which may affect the student's fitness to practise in the relevant profession. These concerns may be brought to the attention of the university by any person or organization. Generally, within assessment structures and processes, practice educators contribute evidence to enable the higher-education institution to judge whether the student is suitable to remain on the educational programme and, ultimately, to enter the NMC and HCPC professional registers. If you suspect, or are aware, that a student's good health and/or good character may be in question, you must inform the university. This is normally done via the university lecturer who liaises with your clinical area.

A student must be of good health and good character before being admitted to the NMC and HCPC professional registers (NMC 2019a; HCPC 2017b). Students are required to make a self-declaration of good health and good character to their regulatory body when applying for registration. In the case of nurses and midwives, good health and good character must be confirmed by the designated registered nurse or midwife at the university (see Appendix 1). For nurses, this is the NMC registrant responsible for directing the preregistration nursing programme and for midwifery programmes; this should be the lead midwife for education. This confirmation of good health and good character does not happen as a matter of course; there are occasions where directors of educational programmes do not support the declaration because of gross misconduct or criminal convictions during the training (Castledine 2000). In the case of students applying for registration with the HCPC, confirmation of good health and good character by the university is not required. Instead, a character reference and a health reference from referees outside the university are accepted by the HCPC. In the case of nurses on the Overseas Nurses Programme, the designated NMC registrant responsible for directing the programme confirms competence, good health and good character to the NMC. In the case of midwives on the Overseas Midwives Programme, the lead midwife for education in the relevant approved educational institution or her designated registered midwife substitute confirms competence, good health and good character to the NMC.

PROFESSIONAL AND LEGAL RESPONSIBILITY AND ACCOUNTABILITY TO THE STUDENT

Professional accountability to the student requires the practitioner to respect and uphold student rights and the higher-education institution's regulations as discussed previously. It also requires the practitioner to be aware of those aspects of accountability when supervising and assessing students. These have been discussed in the section, Responsibility and accountability for what?

The practitioner has a legal duty of care not only for patients/clients, but also for others under her/his care, such as students (HCPC 2016; NMC 2018a). In law, the courts could find a registered practitioner negligent if a person suffers harm because she or he failed to care for that person properly. Lord Atkin (House of Lords 1932) defined the duty of care when he gave judgement in the case of Donoghue v Stephenson:

You must take reasonable care to avoid acts or omissions that you can reasonably foresee would be likely to injure your neighbour. Who, then, in the law is my neighbour? The answer seems to be persons who are so closely and directly affected by my act that I ought to have them in contemplations as being so affected when I am directing my mind to the acts or omissions that are called in question.

This means that a practitioner has a duty in relation to colleagues to ensure that they are reasonably safe from their actions (Dimond 1994). This important duty to safeguard the health and safety of other persons who may be affected by the practitioner's acts or omissions also comes under health and safety at work regulations (Young 1994). For example, if work is delegated, a failure to supervise can lead to the practitioner who delegates being sued for negligence by the less experienced person if they (rather than the patient) suffer harm (Young 1994:58). In addition, under the Health and Safety at Work Act 1974, a practitioner could be prosecuted for any such acts or omissions. Giving students verbal instructions only about safety is not enough, as the level and amount of care and supervision required are generally commensurate with the level and amount of danger of a situation (Goudreau & Chasens 2002).

Under health and safety at work regulations, the employer has a statutory duty to keep employees informed, as well as provide training, on topics that are likely to affect health and safety (Young 1994). Examples of training are the provision of information on particular diseases that have health implications to the practitioner, such as human immunodeficiency virus (HIV) infection and acquired immunodeficiency syndrome (AIDS), and treatments that carry risks to those administering them, such as the toxic effects of certain drugs. Practitioners working in some areas will often face particular risks. For example, the community nurse will need specialist training to enable her/him to move and handle clients safely in their homes, and the nurse in the psychiatric or learning disability areas may need a greater input on preventing and dealing with aggression and violence. Careful record keeping of any training is important under the Health and Safety at Work Act for the protection of both the employer and employee.

Training needs to be given to both qualified and unqualified personnel. This means that students must also receive such training. The higher-education institution must ensure that a student receives sufficient training on health and safety before starting clinical placement. This is to protect the student as well as patients and others. Areas of particular concern are moving and handling, the handling of aggression and violence, firefighting regulations and safety and the control of infection. Subsequently, when the student starts the clinical placement, it is the joint responsibility of the practice educator and the student to ensure that the following training takes place on the student's first working day:

- the student understands their responsibilities in the event of a fire, cardiac arrest and any other emergency;
- the student has been shown the layout of the clinical area, including fire exits and fire and resuscitation equipment;
- the student knows their responsibilities regarding health and safety at work;
- the student has been instructed in moving and handling patients/clients in the clinical area;
- the student knows their responsibilities in respect of data protection and confidentiality.

The training should be documented in the student's records. This is to protect the student, the service provider and the higher-education institution in case of any later legal action for negligence.

STUDENTS WITH SPECIAL NEEDS

Equality Law

In the UK, the Equality Act 2010 became law in October 2010. It consolidates and replaces the numerous arrays of Acts and Regulations that formed the basis of antidiscrimination law. These were, primarily, the Equal Pay Act 1970, the Sex Discrimination Act 1975, the Race Relations Act 1976, the Disability Discrimination Act 1995, much of the Equality Act 2006, the Employment Equality (Religion or Belief) Regulations 2003, the Employment Equality (Sexual Orientation) Regulations 2003, the Employment Equality (Age) Regulations 2006 and the Equality Act (Sexual Orientation) Regulations 2007 (all subsequently updated and amended), plus other ancillary pieces of legislation. The Act bans unfair treatment of people because of protected characteristics (Office for Disability Issues 2013). This means that the legislation protects people with a wide range of disabilities and health conditions from unlawful discrimination. To avoid discrimination and to provide equal opportunities at work, employers and service providers (which include education providers) are under a duty to make reasonable changes for disabled applicants and employees. This is known as *reasonable adjustments*. Reasonable adjustments to their workplaces to overcome barriers experienced by disabled people must be made. Reasonable adjustments apply to any 'provision, criterion or practice' and 'any physical feature of premises'. If any of these things place a disabled person 'at a substantial disadvantage', then the employer must take any steps that are 'reasonable in all the circumstances' to prevent that disadvantage occurring (Equality Act 2010). The duty to adjust is ongoing and, subject to their effectiveness in overcoming the disadvantage, will need to be reviewed and further adjustments made. However, reasonable adjustments need to be made only if the employer is aware, or should reasonably be aware, that a worker has a disability (Equality and Human Rights Commission 2019).

The NMC (2011) and the HCPC (2015) do not have blanket bans on particular impairments or health conditions. When there is a declaration of disability or health condition, impairment of fitness to practise is considered on an individual basis, as individuals may be affected differently. Rowntree (1987:60) says that to 'treat people equally is not necessarily to treat them fairly. Indeed, people being so different, equal treatment probably means injustice for most'. Rowntree's words call for the necessity for reasonable adjustment so that the same treatment is not just meted out to all. There is thus a better chance of providing equal opportunities for all students to be able to learn effectively during clinical placements. As stated, to make reasonable adjustments for students, it is students' responsibility to declare the disability and the extent to which it may affect their learning, and delivery of patient care, in the clinical placement. Disclosure should be without fear of being discriminated against.

The experts in how support may best be given are the students; listen to what they have to say and develop a rapport that will be beneficial to them, the team and patient/client care. Students with particular health problems (e.g., diabetes) should be allocated the appropriate meal breaks to enable them to deal with dietary and medical needs. A student with a hearing impairment may want to sit in a certain place to make best use of hearing aids (e.g., during handovers).

DYSLEXIA

Dyslexia is not uncommon. It can affect 5% to 10% of a given population. It can be inherited, and recent studies have identified a number of genes that may predispose an individual to developing dyslexia (National Institute of Neurological Disorders and Stroke 2019). Dyslexia is perceived to be a learning disability that impairs a person's fluency or accuracy in comprehension with reading, writing or spelling (British Dyslexic Association 2019). It can occur at any level of intellectual ability. Individuals with dyslexia suffer from a weakness in the processing of language-based information, which affects their ability to learn. It is now widely accepted that it can also affect a number of areas of cognitive functioning, including short-term memory, mathematical calculations, personal organization and concentration span. Most people with dyslexia have been identified as having one or more of the following deficiencies in the subskills that are required to acquire and use adequate literacy skills:

- A marked inefficiency in the working of the short-term memory system; this means that a person with dyslexia may have problems with the amount of information that can be held and processed in the real-time, conscious memory.
- Inadequate phonological (pattern of speech sounds) processing abilities, causing problems with connecting the letter patterns with the associated sounds; this is usually caused by problems with the speed in which auditory information can be processed and with accessing the memory of audio sounds to relate them to the letter pattern. This gives rise to spelling inaccuracies.
- Difficulties with automaticity; this can cause problems with sequencing, organizing and prioritizing activities.
- A range of problems connected with visual processing to do with the speed with which visual information can be processed and with accessing the memory of visual patterns.

Some individuals with dyslexia also have a specific learning difference (SpLD) as a comorbidity. SpLD refers to a difficulty that affects a particular process. Amongst SpLD are dyspraxia and dyscalculia. Dyspraxia is an impairment or immaturity of the organization of movement, causing individuals to appear clumsy as the brain sends the wrong signals to parts of the body in the wrong order. Dyscalculia is innate difficulty in learning or comprehending simple mathematics. This gives rise to difficulties in understanding numbers, learning how to manipulate numbers and learning mathematical facts.

The effects of dyslexia can largely be overcome by skilled teaching and support and the use of compensatory strategies (Dyslexia Action 2019). There are students who will not disclose their disability for fear of unfair treatment in the workplace, ridicule or discrimination (White 2007; Illingworth 2005). Students who have dyslexia should be accorded due regard for their condition and provided with any extra support and time they may require to learn (Salkeld 2016). Because of the complexity of the nature of a learning disability, it can be difficult to determine the amount and type of support required. Not all students with dyslexia are the same. Each individual may present a different combination of difficulties: support will need to be tailored to meet the individual's learning needs. The label of the disability is less important than the need to recognize the specific areas of difficulty a student is faced with. Therefore, whether the individual is diagnosed with dyslexia, dyspraxia or dyscalculia is immaterial. All of these are classed as a disability under equality legislation, and individuals with any of these conditions will require understanding and support to help them to reach their potential.

The Equality Act 2010 requires reasonable adjustments to be made.

The range of difficulties encountered by students is wide-ranging. It will be useful for the practice educator to have a working knowledge of what these could be and some strategies to use (see Table 2.1). From the list of what typical problems relate to during clinical placements (RCN 2010; White 2007), some suggested strategies that the practice educator and students may wish to use to help make the placement experience a positive one are put forward. These have drawn upon and been adapted from publications of the RCN and the work of White (2007). These strategies are not exhaustive. Frequently, students will be aware of and have developed self-help strategies.

The reader is directed to the publication by the RCN (2010), which provides a more comprehensive discussion of the strategies and tips to help individuals with a learning disability during clinical practice.

The underpinning philosophy of support is to promote independence (RCN 2010). Remember that you will not be there for the student after the completion of the clinical placement. The student should be encouraged and supported to participate actively and take the responsibility for learning to develop independence. However, the input from the practice educator is crucial to assist the student to learn to achieve placement learning outcomes and to enable the student to reach her/his potential (White 2007).

The following framework has been suggested by Reid and Kirk (2001) to facilitate professional development. Students can be assisted to set, monitor and evaluate their goals of learning. The following questions may be helpful: Questions to help to become self-directing include:
- What is my goal?
- What do I want to accomplish?
- What do I need?
- What is my deadline?

Questions to assist with monitoring progress include:
- How am I doing?
- Do I need other resources?
- What else can I do?

Questions for self-evaluation include:
- Did I accomplish my goal?
- Was I efficient?
- What worked?
- What did not work?
- Why did it not work?

MORAL RESPONSIBILITY AND ACCOUNTABILITY TO THE STUDENT

Moral responsibility and accountability are of special importance, as they pervade the practice educator–student

TABLE 2.1 Difficulties Encountered by Students	
Typical Problems	**Strategies to Help Students**
Literacy skills: e.g. reading and writing reports. Reading and writing speeds are slower; errors in charting and writing patient/client records; late completion of care plans; deadlines missed; difficulty reading other people's handwriting; difficulty with identifying relevant information from case notes.	• Make a nursing and ordinary dictionary available in the clinical area or encourage the student to carry them; a spell check dictionary is invaluable. • Provide more time and a quiet environment free from distractions when doing written tasks or other activities that require concentration. • Encourage students to write drafts of reports to be checked by the practice educator. • Encourage students to take blank forms home and practise writing reports; check the examples. • Show examples of well-written reports; initially, work alongside the student to indicate what needs to be written, withdrawing direct supervision as appropriate. • Assist the student in compiling a list of frequently used phrases which can be used when writing reports; devise a checklist of key areas to include in certain types of documentation.
Dealing with information: difficulty with multitasking, for example, when receiving a handover report, there may be inability to write down key details fast enough; handovers may be incomplete and muddled; difficulty remembering telephone conversations; difficulty with identifying relevant information from case notes.	• Provide a list of common terminology used in your clinical area. • Go over the key points of the patients/clients allocated to the student following the handover; assist the student to develop an action plan/work schedule. • Help the student develop 'shorthand' when taking notes, for example, # for fractures, Rx for treatment. • Encourage the student to write out the handover before giving it – this will require checking initially, but once the student has demonstrated the ability to capture the salient points on paper, stop checking to allow the development of confidence; the student may wish to repeat the information back to the caller. • When the student answers the telephone, remind and empower the student to ask the caller to speak slowly and repeat information; encourage the student to make notes while talking on the telephone. • Encourage the student to use a customized handover sheet developed personally or one that is already in use. • Provide opportunities to discuss case notes with the student.
Administering drugs: reading, spelling or pronouncing drug names; reading doctors' handwriting on prescription charts; students with dyscalculia have greater difficulty doing drug calculations.	• Provide a list of commonly used drugs for your area. • Encourage the student to write out the names of drugs and check the spelling; assist with the development of a personal crib sheet to help identify and learn drugs. • Help with pronunciation of drug names. • Encourage the student to practise saying drug names and listen to their vocalizations. • Assist the student in using the formulas for doing drug calculations. Working out the drug dose methodically on paper followed by using a calculator (if its use is allowed by the Trust), or vice versa, will reinforce learning. • Explain drug administration protocol and encourage the student to study this in her/his own time.
Memory: difficulty remembering information or instruction, for example, passing on inaccurate/incomplete information to another team member following doctors' rounds and at handovers; giving incomplete information to patients/clients; forgetting to do things.	• Provide an orientation pack with outlines of useful information and routines. • Encourage the student to make notes. • Support and empower the student in seeking clarification. • Help the student in devising and using mnemonics.

Continued

TABLE 2.1 Difficulties Encountered by Students—cont'd

Typical Problems	Strategies to Help Students
Sequencing ability: e.g. when undertaking a complex activity or procedure involving many steps, the activity or procedure is carried out in the wrong sequence.	• Before carrying out the procedure, provide written instructions of procedures for the student to study in her/his own time; create flow charts if appropriate and feasible. • Explain and demonstrate the procedure at a pace that is comfortable to the student, as anxiety will be increased if the student feels rushed. • Provide the opportunity to practise as close as possible to the demonstration. • Provide opportunities for repeated practice until the student has mastered the activity.
Visual orientation: confusing left and right or up and down, for example, identifying the right limb for the left limb.	• Provide an orientation pack. • Do a detailed orientation to the clinical area and point out salient landmarks; back-up with a map or a sketch with main landmarks. • Encourage the student to take the same route. • Encourage the student to develop strategies for helping to remember the side of the body being treated, for example, wriggling her left limb when having to label a patient's left limb.
Hand/eye coordination: may result in poor presentation of written work, for example, untidy and difficult-to-read handwritten patient/client records; difficulty in undertaking some clinical skills.	• Check drafts of written reports and indicate where improvements can be made to aid tidiness and clarity. • Provide opportunities to practise activities so that there is repetition. • Provide alternative equipment if this constitutes reasonable adjustment.
Speech: may talk in a disorganized way, especially when the speech has to be spontaneous, e.g. at meetings and on the telephone.	• Work with the student to write down what needs to be said at handovers; rehearse handover reports.
Organizational skills: poor time management and surrounding working environment can be untidy and disorganized.	• Plan work to enable the student to work with small numbers of patients • Provide clear protocols for care; create flow charts if appropriate and feasible. • Keep to a structured routine where possible. • Encourage and assist the student to write out a work schedule – ask the student what the key activities are in the schedule; set achievable tasks for a shorter duration initially, for example, a few hours, gradually increasing to a whole morning and then a whole shift. • After the shift, spend time with the student to reflect on how the student had managed her time and workload.
Emotional factors: a range of emotions may be displayed, such as anxiety, anger and acute embarrassment. Individuals may have lowered self-esteem because of past difficulties with learning and failure; students may fear mispronouncing words; anxiety about negative staff attitude toward the disability.	• Maintain a friendly and relaxed atmosphere; be helpful and supportive without smothering. • Be approachable so that the student is not afraid to ask questions; give regular constructive feedback. • Debrief regularly, for example, at the end of each shift or after a complex caregiving episode. • Encourage other staff members to include the student as a member of the team. • Introduce the student to the team.

relationship. Cox (1982) makes the point that, unless students are adequately supervised and supported during clinical placements, they are getting short-changed in educational terms. What actions can practice educators take so that they do not fall short of fulfilling moral responsibilities and accountability owed to the student?

During the early days of working in a clinical area, the student is a guest in that area. Special efforts should be made to make students feel welcome initially and to help them settle into the area as quickly as possible. A common anxiety of students starting new placements is to feel unwelcome and unwanted (Levett-Jones et al 2009; Papastravrou et al 2016). If students feel safe and that they belong, they will begin to relax and be in a better position to start learning (Maslow 1954). In the hierarchy of human needs, Maslow (1954) postulates that the basic needs must be met first in order for the higher needs to be achieved. Many students lack confidence in their ability to learn and need to be empowered to believe in their ability to succeed (Johnson 2012).

The clinical area is anxiety provoking for students (Simpson & Sawatzky, 2020). The practice educator can help reduce levels of anxiety and stress for students by being aware of situations that may be stressful to students. Action can then be taken to assist students to cope with these stressors. The quality of student–practice educator interactions has the potential to have either positive or negative effects on the outcomes of the educational process by affecting student performance in the clinical setting (e.g. see King et al 2020; Donough & Van der Heever 2018; Levett-Jones et al 2009; Saarikoski & Leino-Kilpi 2002). The practice educator has the responsibility to befriend the student so that a positive relationship can start to be fostered. Other qualities of the practice educator that a student seeks, and which directly affect learning and performance and hence the outcomes of assessment, are discussed at length by authors such as Spouse (2003) and Neary (2000). The practice educator owes it to the student to know what these are so that the student may be assisted in the most effective ways to achieve learning outcomes. This point is developed further in Chapter 8.

As we have seen in Chapter 1, the power for making assessment decisions is firmly in the hands of the practice educator as assessor. The NMC (2018b) states that the practice educator is accountable for summative assessment decisions. To be accountable, one is vested with authority (see earlier discussion). The law also emphasizes the authority of the roles of the teacher and assessor (Young 1992). A student has the right to appeal only against the conduct of the assessment, but not the verdict. Within this assessment practice, several assumptions are made about the assessor (Harding & Greig 1994):

- The assessor is aware of personal limitations and can always be objective in assessment. The discussion in Chapter 5 will show that our assessments can be greatly influenced by personal biases and prejudices. This makes many assessment decisions far from the objectivity we like to espouse.
- There is a universally agreed standard of practice by which to judge a student's practice. However, standards of clinical practice vary among practitioners. Some students, therefore, may be subject to assessments that have been made based on standards of practice falling at either end of the continuum of high to low standards. In either case, the student is treated unfairly.
- Assessors possess the necessary knowledge, skills and attitudes for the supervision and assessment of learners who may be undertaking a course of training different from their own. However, for many years research studies have found that assessors frequently do not understand the learning needs of students they are assessing (White 2007; Duffy 2004; Fraser et al 1997; May et al 1997; Eraut et al 1995; White et al 1994; Bedford et al 1993).
- Students receive sufficient quality teaching and supervision from their practice educators to enable them to achieve learning outcomes so that they pass their assessments. Again, findings from the previously mentioned studies indicate that this is not the case. The student is generally in competition against the patient/client for the practitioner's time, and the student loses out. Practice educators may also not be the best role models (Fowler 2008). The Standards of Conduct, Performance and Ethics (HCPC 2016; NMC 2018a) make it clear that the duty of care to the patient/client must always take precedence over all else.

By virtue of the authority and assumptions vested in assessors, students are owed a high level of moral responsibility and accountability. In the eyes of the law, 'educators have a duty to their students that is greater than they would have to the general public because of the teacher–student relationship' (Goudreau & Chasens 2002:43). Lello (1979:6) makes the point that 'if people are working closely together, they have a continuing and permanent answerability to each other'. Who, then, is on trial, asks Rowntree (1987:9): the assessor or the student? Ponder this question posed by Rowntree in Activity 2.4.

Activity 2.4

A student fails a placement. Has the placement, and by inference the practice educator, failed in their duties towards the student, or has the student failed the placement?

Even if a student has been openly disinterested and has made no effort to learn, Rowntree cautions against placing the entire responsibility for the failure upon the student. There may be no straightforward answers to the question. It is up to the practice educator as assessor to confront the situation after considering the moral responsibility and accountability owed to the student. Issues surrounding professional moral responsibility and accountability are less tangible; it is perhaps easier for the student to obtain redress if they are unfairly treated because there is likely to be overt evidence of this. Moral responsibility and accountability, however, rest very much with the individual's moral code. It may not be possible for the student to obtain any form of redress if unfairness is the result of failure to exercise an appropriate level of moral responsibility and accountability toward the student.

THE TRUST/EMPLOYING AUTHORITY AND THE HIGHER-EDUCATION INSTITUTION

Higher-education institutions enter into contracts with their students to provide such educational experiences as are required to fulfil the aims of the programme. In the case of preregistration health care students, where clinical experience is a requisite component of these programmes, higher-education institutions in the UK enter into contracts with service providers such as the NHS Trusts and private organizations (e.g. nursing homes) to provide the clinical experiences. Such contracts typically specify the management of the educational process for students during clinical practice. The specifications of the service agreement between the University of Sheffield and an NHS Trust (University of Sheffield 2001; reproduced with permission) is provided in detail here as an example. The agreement specifies that the Trust will provide the following:
- A high standard of teaching, learning and assessment.
- A designated supervisor who is responsible for supervising, teaching and assessing student performance.
- The supervisor is also responsible for assigning the relevant duties to the student so that the student is given opportunities to work with a range of patients/clients.
- A liaison officer for the placement area who will liaise directly with the designated university link lecturer.
- Advising students of all local internal protocols, policies and reporting procedures relevant to the area of work.
- Ensuring that the university is notified of any accident or illness sustained by a student on placement within a timescale appropriate to the seriousness of the situation.
- Advising or instructing students to leave clinical areas if, in the Trust's view, the student is at risk or the student's health status is putting colleagues or patients at risk.

- Informing students of the specific approaches and practices for moving and handling people.
- Liability for students during the period of their placement, extending to matters of employers/occupiers' liability and public liability and in respect of acts or omissions of its own employees.
- When undertaking specific procedures, the student will be provided with all protective clothing or equipment necessary for the maintenance of health and safety.
- In the event where there are reasonable grounds to suspect that a student may have committed a criminal offence or an act of serious misconduct, the Trust may immediately suspend, without prejudice, the attachment of the student and remove the student from the work area. Any such suspension must be reported to the university within 24 working hours.
- Where a student is involved in any Trust disciplinary proceedings, the university will be informed.
- There is no discrimination against any student on grounds of race, creed, gender, sexual orientation or disability, and the Trust will apply its equal opportunity policy to students as it does to its own employees.
- Should service developments and changes impact on the placement educational environment in respect of both quality and capacity, the Trust will inform the university in advance of any service changes.
- The Trust will allow access to placement areas for university staff for the purposes of educational audit.

The specifications of these agreements have been provided here in detail to inform practice educators of their direct lines of responsibility and accountability to the Trust, and indirectly to the higher-education institution, when supervising and assessing students. The list of specifications may appear onerous. However, if the practice educator exercises the requisite duty of care owed to students as discussed, and follows assessment regulations laid down by the higher-education institution, there will then be no necessity for concern.

YOURSELF, COLLEAGUES AND YOUR PROFESSION

The NMC's and HCPC's responsibilities are set out in the Nurses and Midwives Order 2001 (NMC 2001) and the Health Professions Order 2001, respectively. The Councils' main responsibility is to protect the interests of the public. To do this, standards for education, training and professional conduct are set for its practitioners. The NMC (2018a), the HCPC (2016) and the law make it clear that standards of clinical practice must be upheld at all times. As a practice educator then, failure to uphold standards of clinical practice may compromise not only yourself professionally and legally but also your colleagues and the profession because your personal standard of practice is frequently reflected in your assessment decisions. Stated simplistically, a lower standard of clinical practice may result in the practice educator expecting a lower, maybe even unsafe, standard of performance of their student. You would not have fulfilled moral and professional responsibilities and accountability toward your colleagues and the profession if these compromised standards were not recognized, resulting in a failure to correct such deficits or to remove the student from training. Such unsafe students are likely to become registered practitioners on the NMC's and HCPC's professional registers. As practitioners and practice educators, we need to uphold the role of the NMC and HCPC in protecting the public by maintaining a register of people who are recommended to be practitioners who are fit to practise and who have demonstrated fitness to practise through a qualification registered with the NMC or the HCPC. Fowler and Heater (1983:404) stated very strongly that practice educators are: 'bound by a moral responsibility to the profession of nursing to give passing grades to only those students who have demonstrated clinical competence'.

In accepting the role of practice educator, the practitioner implicitly accepts the professional (NMC 2018b) and moral responsibility and accountability for maintaining standards of supervision and assessment in order that the standards of professional colleagues and the profession are protected.

ISSUES AND DILEMMA OF THE MENTOR–ASSESSOR INTERFACE

Holloway (1985) found that moral accountability to students (see earlier discussion) emphasizes the importance of a special relationship between teacher and student. This special relationship is permeated by empathy, trust and affinity. Staff–student relationships are an important influence on students' experience of belonging and the achievement of positive clinical experiences (Levett-Jones et al 2009).

The special relationship that many students expect of their practice educators is more likely to develop if students have confidence in their practice educators (Gray & Smith 2000). At the same time, students look to their practice educators for constructive feedback, which requires some judgement to be made about their performance. These challenging student expectations mean that the practice educator has to be able to maintain a professional/friend balance (Fraser et al 1997) to meet the dichotomous demands of the role of a practice educator as mentor and assessor. Good mentoring practices (discussed

in Chapters 8 and 9) on the part of the practitioner as practice educator are required for the development of this special relationship. At the same time, the practice educator as practitioner has professional accountabilities to fulfil. Professional accountability stresses the importance of maintaining standards of professional practice to safeguard patient/client care. The practitioner working with a student is thus required to be an assessor to judge the student's clinical competence. This demands good supervision and assessing practices to fulfil the role of assessor. The formal role of assessor is generally not as well acknowledged as the role of mentor. Is this because practice educators are avoiding their role of assessor? In a study that examined the mentoring and assessing practices of practice educators in nursing, midwifery and medicine, Bray and Nettleton (2007) found that practice educators identified assessment as having less of a priority than the more pastoral aspects of teaching and supporting students. Likewise, practitioners failed to identify that assessment is central to being a practice educator (Chow & Suen 2001; in Bray & Nettleton 2007). Current standards require a cultural shift from mentor to assessor.

Can both moral accountability to students and professional accountability be fulfilled without causing anguish to both parties? In developing a special relationship, the practitioner as mentor is a friend to the student (Neary 1997; Darling 1984). Enacting the role of assessor requires the practitioner to be a judge (Neary 1997). Is a friend capable of being an objective judge? Students in Neary's (1997) study saw the assessor as not forming any special relationship with them but as having the formal tasks of assessing skills and progress, completing assessment booklets and keeping records. They thought that practice educators took responsibility for students and provided guidance, gave support, assisted the student in setting learning outcomes and subsequently acted as facilitator for learning and created learning opportunities.

Whereas it is already accepted in many practice settings that the practice educator can act as an assessor and vice versa (HCPC 2018a; NMC 2018b; Andrews & Wallis 1999; Neary 1997), should a clinician who supervises the student while in clinical practice and an assessor be the same person? The student nurses interviewed in Neary's study had opinions that ranged from being happy with the same practitioner in both supervision and assessor roles to the opposing view that they should be separate.

Many of the students did not wish to be assessed summatively by their mentor, especially if the relationship was not a comfortable or relaxed one. They referred to the necessity of a good relationship for the assessment to be fair. Others have emphasised the need to 'keep the assessor sweet' which means they may not raise concerns in practice (Brown et al 2020). However, when the relationship developed into friendship, some students felt that the assessor could not remain unbiased. Brown (2000) found that students' personal qualities and attributes had considerable influence on the judgements made about student performance, suggesting that judgements may be have been made based on the liking for the student. Students in White et al's (1994) study also thought that the nature of the relationship between assessor and student affected the assessment process – positively in the event of a good relationship or negatively in the event of a poor relationship. However, there were students in Neary's study who expected all practice educators to remain professional and to be able to assess against agreed criteria without bias or prejudice. The practitioners in Neary's study were more definite in their view about being both mentor and assessor; many found it difficult to wear two hats and experienced role conflict.

Recent guidelines from the NMC (2018b) state clearly that the practice supervisor has the responsibility to supervise students and facilitate their learning in practice, whereas the practice assessor assesses their overall performance and makes judgements about fitness to practise and, as such, are accountable for such decisions. This is not to say that a suitable prepared individual cannot take on both roles but rather that they cannot wear both hats for the same student.

Assessment of clinical practice is a complex activity and has always been fraught with difficulties. Is it ever possible to remain professional and at the same time be a friend, to be able to assess against agreed criteria without bias or prejudice? What does it take to be a competent practice educator who is able to maintain the correct professional–friend balance with a student? The model of a competent midwife in Fraser et al's study (1997) comprises three main closely interlinked dimensions. These dimensions may provide some helpful parallel processes for the practice educator to draw upon in attempts to achieve the appropriate professional–friend balance.

1. **Professional–friend approach**: the midwife's ability to be autonomous and professional but with women. The competent practice educator will be responsible and accountable for mentoring and assessing practices, making formative and summative assessment decisions (see Chapter 7). The competent practice educator is pragmatic and rigorous and maintains diplomacy. In being 'with student', the practice educator advocates for students and inspires them with confidence.
2. **Individualized approach**: the midwife's ability to provide individualized care. The competent practice educator works in partnership with students and exercises

nonjudgemental appreciation of the differences in the personal backgrounds of students.
3. **Clinical competence**: a sound knowledge base and appropriate skills for the provision of midwifery care. The competent practice educator will have the knowledge base and skills to act in the role of practice supervisor, or as the situation dictates, practice assessor to students.

In this model, it can be seen that the competent midwife is one who is aware of the importance of the professional–friend balance. Likewise, the competent practice educator needs to achieve this professional–friend balance in the roles of being both supervisor and assessor. What is important is that supervision and assessment processes assist learning while retaining a focus on procedures (Torrance & Pryor 1998). If learning is facilitated through our assessment processes, then the products of assessment – in this case, the students – are more likely to be positive.

CONCLUSION

Inherent in professional practice are professional responsibilities and accountability. The nursing and midwifery professions, along with other professional groups serving our society, are increasingly held accountable for the quality of service they provide. Is society receiving the care it needs, or is it receiving the care we think it needs or deserves (Reilly 1980)? This requires an assessment of our goals, our actions, resources and outcomes of care in light of society's needs. As mentors and assessors in whatever setting we practise, we too will be held more and more accountable for our actions. We must answer to the student, to society, to our profession, to our colleagues, to our employer, to the higher-education institution offering the programme and to ourselves.

Students are the direct consumers and beneficiaries of our educational programmes. Are they getting the kind of learning that is needed, or are they getting short changed in educational terms? Before we claim that the student is indeed the beneficiary, we should try to answer the following question posed by Reilly (1980:3): 'How well do we meet our contract with the learner?'

Assessment of clinical practice is a significant responsibility and can be both challenging and time-consuming. It also carries professional, contractual and moral accountability. Lello (1979) acknowledges the burden of being answerable and responsible. The strain results from the amount of responsibility shouldered rather than from the amount of work done. To achieve the purposes of clinical assessment, we need to recognize and accept the responsibilities and accountability of an assessor. Reilly (1980:3) challenges us most succinctly by posing the following questions:

> We are the gatekeepers of our profession, with the power to determine who enters the profession and to define the nature of professional practice. How well are we using the power bestowed upon us?

> How well do we meet the test of accountability to ourselves? Are we authentic individuals? Have we formalized for ourselves values and beliefs that guide our actions? Are we true to those values, and are we real and genuine human beings?

Reilly raised these questions to remind nursing educators in higher-education institutions and practice educators involved with the evaluation of nursing and midwifery programmes that, to achieve quality in any plan for accountability, they must incorporate the concept of responsibility. Our role as assessors carries the ultimate responsibility: that of ensuring that only practitioners who are competent are allowed to register with the statutory professional body so that the public is safeguarded against unsafe and incompetent practice.

KEY POINTS FOR REFLECTION

Health care practitioners are responsible and accountable for the quality of service they provide. Within their additional role as assessors of health care students, practitioners are also responsible and accountable for the quality of the supervision and assessment of students through the exercise of educational processes. They have a gatekeeping role in the determination of who enters the profession through assessment decisions made.

In relationship to responsibility and accountability for the assessment of clinical practice, two key questions are posed:
- What are practice educators responsible and accountable for?
- Who are practice educators responsible and accountable to?

WHAT ARE PRACTICE EDUCATORS RESPONSIBLE AND ACCOUNTABLE FOR?

It is suggested here that the practice educator can be answerable for the following aspect of personal professional practice with its inevitable impact on learning and the following aspects of supervision and assessment:
- Personal standards of practice because these frequently form the basis of how and what are assessed.
- Standards of care delivery by learners through supervision of learners' practice and appropriate delegation of tasks. Students are never professionally accountable, and practice educators are professionally responsible for the consequences of students' actions and omissions.
- What is taught, learned and assessed by having a full understanding of relevant aspects of the curriculum so that learners can be assisted to achieve the programme learning outcomes.
- Standards of teaching and assessing because learners are entitled to the best instruction available. Failure to instruct properly could be construed as a negligent act.
- Professional judgements about student performance and accountability for the summative assessment decision;

practice educators have a moral responsibility to fail incompetent students.

WHO ARE PRACTICE EDUCATORS RESPONSIBLE AND ACCOUNTABLE TO?

Practice educators are answerable to the following individuals and organizations:
- The patient/client for both a legal and professional duty of care whose rights as a patient/client supersede at all times the student's rights to knowledge and experience.
- Students through upholding their rights as learners for the teaching, supervision and support to facilitate their learning. Assessors also have a duty of care to students.
- The Trust/employing authority and the higher-education institution for upholding the conditions of the contract between these organizations to support the clinical learning of students.
- Yourself, colleagues and your profession by upholding the standards for education, training and professional conduct laid down by the statutory professional body.

REFERENCES

Allan HT, Smith P, O'Driscoll M. Experiences of supernumerary status and the hidden curriculum in nursing: a new twist in the theory–practice gap? *J Clin Nurs*, 2011;20:847–855.

Allen J, Dennis M. Leadership and accountability. *Nurs Manag*, 2010;17(7):28-29.

Andrews M, Wallis M. Mentorship in nursing: a review of the literature. *J Adv Nurs*, 1999;29(1):201–207.

Armstrong N. Clinical mentors' influence on student midwives' clinical practice. *Br J Midwifery*, 2010;16(2):114–123.

Ashworth P, Morrison P. Problems of competence-based nurse education. *Nurse Educ Today*, 1991;11:256-260.

Bachmann L, Utheim Groenvik C, Hauge K, Julnes S. Failing to fail nursing students among mentors: a confirmatory factor analysis of the failing to fail scale. *Nursing Open*, 2019;6:966–973.

Baker R. Harold Shipman's Clinical Practice 1974-1998: A Review Commissioned by the Chief Medical Officer. Stationery Office, London:2001.

Bandura A. Social Learning Theory. Prentice Hall, Englewood Cliffs, NJ:1977.

Beaumont S. Stop incompetent nurses. *Br J Nurs*, 2004;13(11):663.

Becher T, Eraut M, Knight J. Policies for Educational Accountability. Heinemann Educational Books, London:1981.

Bedford H, Phillips T, Robinson J. Assessment of Competencies in Nursing and Midwifery Education and Training. The English National Board for Nursing, Midwifery and Health Visiting, London:1993.

British Dyslexic Association. Offering dyslexia information, advice and services online. 2019. Available: https://www.bdadyslexia.org.uk. Accessed June 2019.

Bergman R. Accountability – definition and dimensions. *Int Nurs Rev*, 1981;28(2):53–59.

Bray L, Nettleton P. Assessor or mentor? Role confusion in professional education. *Nurse Educ Today*, 2007;27:848–855.

Brown N. What are the criteria that mentors use to make judgements on the clinical performance of student mental health nurses? An exploratory study of the formal written communication at the end of clinical nursing practice modules. *J Psychiatr Ment Health Nurs*, 2000;7(5): 407–416.

Brown P, Jones A, Davies J. Shall I tell my mentor? Exploring the mentor-student relationship and its impact on students' raising concerns on clinical placement. *J Clin Nurs*. 2020; 29:3298–3310. doi:10.1111/jocn.15356

Brykczynska G. Working with children: accountability, paediatric nursing Accountability in Nursing Practice. In: Watson R Accountability in Nursing Practice. Chapman & Hall, London:2003, pp. 147–160.

Cassidy S. Seeking authorisation: a grounded theory explanation of mentor's experiences of assessing nursing students on the borderline of achievement of practice competence. *J Adv Nurs*, 2017;73(9):2167–2178.

Castledine G. Professional misconduct case studies: nursing students' accountability. *Br J Nurs*, 2000;9(15):965.

Castledine G. Accountability in delivering care. *Nurs Stand*, 1991;5(25):28–31.

Caulfield H. Vital notes for nursing: accountability. *Nurs Manage*, 2005;17(3):18–20.

Champion R. Educational accountability – what ho the 1990s! *Nurse Educ Today*, 1991;11:407–414.

Charters A. Encouraging student centred learning in a clinical environment. *Emerg Nurs*, 2000;7(10):25–29.

Clothier C. The Allitt Inquiry: Independent Inquiry Relating to Deaths and Injuries on the Children's Ward at Grantham and Kesteven General Hospital During the Period February to April 1991. Stationery Office, London:1994.

Competition and Markets Authority UK higher education providers – advice on consumer protection law. Available: https://assets.publishing.service.gov.uk/government/uploads/system/uploads/attachment_data/file/428549/HE_providers_-_advice_on_consumer_protection_law.pdf. Accessed June 2019.

Cornock M. Legal definitions of responsibility, accountability and liability. *Nurs Child Young People*, 2011;23(3):25–26.

Cox C. The seeds of time. *Nurse Educ Today*, 1982;2(6):4–10.

Darling LAW. What do nurses want in a mentor? *J Nurs Admin*, 1984;42–44.

Department of Health. Making a Difference. Department of Health, London:1999.

Department of Health & Social Care. The NHS Constitution for England. 2015. Available: https://www.gov.uk/government/publications/the-nhs-constitution-for-england/the-nhs-constitution-for-england#patients-and-the-public-your-rights-and-the-nhs-pledges-to-you. Accessed June 2019.

Dimond B. Dimond's Legal Aspects of Nursing: A Definitive Guide to Law for Nurses. 8th ed. Pearson Education, Harlow, Essex:2019.

Dimond B. The Legal Aspects of Midwifery. Books for Midwives Press, Cheshire:1994.

Dolan G. Assessing student nurse clinical competency: will we ever get it right? *J Clin Nurs*, 2003;12:132–141.

Donough G, Van der Heever M. Undergraduate nursing students' experience of clinical supervision. *Curationis*. 2018;41(1):e1–e8. doi:10.4102/curationis.v41i1.1833

Duffy K. Failing Students Report. Nursing and Midwifery Council, London:2004.

Dyslexia Action. Dyslexia Action Training. 2019. Available: https://dyslexiaaction.org.uk. Accessed June 2019.

Earnshaw GJ. Mentorship: the students' views. *Nurse Educ Today*, 1995;15 274–279.

Emerton A. Professionalism and the UKCC. *Br J Nurs*, 1992;1(1):25–29.

Eraut M, Alderton J, Boylan A. An Evaluation of the Contribution of the Biological and Social Sciences to Pre-registration Nursing and Midwifery Programmes. The English National Board for Nursing, Midwifery and Health Visiting, London:1995.

Equality Act. Equality Act 2010. 2010. Available: http://www.legislation.gov.uk/ukpga/2010/15/pdfs/ukpga_20100015_en.pdf. Accessed August 2011.

Equality and Human Rights Commission. Employing People: Workplace Adjustments. 2019. Available: https://www.equalityhumanrights.com/en/multipage-guide/employing-people-workplace-adjustments. Accessed June 2019.

Fowler D. Student midwives and accountability: are mentors good role models? *Br J Midwifery*, 2008;16(2):100–104.

Fowler G, Heater B. Guidelines for clinical evaluation. *J Nurs Educ*, 1983;22(9):402–404.

Fraser D, Murphy R, Worth-Butler M. An Outcome Evaluation of the Effectiveness of Pre-registration Midwifery Programmes of Education. The English National Board for Nursing, Midwifery and Health Visiting, London:1997

Gainsbury S. Nurse mentors still 'failing to fail' students. *Nurs Times*, 2010;106(16):7

Goclowski J. Legal implications of academic dismissal and educational malpractice for nursing faculty. *J Nurs Educ*, 1985;24(3):104–108.

Goudreau KA, Chasens ER. Negligence in nursing education. *Nurse Educ*, 2002;27(1):42–46.

Gopee N. Assessing student nurses' clinical skills: the ethical competence of mentors. *Int J Ther Rehabil*, 2008;15(9):401–407.

Graveley EA, Stanley M. A clinical failure: what the courts tell us. *J Nurs Educ*, 1993;32(3):135–137.

Gray MA, Smith LN, The qualities of an effective mentor from the student nurses perspective: findings from a longitudinal qualitative study. *J Adv Nurs*, 2000;32:1542–1549.

Griffith R, Tengnah C. Law and Professional Issues in Nursing. 4th ed. Learning Matters, Exeter:2016.

Gunby S. Legal issues in teaching nursing. In: Penn BK, Mastering the Teaching Role: A Guide for Nurse Educators. FA Davis, Philadelphia:2008. pp. 411–421.

Hager A, Gonczi R. Professions and competencies. In: Edwards R, Hanson A, Raggatt P, Boundaries of Adult Learning. Routledge, London:1995. pp. 246–260.

Han S, Kim O, Choi E, Han J. Effects of nurses' mentoring in turnover intention: focused on the mediating effects role stress and burnout. *J Korean Acad Nurs*, 2013;43(5):605–612.

Hughes L, Mitchell M, Johnston A. Failure to fail in nursing – a catch phrase or a real issue? A systematic integrative literature review. *Nurse Educ Pract*, 2016;(20):54–63.

Harding C, Greig M. Issues of accountability in the assessment of practice. *Nurse Educ Today*, 1994;14:118–123.

The Health Professions. Consolidated Text Incorporating Repeals and Amendments Made up to 1st April 2010. HCPC, London: 2001.

Hepworth S. The assessment of student nurses. *Nurse Educ Today*, 1991;11(1):46–52.

Health and Care Professions Council. Health, Disability and Becoming a Health and Care Professional. 2015. Available: https://www.hcpc-uk.org/globalassets/resources/guidance/health-disability-and-becoming-a-health-and-care-professional.pdf. Accessed June 2019.

Health and Care Professions Council. Standards of Conduct, Performance and Ethics. 2016. Available: https://www.hcpc-uk.org/standards/standards-of-conduct-performance-and-ethics/. Accessed June 2019.

Health Care Professions Council. Standards of Education and Training. 2017a. Available: https://www.hcpc-uk.org/globalassets/resources/standards/standards-of-education-and-training.pdf

Health and Care Professions Council. Guidance on Health and Character. 2017b. Available: https://www.hcpc-uk.org/globalassets/resources/guidance/guidance-on-health-and-character.pdf. Accessed June 2019.

Health and Care Professions Council. Standards of Education and Training Guidance. 2018a. Available: https://www.hcpc-uk.org/standards/standards-relevant-to-education-and-training/. Accessed June 2019.

Health and Care Professions Council. Standards of Proficiency. 2023. Available: https://www.hcpc-uk.org/standards/standards-of-proficiency/. Accessed September 2023.

Health and Care Professions Council. Fitness to Practise Annual Report. 2018c. Available: https://www.hcpc-uk.org/globalassets/resources/reports/fitness-to-practise/hcpc-fitness-to-practise-annual-report-2018.pdf. Accessed June 2019.

Health and Care Professions Council Tribunal Service. Welcome to the Health and Care Professions Tribunal Service. 2019. Available: https://www.hcpts-uk.org. Accessed June 2019.

Health Professions Order. 2001. Available: https://www.legislation.gov.uk/uksi/2002/254/contents

Holloway D. Accountability in further education: teachers' perceptions. *J Further High Educ*, 1985; 9(2):31–45.

Ilott I, Murphy R. Success and Failure in Professional Education: Assessing the Evidence. Whurr, London:1999.

Illingworth K. The effects of dyslexia on the work of nurses and healthcare assistants. *Nurs Stand*, 2005;19(38):41–48.

Jack K, Hamshire C, Chambers A. The influence of role models in undergraduate nurse education. *J Clin Nurs*, 2017;26 (23-24):4707–4715.

Johnson EJ. The academic performance of students In: Billings DM, Halstead JA, Teaching in Nursing: A Guide for Faculty. 4th ed. WB Saunders, Philadelphia:2012. Chapter 3: 34–66.

Killam LA, Montgomery P, Luhanga FL. Views on unsafe nursing students in clinical learning. *Int J Nurs Educ Scholarsh*, 2010;7(1):1–17.

King C, Edlington T, Williams B. The "Ideal" Clinical Supervision Environment in Nursing and Allied Health. *J Multidiscip Healthc*. 2020;13:187–196. doi:10.2147/JMDH.S239559

Lawson L. Supporting Mentors and Clinical Educators: A Collaborative Project Into the Development of Knowledge and Skills to Enhance Clinical Education Practice. University of Hertfordshire: unpublished report.

Lello J. Accountability in Education. In: Lello J, Accountability in Education. Ward Lock Educational, London:1979.

Levett-Jones T. Lathlean J, Higgins I. Staff-student relationships and their impact on nursing students' belongingness and learning. *J Adv Nurs*, 2009;65(2):316–324.

McAllister M, Tower M, Walker R. Gentle interruptions: transformative approaches to clinical teaching. *J Nurs Educ*, 2007;46(7):304–312.

McGaghie WC. Professional competence evaluation. *Educ Res*, 1991;20:3–9.

Marks-Maran D. Accountability in nursing education. In: Watson R, Accountability in Nursing Practice. Chapman & Hall, London:2003, pp. 232–240.

Maslow A. Motivation and Personality. Harper and Row, New York:1954.

May N, Veitch L, McIntosh J. Evaluation of Nurse and Midwife Education in Scotland. The National Board for Nursing, Midwifery and Health Visiting for Scotland, Edinburgh:1997.

Neary M. Teaching, Assessing and Evaluation for Clinical Competence. Stanley Thornes, Cheltenham:2000.

Neary M. Defining the role of assessors, mentors and supervisors: part II. *Nurs Stand*, 1997;11(43):34–38.

Nicklin PJ, Kenworthy N. Teaching and Assessing in Clinical Practice. Baillière Tindall, London:2000.

National Institute of Neurological Disorders and Stroke. Dyslexia Information. 2019. Available: https://www.ninds.nih.gov/Disorders/All-Disorders/Dyslexia-Information-Page. Accessed June 2019.

Nursing and Midwifery Council. The Nursing and Midwifery Order (SI 2002/253). 2001. The Stationery Office, Norwich.

Nursing and Midwifery Council. Nursing and Midwifery Council (Education, Registration and Registration Appeals) Rules 2004. 2004. Statutory Instrument 2004/1767. The Stationery Office, Norwich.

Nursing and Midwifery Council. Standards to Support Learning and Assessment in Practice. 2008. Available: https://www.nmc.org.uk/globalassets/sitedocuments/standards/nmc-standards-to-support-learning-assessment.pdf. Accessed June 2019.

Nursing and Midwifery Council. NMC Equality and Diversity Strategy. 2011. Available: https://www.nmc.org.uk/globalassets/siteDocuments/Annual_reports_and_accounts/NMC_Equality-and-diversity-strategy-2012.pdf. Accessed June 2019.

Nursing and Midwifery Council. Nursing and Midwifery Council, The Code: Professional Standards of Practice and Behaviour For Nurses, Midwives and Nursing Associates. 2018a. Available: https://www.nmc.org.uk/standards/code/. Accessed July 2019.

Nursing and Midwifery Council. Standards for Student Supervision and Assessment. 2018b. Available: https://www.nmc.org.uk/standards/standards-for-nurses/. Accessed June 2019.

Nursing and Midwifery Council. Delegation and Accountability: Supplementary Information to the NMC Code. 2018c. Available: https://www.nmc.org.uk/globalassets/sitedocuments/nmc-publications/delegation-and-accountability-supplementary-information-to-the-nmc-code.pdf. Accessed June 2018.

Nursing and Midwifery Council. Standards of Proficiency for Registered Midwives. 2018d. Available: https://www.nmc.org.uk/standards/standards-for-nurses/standards-of-proficiency-for-registered-nurses/. Accessed June 2019.

Nursing and Midwifery. Guidance on Health and Character. 2019a. Available: https://www.nmc.org.uk/globalassets/sitedocuments/registration/guidance-on-health-and-character.pdf. Accessed June 2019.

Nursing and Midwifery Council. Fitness to Practice Committee: Who Sits on the Fitness to Practice Committee and how does it Work? 2019b. Available: https://www.nmc.org.uk/concerns-nurses-midwives/hearings/our-panels-case-examiners/fitness-to-practise-committee/. Accessed June 2019.

Nursing and Midwifery Council. Annual Fitness to Practise Report 2018-2019. 2019c. Available: https://www.nmc.org.uk/globalassets/sitedocuments/annual_reports_and_accounts/ftpannualreports/nmc-fitness-to-practise-report-2019-singles-linked-contents.pdf. Accessed October 2019.

Orchard C. The nurse educator and the nursing student: a review of the issue of clinical evaluation procedures. *J Nurs Educ*, 1994;33(6):245–251.

Office for Disability Issues. Equality Act 2010: Guidance. 2013. Online. Available: https://www.gov.uk/guidance/equality-act-2010-guidance. Accessed June 2019.

Ormerod JA. Accountability in nurse education. *Br J Nurs*, 1993;2(14):730–733.

Papastavrou E, Dimitriadou M, Tsangari H, Andreou C. Nursing students' satisfaction of the clinical learning environment: a research study. *BMC Nursing*, 2016;15:44.

Parkes R. Stressful episodes reported by first-year student nurses: a descriptive account. *Soc Sci Med*, 1985;20(9):945–953.

Pollard KC. Non-formal learning and interprofessional collaboration in health and social care: the influence of the quality of staff interaction on student learning about collaborative behaviour in practice placements. *Learn Health Soc Care*, 2008;7(1):12–26.

Reid G, Kirk J. Dyslexia in Adults: Education and Employment. John Wiley, Chichester:2001.

Reilly DE. Behavioral Objectives: Evaluation in Nursing. Appleton-Century-Crofts, Norwalk:1980.

Rowntree D. Assessing Students: How Shall We Know Them? 2nd ed. Kogan Page, London:1987.

Royal College of Nursing. Dyslexia, Dyspraxia and Dyscalculia: A Toolkit for Nursing Staff. 2010. Available: https://www.nottingham.ac.uk/studentservices/documents/rcn—-dyslexiadyspraxiadyscalculia—-toolkit-for-nursing-staff.pdf. Accessed July 2019.

Royal College of Nursing. Accountability and Delegation. 2023. Available: https://rcni.com/hosted-content/rcn/first-steps/accountability-and-delegation. Accessed June 2023.

Saarikoski M, Leino-Kilpi H. The learning environment and supervision by staff nurses: developing the instrument. *Int J Nurs Stud*, 2002;39:259–267.

Salkeld J. A model to support nursing students with dyslexia. *Nurs Stand*, 2016;30(47):46–51.

Simpson MG, Sawatzky JV. Clinical placement anxiety in undergraduate nursing students: A concept analysis. *Nurse Educ Today*. 2020;87:104329. doi:10.1016/j.nedt.2019.104329

Spink LM. Due process in academic dismissal. *J Nurs Educ*, 1983; 22(7):305–306.

Spouse J. The effective mentor: a model for student-centred learning in clinical practice. *Nurs Times Res*, 1996;1(2):120–132.

Spouse J. Learning through legitimate peripheral participation. *Nurse Educ Today*, 1998;18(5):345–351.

Torrance H, Pryor J. Investigating Formative Assessment: teaching, learning and assessment in the classroom. McGraw-Hill Education UK; 1998.

UKCC. Issues Arising from Professional Conduct Complaints. United Kingdom Central Council for Nursing, Midwifery and Health Visiting, London:1996.

University of Sheffield. University of Sheffield, Service Agreement for the Provision of Clinical Placement Services and Facilities. The University of Sheffield:2001.

Vinales J. Exploring failure to fail in pre-registration nursing. *Br J Nurs*, 2015; 24(5):284–288.

White J. Supporting nursing students with dyslexia in clinical practice. *Nurs Stand*, 2007;21(19):35–42.

White E, Riley E, Davies S. A detailed study of the relationship between teaching, support. Supervision and Role Modelling in Clinical Areas within the Context of P2000 Courses. The English National Board for Nursing, Midwifery and Health Visiting, London:1994.

Wisdom H. Mentor's Experience of Supporting Pre-registration Nursing Students: A Grounded Theory Study. 2011. EdD thesis, The Open University. Available: https://oro.open.ac.uk/49150/1/577997.pdf. Accessed July 2019.

Wood V. The nursing instructor and the teaching climate. *Nurse Educ Today*. 1987;(7):228–234.

Young A. Review: the legal duty of care for nurses and other health professionals. *J Clin Nurs*, 2009;(18): 3071–3078.

Young AP. Case Studies in Law and Nursing. Chapman & Hall, London:1992.

Young AP. Law and Professional Conduct in Nursing and Health Scutari, London Hall, London 1994

What Do We Assess?

INTRODUCTION

The health care professions have a responsibility to, and are accountable to, the public. They serve to train health care practitioners who are clinically competent and fit to practise (HCPC 2010; NMC 2001). Fraser et al (1997:51) put it very simply:

The public needs to be assured that those about to become midwife (or nurse) practitioners have developed the right blend of knowledge, skills and attitudes to become competent.

However, there have been much discussion over the years that nursing and midwifery education does not produce competent nurses and midwives (Bradshaw 2000; Castledine 2000 (Jervis & Tilki 2011; Rutkowski 2007). It is essential that preregistration health care students achieve the learning outcomes that will satisfy the UK Nursing and Midwifery Council (NMC) and the Health and Care Professions Council (HCPC) training requirements (HCPC 2017; NMC 2023). It is necessary to measure and assess the standards of proficiency so that the practitioner who qualifies is clinically competent and fit to practise.

The issue of being clinically competent is not just restricted to newly qualified practitioners. Nurses and midwives and registrants on the HCPC register are required to maintain their professional knowledge and competence (HCPC 2008; NMC 2008). However, the NMC (2011a) reported that approximately 37% of cases referred when the registrant's fitness to practise is in doubt related to a lack of competence of the practitioner and not to professional misconduct. Over 20 years ago, the UK Central Council (UKCC 1999) reported similar findings: there was lack of competence in a significant number of cases. In the case of registrants on the HCPC register (HCPC 2011), 19% of allegations concerned issues of lack of competence.

It is therefore important to consider carefully what it means to be clinically competent.

In this chapter, the use of competency statements and a competency-based model of assessment are suggested as means to be clear about what we want to assess (Hager & Gonczi 1996). The key features of the National Vocational Qualification (NVQ) system are described to illustrate how a prescribed structure and format for assessment can be constraining yet has the potential advantages of validity and reliability of assessment. The nature of competencies, what it means to be clinically competent and their assessment in professional practice are explored. The competency-based model of assessment is critically evaluated as an assessment tool for assessing professional practice.

PREREGISTRATION HEALTH CARE EDUCATION REQUIREMENTS IN THE UK

The nursing and midwifery professions in the UK regulated by the NMC, and professions in the UK regulated by the HCPC, came into being through Acts of Parliament. The Nursing and Midwifery Order (2001) and the Health and Care Professions Order (2001) require these statutory bodies to establish standards of education and training necessary to achieve the standards of proficiency to be admitted to the professional registers. The standards of proficiency are set at a 'threshold' level, as this is the minimum level for safe and effective practice to protect the public.

Before a higher education institution (HEI) can provide and deliver a preregistration health care course of the professions regulated by the NMC and the HCPC, the course must be validated by the relevant statutory body and the HEI. The process of conjoint validation frequently brings competing sets of demands in relation to course assessment strategies (Bedford et al 1993). The NMC and HCPC are concerned that assessment strategies are sensitive to the demands of professional practice. On the other hand, the HEIs' concerns focus on academic credibility and the extent to which assessment strategies are sensitive to intellectual competence. In the case of nursing and midwifery, in the document *Fitness for Practice*, the UKCC (1999) set out a radical agenda to refocus nursing and midwifery education to meet the needs of the rapidly changing health service by ensuring that nurses and midwives are fit to practise. The Commission recommended that preregistration nursing and midwifery education should use: 'outcomes-based competency principles to ensure that students develop not only higher-order intellectual skills and abilities but also the practice, knowledge and skills essential to the art and science of nursing and midwifery' (p. 4).

This agenda is endorsed by the NMC. By refocusing preregistration education on outcomes-based competency principles, the NMC believes that the needs of the three key stakeholders of preregistration education – namely, the NMC, the prospective employers and the HEIs – are more likely to be met. These needs underpin the NMC and HCPC's requirements for preregistration programmes (HCPC 2011; NMC 2010a, 2009). The needs of each of the stakeholders are set out here:

- **Fitness to practise**. The NMC and HCPC are primarily concerned about fitness to practise. Should the student be issued with a 'licence' to practise?
- **Fitness for purpose**. Prospective employers are primarily concerned about fitness for purpose. Is the newly qualified practitioner able to function competently in clinical practice?
- **Fitness for award**. HEIs are primarily concerned about fitness for award. Has the student attained the appropriate level, breadth and depth of learning to be awarded a diploma or degree?

Gilbert Jessup, who is viewed as the most prominent English advocate of competency-based testing, argued that 'the measure of success for any education and training system should be what people learn from it, and how effectively. Just common sense you might think…' (Jessup 1991:3). Jessup suggests that professional training frequently fails to make explicit statements as to what professionals should know, understand and be able to do. Practitioners need to know, with confidence, the 'right blend of knowledge, skills and attitudes to become competent' (Fraser et al 1997:51) and the standard at which they are safe and effective. This knowledge will enable practice educators to conduct assessments and make assessment decisions with the assurance that students who qualify are fit for both practice and purpose.

The use of an outcomes-based competency approach allows the different stakeholders to agree on a set of competencies and outcomes for preregistration programmes to cover the knowledge, understanding, skills, abilities and values expected of newly qualified practitioners (UKCC 1999). Using these competencies and outcomes, referred to as *Standards* by the NMC (NMC 2023), there is a requirement for preregistration nursing and midwifery programmes to be designed to prepare the student to be a practitioner who can apply knowledge, understanding and skills to perform to the standards required in employment and to provide care safely and competently, thereby assuming the responsibilities and accountability necessary for public protection. Jessup's measure of success may thus be fulfilled!

Although the HCPC does not state explicitly that an outcomes-based competency principle is used in its preregistration courses, like the NMC, it requires *Standards* to be achieved in all the preregistration courses of the professions it regulates. An examination of these standards indicates that all the elements of outcomes-based competency principles (to be discussed later) are implicit in the *Standards* (HCPC 2017).

THE NATURE OF COMPETENCE

Two major concepts now require exploring: the nature of competence and the outcomes-based competency approach. I start this discussion by posing the question: What does it mean to be professionally competent? The NMC (2015) stipulates that competence is the individual practitioner's responsibility. On completion of a nursing updating course to return to practise after a career break, Bradshaw (2000:319) came to this conclusion:

> … *I had no objective measures or standards by which to judge what I knew, what I should know, and most importantly, what I did not know … [it] left me unsure about my competence in the practicalities of caring for patients … gradually I realized that I had no idea whether I was competent in the new techniques and technology which I was expected to use [original emphases].*

What, indeed, does it take to be a professionally competent nurse or midwife, or paramedic, or occupational therapist? You may wish to discuss the questions in Activity 3.1 with your colleagues.

Activity 3.1

What does professional competence mean and entail?
What does it mean to be professionally competent?
What does it take to be a professionally competent nurse or midwife, paramedic or allied health professional?

You may have discovered that the concept of professional competence resists straightforward answers or categorization. Debates that I held with groups of nurses and midwives about the meaning of professional competence gave me much room for thought. The main aspects elicited are shown in Fig. 3.1. These aspects point to the multifaceted and complex nature of competence and what it means to be a professionally competent health care practitioner. Research in the nursing and midwifery professions by Watson et al (2002), Fraser et al (1997) and Bedford et al (1993) concluded that there is no commonly shared definition of a competent nurse or a competent midwife. Bedford et al (1993:40) think that there are:

> *many different aspects of this wide-ranging and complex concept … there is more to competence than simply what can be easily observed and measured.*

Wolf (1995), who is viewed as one expert in the field of competency-based assessment, wrote that 'competence' and 'competencies' are vexed terms – acres of print continue to be expended over their definitions. Rather than take the reader on a trawl of these definitions, I have selected those that I see are pertinent to the discussion of competence in the health care professions.

Jessup (1991:26) defines both occupational and job competence. Note that his concept of occupational competence is broader:

> *A person who is described as competent in an occupation or profession is considered to have a repertoire of*

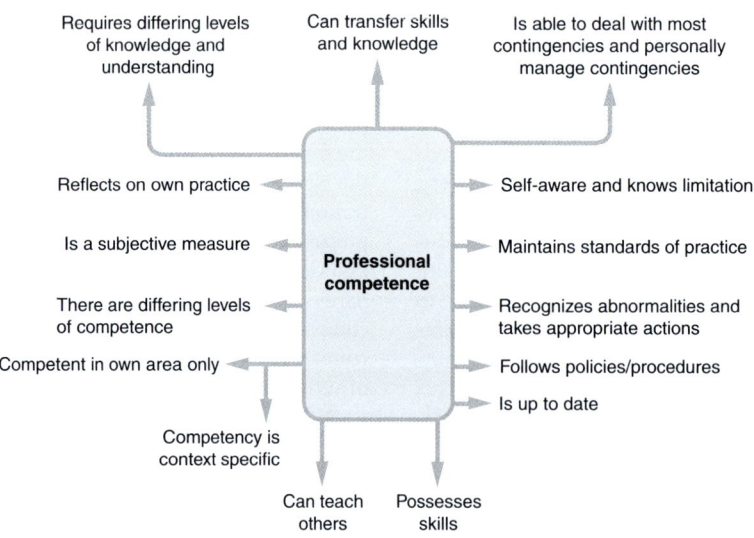

Fig. 3.1 Aspects of professional competence.

skills, knowledge and understanding that he or she can apply in a range of contexts and organizations. To say that a person is competent in a 'job', on the other hand, may mean that their competence is limited to a particular role in a particular company.

Jessup's definition of competence is stated simply as 'the ability to perform to recognized standards' (1991:10). He goes on to say that 'these standards are those used to maintain or improve "quality" in the relevant occupation or profession'. Here, Jessup reiterates the expectation of the Manpower Services Commission (1985, in Wolf 1995:31) of someone who is competent – 'by competent we mean performing at the standards expected of an employee doing the same job'.

Eraut's (1998:135) definition of competence as 'the ability to perform the tasks and roles required to the expected standard' reflects the definition of competence that underpins the thinking of those professions in Australia that have established competency standards. Gonczi et al's (1993:5) definition is as follows:

A competent professional has the attributes necessary for job performance to the appropriate standards.

The definition of competence by Gonczi et al (1993) possesses three key components:

* attributes
* performance
* standards

ATTRIBUTES

Professionals are competent as a result of possession of a set of relevant attributes such as knowledge, understanding, skills, personal traits, attitudes and values. These attributes, which jointly underlie and determine competence, are referred to as *competencies*. A competency is therefore a combination of attributes underlying some aspect of successful professional performance.

PERFORMANCE

In competency-based assessments, competence is focused on *performance* of a role or sets of tasks (Gonczi et al 1993). Performance is directly observable, whereas competence is not; rather, it is inferred from performance, which is why competence is defined as a combination of attributes that underlie successful performance. There are numerous professional roles, such as nurses, midwives, doctors, pharmacists, physiotherapist,

teachers and so on. Roles consist of a multitude of tasks, which can be further divided into subtasks. The approach taken by the NVQ movement in the UK focuses on the performance of discrete tasks and subtasks: each NVQ covers a particular area of work at a specific level of achievement (Wolf 1995). The professions in Australia have taken what Gonczi et al (1993) describe as the 'integrated approach' – analysis into tasks ceases at the level of relatively complex and demanding professional activities. Competency standards consider the complex combinations of attributes that are required for effective professional activities.

Gonczi et al (1993) stress that both the attributes of the practitioners and their performance of key professional tasks are essential to their definition of competence; this means that attributes of individuals do not in themselves constitute competence. Nor is competence the mere performance of a series of tasks. Rather, the notion of competence integrates attributes with performance; that is, the competent practitioner is not only able to perform but is also capable (Worth-Butler et al 1994). Competence assessment that incorporates both performance and capability underpin the notion of 'fitness to practise'.

The NMC (2015) and the HCPC (2008) require health care practitioners to integrate attributes with performance in their definition of 'fitness to practise'. Their notion of fitness to practise means having the skills, knowledge, good health and good character to practise safely and effectively (HCPC 2010, NMC 2010b). The NMC adds that this practice is to be without supervision.

STANDARDS

The judgement of the performance of a role and its associated tasks is either competent or incompetent – competence therefore requires that the performance be judged against prespecified standards. Standards specify the skills, knowledge and understanding that underpin performance in the workplace (Wolf 1995). The standards embody and define competence in the relevant occupational context. A competency standard consists of a unit of competence (representing a wide work function), which is subdivided into smaller elements of competence (tasks within the wider function) with their associated performance criteria (the standards by which the competence in the task will be judged) (Hager & Gonczi 1996). This is the framework in both England and Australia. This framework is illustrated in Fig. 3.2.

An example of a unit of competency and its associated elements of competency is shown in Appendix 2.

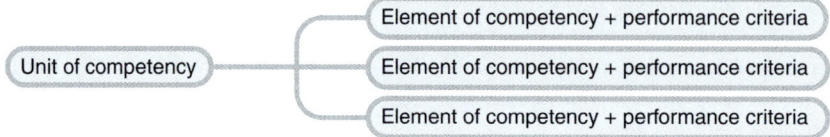

Fig. 3.2 A competency standard.

THE OUTCOMES-BASED COMPETENCY APPROACH TO PROFESSIONAL EDUCATION AND ASSESSMENT

An Outline of the Background of Competency-Based Assessment

Modern competency-based assessment (in association with competency-based education) first became important in the early 1970s in the context of American teacher education and certification (Wolf 1995). In response to mounting public attacks on the quality of teacher education, the federal government became involved in education reform– competency-based teacher education was seen as a major panacea for the improvement of American education. In the late 1980s in Australia, there was considerable pressure from the national government on industry and the professions to adopt a competency-based approach to education, staff development and performance appraisal (Sutton & Arbon 1994). Consequently, most of the professions have developed competency-based standards (statements) and competency-based assessment strategies (Hager & Gonczi 1996). In the UK in the 1980s, following a Scottish lead, the government launched a huge programme of standards development; this produced 'standards of competence' in a big range of occupational sectors, each with its associated NVQ award, or in Scotland, the Scottish Vocational Qualification (SVQ). Although NVQs were approved by a national body, the Qualifications and Curriculum Authority, the actual processes of supervision and assessment were carried out by awarding bodies such as the City and Guilds of London Institute. The new qualifications framework for England, Wales and Northern Ireland, the Qualifications and Credit Framework (QCF), has developed new qualifications to replace the Health and Health and Social Care suite of NVQs (Skills for Health 2012). Although the qualifications in the QCF units are competence based, QCF units differ from NVQ units in that they contain learning outcomes instead of knowledge and performance criteria statements. The reader is directed to the work of Wolf (1995), who gives a critique of competency-based assessment and the NVQ system.

Competency-based assessment is a form of assessment that emphasizes the outcomes of achievement. These outcomes are specified to the point where they are clear and transparent so that assessors, assessees and third parties can all make reasonably objective judgements with respect to their achievement or nonachievement. Certification is made on the basis of demonstrated achievement of these outcomes (Wolf 1995).

USING COMPETENCY-BASED ASSESSMENT IN PROFESSIONAL HEALTH CARE EDUCATION

Can a case be made for using the competency-based approach in the health care professions? Forty years ago, Patricia Benner (1982:303, 309) had this to say about using this approach in nursing education:

> The quest for competency statements and competency-based exams in nursing has led to what seems to be a premature faith in the current state of the art and capability of competency-based performance examinations in nursing. Carried along by a technological, measurement-oriented age, we have been convinced that many of our problems in nursing education and practice will be solved when we have mastered the current measurement technology available – when we can simply and unequivocally describe the competencies involved in the practice of nursing and measure them. Some of us have gone so far as to say that any area of practice that cannot be so defined, described and measured does not legitimately belong in the arena of professional practice.

Unfortunately, this faith in the feasibility of competency examinations does not come to grips with the difficulties and issues inherent in the methodology . . .

Notwithstanding Benner's warning about competency-based education in nursing, one recommendation made in the reports *Making a Difference* (Department of Health 1999) and *Fitness for Practice* (UKCC 1999) was to refocus preregistration nursing and midwifery education on an outcomes-based competency approach. This recommendation is endorsed by the HCPC (HCPC 2023) and the NMC (NMC 2010a, 2023). Is this recommendation justified? What are the implications of using competency-based assessment of clinical practice? An examination of two particular ways of using competency-based assessment may provide some answers: these are the NVQ system in the UK and the 'integrated' approach used by the professions in Australia.

COMPETENCY-BASED ASSESSMENT FOR NATIONAL VOCATIONAL QUALIFICATIONS

The NVQ framework represents a very particular application of competency-based assessment (Wolf 1995). This section will provide an outline of the basic structure of NVQs and discuss the principles underlying competency-based assessment for NVQs. The process of assessment within the competency-based framework is discussed in Chapter 6. Inferences will then be drawn about the appropriateness of the NVQ system for the assessment of professional practice, such as in the nursing and midwifery professions.

An NVQ comprises several units and their associated elements to be achieved at one of the five prespecified levels (DfES 2005). A unit consists of a group of 'elements of competence' and its associated performance criteria and knowledge specification. Each unit reflects a discrete activity or subarea of competence – each is worthy of separate accreditation, much like an academic module in fact (NCVQ 1991). An element of competence is a description of something that a person who works in a given occupational area should be able to do; it encompasses some action, behaviour or outcome. Competency-based assessment for NVQs is made concrete through highly specified performance criteria and knowledge specification. The element of competence is assessed and validated against these performance criteria and knowledge specifications. Appendix 2 provides an example of a unit, its associated elements and one element of competence with its performance criteria.

Assessment requires that the individual demonstrates successfully that they have met every one of the performance criteria and knowledge specification because these are the statements by which an assessor judges whether the evidence provided by the individual is sufficient to demonstrate competent performance (Wolf 1995). The NVQ approach requires assessment to be centred on whether performance meets the prespecified standards. Performance is judged to be either competent or not yet competent only – the individual has either consistently demonstrated workplace performance that meets the specified standards or has not yet been able to do so.

Up until 2005, each element of competence with its associated performance criteria had an associated range. These ranges officially 'elaborate the statement of competence by making explicit the contexts to which the element [of competence] and performance criteria apply. Also, they put limits on the specification to ensure a consistent interpretation' (NCVQ 1991:14). Contextualizing the performance criteria identifies the different contexts in which the individual is expected to achieve competent performance. This means that competence must also be assessed 'across the range', and performance evidence is 'normally required for every performance criteria [sic] across as much of the range as possible' (City and Guilds 1992). Following the review of the National Occupational Standards in Health and Social Care and the launch of the new Health and Social Care N/SVQs in February 2005 (Skills for Health 2005), the range has been replaced by the scope. The statements in the scope do not appear to be as specific as the range statements. The scope is intended to give guidance on possible areas to be covered in the unit. It specifies a list of options linked with items in the performance criteria. Evidence is required for any option related to the candidate's work area. The specification of the scope for the unit HSC35 can be found in Appendix 2.

In its early years, NVQs were criticized for producing people who might be able to demonstrate performance but would have no understanding of what they were doing (Norris 1991). To fend off mounting attacks on NVQs as undemanding, and to ensure that individuals have an understanding of what they are doing (Wolf 1995), the National Council for Vocational Qualifications added a separate 'knowledge/understanding' list to every element of competence. Candidates are required to demonstrate that they understand all the items listed under knowledge evidence and supporting evidence. From 2005, knowledge and understanding are specified at unit level. Appendix 2 contains the knowledge and understanding statements required for unit HSC35.

NVQs are offered at five levels to cover progression from routine and predictable work activities to the complex and unpredictable (Department of Education 2012; DfES 2005). Box 3.1 details the summary of each level.

It can be seen that the NVQ system applies competency-based assessment in a very tightly defined format. It embraces the performance philosophy of competency-based systems to the very core (Wolf 1995). Thus its notion of competence is 'the ability to perform the activities within an occupation' (Wolf 1995:31). Although competency-based systems vary in their interpretation of what outcomes may be (e.g. see Gonczi et al 1993), the learning outcomes in NVQs relate directly to performance – what counts as an outcome is thus very highly constrained. An element of competence must encompass some action, behaviour or outcome that is contextually related to that occupational sector through its range statement. The elements of competence referred to in Unit HSC35 are legitimate as being outcome-based because they involve an active verb and an object and relate directly to performance. Each element of competence is specified in such a way that there can be no doubt about what constitutes satisfactory performance. For example, competence in Element HSC35a requires the person to be able to 'develop supportive relationships that promote choice and independence'.

BOX 3.1   Summary of the Five National Vocational Qualification Levels

- **Level 1:** Competence that involves the application of knowledge in the performance of a range of varied work activities, most of which may be routine and predictable.
- **Level 2:** Competence that involves the application of knowledge in a significant range of varied work activities, performed in a variety of contexts. Some of these activities are complex or nonroutine, and there is some individual responsibility or autonomy. Collaboration with others, perhaps through membership of a work group or team, may often be a requirement.
- **Level 3:** Competence that involves the application of knowledge in a broad range of varied work activities performed in a wide variety of contexts, most of which are complex and nonroutine. There is considerable responsibility and autonomy, and control or guidance of others is often required.
- **Level 4:** Competence that involves the application of knowledge in a broad range of complex, technical or professional work activities performed in a variety of contexts and with a substantial degree of personal responsibility and autonomy. Responsibility for the work of others and the allocation of resources is often present.
- **Level 5:** Competence that involves the application of a range of fundamental principles across a wide and often unpredictable variety of contexts. Very substantial personal autonomy and often significant responsibility for the work of others and for the allocation of substantial resources feature strongly, as do personal accountabilities for analysis, diagnosis, design, planning, execution and evaluation.

ARGUMENTS FOR AND AGAINST THE NATIONAL VOCATIONAL QUALIFICATION SYSTEM FOR ASSESSING PROFESSIONAL PRACTICE

As stated earlier, the NVQ framework represents a very particular application of competency-based assessment that can be summarized as follows:

- the elements of competence define the performance requirements
- the performance criteria describe competent performance
- the scope specifies the list of options for which assessment evidence is required
- statements of knowledge and supporting evidence define the underpinning knowledge and understanding required
- levels specify the nature of work activities for competent performance, ranging from the routine and predictable to the complex and unpredictable.

A contentious issue about what is to be assessed concerns the optimum level of specificity. Storey et al (1995:382) say that 'if there is too little specificity, the result may be a lack of clarity, poor communication and diminished credibility'. This is the criticism directed at earlier preregistration nursing and midwifery competencies and outcomes. On the other hand, too much specificity can lead to assessment criteria that take too long to read and are cumbersome to use by busy practitioners. This criticism has been directed at the NVQ system. However, you may agree that the NVQ approach has the attraction of precision and clarity as to what is to be assessed to achieve competence. Advocates of this approach also emphasize its potential contribution to effective training and learning. Storey et al (1995) and Fletcher (1991), for example, argue that specific criteria for assessing competence are provided, thereby giving the much-desired guidance for assessees and assessors. Individuals know exactly what they have to achieve, and assessors can provide specific guidance and feedback. Educational provisions and employment needs can be brought together.

The appropriateness of the NVQ approach for assessing professionals such as in nursing and midwifery has been criticized (Le Var 1996, Norris 1991). What could be the trouble with an approach where the assessment of competence is grounded in performance in the workplace? The NVQ model is seen by Norris (1991:334) to be 'highly reductive, providing atomised lists of tasks and functions'. He elaborates further: 'the sum of the parts rarely if ever represents the totality of good practice … in their tidiness and precision, far from preserving the essential features of expertise, they distort and understate the very things they are trying to represent'.

Competence is conceived of in terms of the discrete behaviours associated with the ability to complete individual tasks. This approach is unconcerned with the connections between tasks and ignores the possibility that the coming together of tasks could lead to their transformation (Hager & Gonczi 1996). Le Var (1996) feared that the care activities in nursing and midwifery would become fragmented if students were trained within this approach. If holistic care is to be valued and provided, care activities need to be designed and integrated around the needs of the client at that particular time. Unless professionals are involved in the planning and evaluation of total care, they cannot engage in the processes of critical analysis and synthesis that lead to the development of theories and

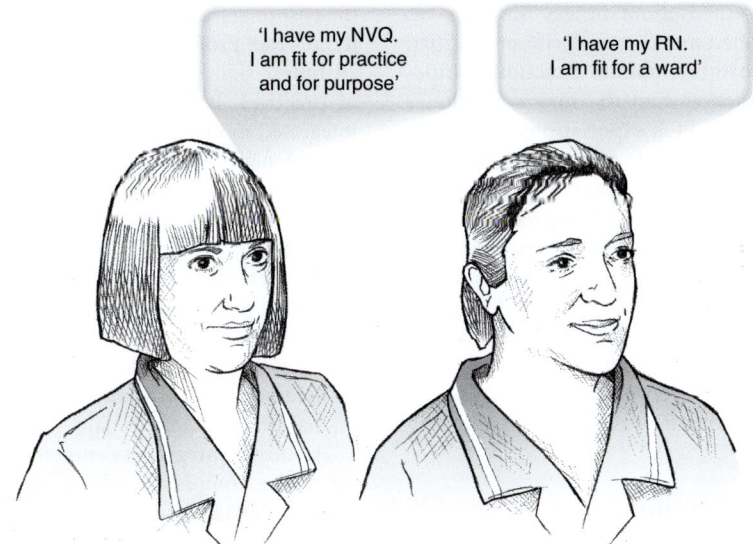

Fig. 3.3 The National Vocational Qualification (NVQ) represents a very particular application of competency-based assessment. *RN*, Registered nurse

principles of practice. If this 'atomized' approach of the NVQ system is used by professionals, qualifications could be in danger of being reduced to a list of technical skills (Storey et al 1995). Hager and Gonczi (1996) and Le Var (1996) echo this concern when they point out that this approach ignores the complexity of performance in the real world and the role of professional judgement. Furthermore, the practice and assessment of 'components of care' do not engender the development of problem-solving skills. Watson et al (2002) also argue that being competent requires something greater than the demonstration of correct procedure, as the competent practitioner needs to be able to intertwine the unpredictable and elusive aspects of human care with the flexible application of technical and psychological skills.

So far, a number of general concerns have been raised about the use of a competency-based approach to nursing and midwifery education. The degree to which competencies can be used to describe professional practice is questionable (Watson et al 2002; Sutton & Arbon 1994; Benner 1982). The practice of health care professionals is undeniably complex, and competency-based statements can provide only a limited view of this practice; they cannot be used to reflect the complexities of practice with accuracy. They must, by their very nature, provide a reductive analysis of practice (Sutton & Arbon 1994), which excludes learning derived from a whole performance (Benner 1982). Although competency statements purport to describe the attributes, including knowledge and skills necessary for effective and/or superior performance,

the testing of intangible attributes such as attitudes is still subjective (Ashworth & Morrison 1991; Benner 1982). Benner pointed out the difficulties of testing some attributes and abilities such as empathy and the ability to relate to others, as learning the behaviour does not guarantee the possession of the accompanying attitude and/or values.

If we return to the definition of a competent professional offered by Gonczi et al (1993), you will notice that the competent professional should also possess the appropriate underlying personal attitudes and traits. The assessment of these aspects of competence is not given due consideration in the NVQ system. The Training Agency (1988) states that competence should take into account the 'qualities of personal effectiveness that are required in the workplace to deal with co-workers, managers and customers'. Underlying attributes and qualities may include interpersonal and social skills, attitudes, perceptiveness, receptivity, creativity and maturity as well as knowledge, understanding and critical thinking capacity (Ashworth & Morrison 1991). These underlying attributes of the practitioner are crucial to effective performance (Hager & Gonczi 1996) and are fundamental to excellence in clinical practice (Novak 1988).

If the NVQ system for assessing professional practice is used, the reader is left to ponder the answers to the following questions:

- The NMC and HCPC are concerned about fitness to practise. Will the student who is assessed using this system be 'fit for practice' and be allowed to register?

- Employers are concerned about fitness for purpose. Will the newly qualified nurse or midwife or dietitian or orthoptist and so on be able to function competently in clinical practice? Can the new practitioner fulfil the NMC's and HCPC's expectations of competence – that is, possess the 'skills and abilities required for lawful, safe and effective professional practice without direct supervision'? Because of the speed of change in the context and content of health care, fitness for purpose is an evolving entity: it is not fixed, and depends on the 'commitment of employers and employees to constant updating' (UKCC 1999:34). Having trained and been assessed using the NVQ system during clinical practice, how likely is the new practitioner in making this commitment?

THE CASE FOR AN INTEGRATED COMPETENCY-BASED APPROACH FOR ASSESSING HEALTH CARE PRACTICE

The UKCC Education Commission recommended refocusing preregistration education on 'outcomes-based competency principles to ensure that students develop not only higher order intellectual skills and abilities but also the practice knowledge and skills essential to the art and science of nursing and midwifery' (UKCC 1999:4). These recommendations are endorsed by the NMC (2023, 2023).

In refocusing preregistration education on outcomes-based competency principles, the NMC believes that the needs of the three key stakeholders of preregistration education—the NMC, the prospective employers and the HEIs—are more likely to be met. This belief reinforces Hager and Gonczi's (1996) views that a competency-based approach to education and training potentially provides a framework for bringing together professional policies for training and employment requirements. Competencies provide consumers and professionals with some common understanding of standards expected of professionals, and may thereby enable both parties to relate to each other more successfully.

The nursing profession of Australia (Sutton & Arbon 1994) views competency development as one means by which the profession can monitor and maintain its own professional standards and thus enhance its accountability to the public. Hager and Gonczi (1996), however, recommended that any assessment strategy that uses the outcomes-based competency model should be holistically orientated–a holistic/integrated competency-based model is more valid and reliable than current ways of assessing professionals. It enables us to come closer than we have in the past to assessing what we want to assess (i.e. the capacity of the professional to integrate knowledge, values, attitudes, skills and other attributes in the real world of practice). It is therefore important that any holistic/integrated model of assessment using the outcomes-based competency approach to the assessment of professional practice takes into account the following:

- effective performance of work activities in a range of contexts
- the exercising of cognitive skills such as integration of theory with practice, critical analysis, problem-solving and synthesis
- the ability to provide holistic care
- the underlying attitudes and traits of the learner
- that practice is up to date.

A holistic/integrated competency-based approach considers the complex combinations of attributes (knowledge, understanding, skills, personal traits, attitudes and values) that are used to understand and function within the particular situations in which professionals find themselves. The abilities of practitioners are considered in relation to the tasks that need to be performed in particular situations. The notion of competence is relational; it is conceived of as the complex structuring of attributes needed for intelligent performance in specific situations. It incorporates the idea of professional judgement. Many authors (e.g. Eraut 1998; Jessup 1991; McGaghie 1991; Black & Wolf 1990) also consider that, other than practical skills and knowledge, professional judgement is an important underpinning of competence. Jessup (1991:127) describes it thus: 'An analysis of the knowledge which people actually draw upon, and need to draw upon, to perform competently, may not appear in what is taught as the body of knowledge underpinning a profession or occupation, or if it is covered, may not be accorded the priority it deserves. Competent professionals tend to acquire a set of guiding principles, of which they are often partially conscious, derived largely from their experience. These may build upon 'academic' theories and knowledge or be only loosely related. Although this is recognized in areas such as management, it also appears to be true in well-established professions such as medicine'.

The NVQ represents a very particular application of competency-based assessment.

The holistic/integrated approach is to conceive of competent care as the capacity of the practitioner to employ a complex interaction of attributes in a range of contexts. Thus a knowledge base and possession of a repertoire of practical skills will need to mesh with, among other things, ethical values and interpersonal skills. Practitioners may then be able to 'perform the task with desirable outcomes under the varied circumstances of the real world' (Benner

1982:304). Adapting the definition of competence used by Queensland Nursing Council 2009, the NMC (2023) states that competence is a requirement for entry to the NMC register. It is a holistic concept that may be defined as "the combination of skills, knowledge and attitudes, values and technical abilities that underpin safe and effective nursing practice and interventions". It can be seen that there is thus a common expectation of a practitioner who is supposed to be competent.

The real world of health care is dynamic, complex and unpredictable. Health care professionals face challenging and unique situations within practice and need flexible ways of responding to, and learning from, these situations. It follows then that competence is also developmental in orientation – never a total accomplishment, always looking forward to better performance, improved decision-making and greater quantity of outcome (Bedford et al 1993). The holistic/integrated competency-based approach allows the incorporation of ethics and values as elements in competent performance, the need for reflective practice, the importance of context and the fact that there is more than one way of conceptualizing competence. In the nursing context, the holistic/integrated approach views that competence is (Percival et al 1994:139):

An inner, highly differentiated characteristic of a person, which is applicable to the very demanding and very specific context of nursing. It is an ability that effectively encompasses the entire demands of the nursing role, and therefore nursing competence itself possesses a complexity that increases with experience and as responsibilities become more intricate.

The qualities expected by practising nurses and midwives of the competent professional nurse or midwife (see Fig. 3.1) have many similarities to the holistic/integrated way of conceptualizing competence. Another inference that can be drawn from the information in Fig. 3.1 is what Gonczi et al (1993:13) said of clinical competence–that is: 'clinical competence is a complex phenomenon, which almost always requires the practitioner to use a combination of attributes simultaneously and, in addition, that the practitioners need to adapt their practices to different contexts' It seems that if a competency-based model for assessing health care practice is used, then adopting the concepts of competence inherent in the holistic/integrated approach is the way forward. In her critique of the use of the competency-based model for the nursing profession, Le Var (1996) concluded that the holistic/integrated approach is in keeping with, and will also help fulfil, the current assessment philosophy and practice in professional nursing.

The components of the holistic/integrated competency-based model can be summarized as:
- a complex combination of attributes – knowledge, attitudes, personal traits, values, skills and understanding
- exercising cognitive skills – for example, using professional judgement in specific situations
- effective performance on different occasions in different contexts
- developmental in orientation to emphasize the need for reflective practice.

Using these components, an integrated competency-based model for assessing nursing and midwifery practice can be constructed, as shown in Fig. 3.4.

It is suggested here that, if assessment is unified by using the holistic/integrated competency-based model, health care practitioners are more likely to develop the requisite technical competence and scientific rationality, as well as fulfil the paradoxical expectation of meeting the holistic care needs of patients and clients (Department of Health 1999). Practitioners will thus achieve

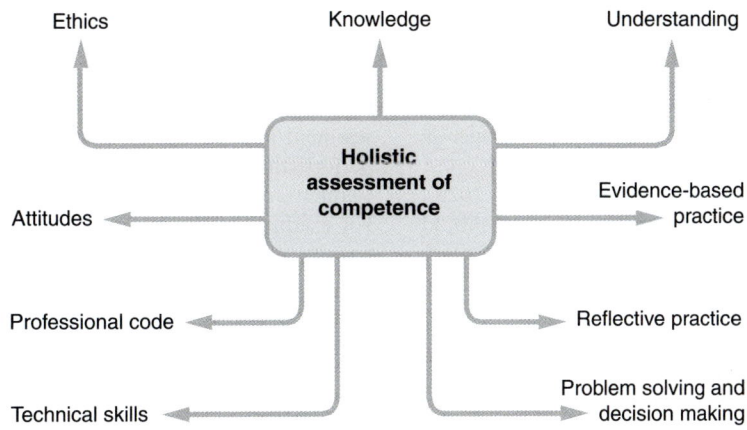

Fig. 3.4 The components of a holistic/integrated competency-based model of assessment.

fitness to practise and not just be fit for practice, because according to Moore (2005), there is a fundamental difference between the two terminologies. Moore suggests that the term fitness for practice appears to be used to refer to the professional who has sufficient knowledge and skills to be able to practise safely, and the term fitness to practise is more frequently associated with health and conduct. Therefore, it seems reasonable to assume that someone who is not fit for practice is not fit to practise. On the other hand, someone who is not fit to practise may still be fit for practice (Moore 2005). More recently, both the NMC and HCPC have defined fitness to practise as having the skills, knowledge, good health and good character to practise safely and effectively (HCPC 2010; NMC 2010b).

For the purposes of the discussion on assessment methodology, the components of professional competence are grouped into the category of reflective practice and the three domains of learning classified by Bloom et al (1956):

- cognitive domain: knowledge, understanding, problem solving, decision making, professional code
- affective domain: attitude, ethics, professional code
- psychomotor domain: technical skills.

USING THE HOLISTIC/INTEGRATED APPROACH FOR COMPETENCY-BASED ASSESSMENT OF CLINICAL PRACTICE

The holistic/integrated approach to competency-based assessment used by the professions in Australia seeks to identify attributes as well as key functions and activities, and to combine these in an integrated set of competency statements (Gonczi et al 1993). This has meant that analysis into tasks has ceased at the level of relatively complex and demanding professional activities – typically, a profession does not develop more than 30 to 40 competencies.

Competencies should be designed to reflect the holistic nature of a profession and should represent the practice repertoire of the newly qualified practitioner (Hager & Gonczi 1996).

The UKCC (1999), endorsed by the NMC (2023), provided the following guiding principles that should be reflected in preregistration nursing and midwifery programmes:

- Nursing and midwifery are practice-based professions that recognize the primacy of patient and client well-being and respect for individuals.
- *The Code: Professional standards of practice and behaviour for nurses, midwives and nursing associates* (NMC 2018) applies to all practice interventions.

- The importance of lifelong learning and continuing professional development are recognized.
- Skills and knowledge are transferable.
- Practice is based on the best available evidence.

Additionally, the Department of Health (1999) called for an increase in practical skills within training programmes. Thus a strategy similar to that used by the nursing profession in Australia has been used by the NMC in developing the standards for both the preregistration nursing and midwifery programmes (NMC 2023). Adapting the definition of competence used by Queensland Nursing Council 2009, the NMC states that competence is a requirement for entry to the NMC register. It is a holistic concept that may be defined as 'the combination of skills, knowledge and attitudes, values and technical abilities that underpin safe and effective nursing practice and interventions'. The NMC has defined a competency framework for preregistration nursing education. Within this framework, there are 'sets of competency' requirements for each field (branch) of nursing. Each set of competency comprises generic and specific standards for competence plus related generic and specific competencies for that field of nursing. Each set of competency is laid out under the four domains of professional values, communication and interpersonal skills, nursing practice and decision-making and leadership, management and team working. Proficiencies support the development and achievement of learning outcomes in each set of competency. Although the competency framework for the preregistration midwifery programme does not specify the standard for competence, it specifies competencies, which are laid out under the four domains of effective midwifery practice, professional and ethical practice, developing the individual midwife and others and achieving quality care through evaluation and research. Proficiencies support the development and achievement of learning outcomes in the competencies.

The need for an integrated competency-based approach for the assessment of clinical practice has been highlighted. This has now been adopted by the NMC as previously described. Within an integrated assessment framework, assessment approaches can assess a range of elements and performance criteria, rather than collect evidence for each element and performance criterion (Gonczi et al 1993). For example, in the case of a student midwife on a community placement, home visits of women and their babies can be used to assess elements such as the practical skills of examination of the woman and/or baby, conducting interviews, monitoring progress and compiling case records and reports. The performance on these visits can also be used to measure a number of attributes at the same time, such as communication and interpersonal skills, underpinning knowledge, understanding, problem solving and so on.

There is a consideration of assessment methods that are available and how these may be used to generate the assessment evidence required to infer, and confer, competence. There is a discussion of how the components of the holistic/integrated competency-based model of the assessment of clinical practice can be incorporated and used within a learning contract.

A 'CLINICAL SKILLS CHECKLIST' FOR PREREGISTRATION NURSING AND MIDWIFERY EDUCATION

Although the holistic/integrated competency-based approach to the assessment of clinical practice will concomitantly assess practical skills, it may not identify the nature and repertoire of the skills which the student has become competent in. Moreover, the acquisition of skills is not straightforward during clinical practice. Farley and Hendry (1997) suggested that the presence of a patient will detract from the focus on the technical aspect of the procedure because the student has to interact with the client/patient. Having to concentrate on two separate and different aspects of care may affect the student's ability to do both well. In 1999, the UKCC expressed concern and unease about the lack of essential practical nursing skills of newly qualified nurses (UKCC 1999). Although concerns about the practical skills of newly qualified midwives were not as marked as those for nursing, they remain significant because of the requirement of midwives to practise autonomously on registration. Both the UKCC (1999) and the Department of Health (1999) then called for an increase in the level of practical skills during preregistration training. Similar concerns were still expressed by the NMC (2005). This concern has resulted in the introduction of essential skills clusters in preregistration nursing and midwifery programmes in 2007 and proficiencies in 2018. These proficiencies give specific guidance on the skills development required at specified progression points in the programme and for entry to the register. The proficiencies for nursing relate to

- being an accountable practitioner
- Promoting health and preventing ill health
- Assessing needs and planning care
- Providing and evaluating care
  Leading and managing nursing care and working in teams
- Improving safety and quality of care
- Coordinating care
  Those for midwifery are:
- communication
- initial consultation between the woman and the midwife
- normal labour and birth

- initiation and continuance of breastfeeding
- medical products management.

These proficiencies are complemented by lists of skills that must be achieved to create nurses fit for purpose in the 21st century. The use of a clinical skills checklist will help both the student and the practice educator keep track of clinical experiences and caregiving situations that the student needs to engage in to acquire the proficiencies for registration. It is emphasized that the checklist should not fragment the clinical experience and assessment of the student – rather, it should be used as a guide to planning clinical experiences so that the student has the opportunity to engage in those clinical activities to enable the development of the skills required for the achievement of the statutory standards of preregistration programmes. The checklist should be seen as a formative tool used toward the achievement of these statutory standards because the 'assessment of competence cannot be reduced solely to an assessment of a student's ability to carry out certain tasks' (UKCC 1999:38).

Following an extensive review of the literature and consultation with assessors, mentors, students and newly qualified staff nurses, Hilton (2004) developed several checklists of clinical skills to help students' and practice educators' direct learning in relation to the development of these essential skills. These checklists will also assist in the keeping of a record of achievement and progress. The clinical skills are framed around the 12 Activities of Living model of Aggleton and Chalmers (Hilton 2004) and are to be achieved at five levels:

- Level 1: have observed the procedure in the practice setting
- Level 2: have participated in the skill under direct supervision
- Level 3: have performed the skill on a number of occasions and required minimal supervision
- Level 4: can perform the skill safely and competently, giving the rationale for their actions
- Level 5: have taught the skill to others.

Hilton (2004) makes the important point that the lists of skills are not exhaustive, and students and practice educators are encouraged to include skills that are unique to a particular clinical setting. The checklists of clinical skills developed by Hilton (2004) around the 12 activities of living can be found in Appendix 3.

LEVELS OF PERFORMANCE

Phillips et al (2000) and Gerrish et al (1997) raise many issues surrounding the assessment of levels of clinical practice. Some of these are framed in the following questions:

- Is there any purpose in attributing levels to practice in nursing and midwifery education?

- If we accept the viability of the use of levels criteria to differentiate practice, what constitutes evidence of movement from one level of practice to another?
- Does learning in the practice setting progress in a linear fashion, as implied by assessment tools which apply Steinaker and Bell's (1979) taxonomy of experiential learning?
- If practice is assessed only in relation to a competent/incompetent distinction, as in the NVQ system, what are the criteria that constitute competent versus incompetent performance?

Preregistration nursing and midwifery curricula generally prescribe the expected level of competent performance at prespecified points of the programme (Phillips et al 2000; Gerrish et al 1997). Within a consideration of what to assess in clinical practice of a preregistration programme is the necessity to determine whether a student is achieving competent practice as the training progresses. Bradshaw (1998) is concerned that we are able to state that the nurse or midwife has reached certain minimum standards of competence in the practical knowledge and skills needed to care for patients. It is necessary to decide whether the student is learning, and therefore achieving, the competencies within the student's expected capability; this is generally determined by the stage of training the student is at. This assessment necessarily involves the use of criteria to decide how a competent/incompetent distinction can be made and whether the student has made the requisite progress at the level specified at a particular stage of the course. These aspects of assessment are seen as part and parcel of the monitoring of progress of students and are discussed in detail in.

PROFESSIONAL CONDUCT, VALUES AND ETHICS

In the health care professions, competence to perform complex and technical problems only is now increasingly challenged by the public and the professions themselves. There is an expectation that the personal attributes of practitioners are also developed because these are necessary for effective professional practice (NMC 2023; HCPC 2009; Toohey 2002). It is universally argued that whatever knowledge and skills students possess on qualification are no good without the right values and attitudes (Roberts 2009). The issue of impairment of fitness to practise in preregistration health care students is complex. Fitness to practise means having the skills, knowledge, good health and good character to practise safely and effectively (NMC 2010c; HCPC 2009). Fitness to practise is questioned when there are allegations of misconduct, lack of competence and ill health. This means that a student's professional conduct, values and ethics can be questioned. There is little published research on allegations of undesirable professional conduct, values and ethics in preregistration health care students where future professional suitability is in doubt. From the nursing literature in the UK, Braithwaite et al (1994) and Hutt (1988) reported disciplinary proceedings for students discontinuing their course. Also of interest is personality disorders as a reason for discontinuation of the course (Lindop 1987).

More recent studies on undesirable professional conduct, values and ethics come from the United States in the field of medicine. One study reported that over a 10-year period from 1990 to 2000, 95% of disciplinary actions taken by the Medical Board of California were for deficiencies in professionalism (Papadakis et al 2004). Compared with a control group, the disciplined doctors were twice as likely to have had 'concerns/problem/extreme' excerpts recorded in their medical school profiles. In a later study, three types of unprofessional behaviour were identified in medical students which had a significant association with those individuals being disciplined as practising doctors (Teherani et al 2005). The unprofessional behaviours reported were poor reliability and responsibility, lack of self-improvement and adaptability and poor initiative and motivation. Another study in the United States also found that disciplinary action by a medical board was strongly associated with prior unprofessional behaviour in medical schools (Papadakis et al 2005). Severe irresponsibility and severe diminished capacity for self-improvement were most strongly linked to disciplinary action.

The argument for formalizing the development and assessment of personal attributes is that these translate into certain kinds of desirable professional values and ethics, which then ensure that the student achieves fitness to practise (Miller 2010; Hilton & Slotnick 2005; Toohey 2002). Practitioners who are willing to look carefully and analytically at their own practice and mistakes; professionals who are prepared to acknowledge their limitation and call in a second opinion; and practitioners who can work within a team so that care is coordinated with the patient/client in mind. In the main, opportunities for students to learn about such aspects of professional practice are informal and opportunistic (e.g. by learning from role models in the workplace). Although the learning from positive role models may be significant, it may not be sufficient. It would also be naïve to think that all role models are positive ones.

In their studies, Fraser et al (1997) and Hart et al (2001) identified some key personal attributes that professional midwives should possess. There are many similarities between these and those identified by Hilton and Slotnick (2005) in the medical profession; these authors have grouped these personal attributes into the two broad categories of personal (intrinsic) attributes and cooperative attributes. Each category encompasses three domains, as shown here.

PERSONAL (INTRINSIC) ATTRIBUTES

- Ethical practice: the foundation on which agreement exists between patient/client expectations and what professionals expect to provide.
- Reflection/self-awareness: necessary to deal with complex clinical problems.
- Responsibility/accountability for actions (commitment to excellence, lifelong learning, critical reasoning): must be well developed to fulfil the high expectations placed on professionals.

COOPERATIVE ATTRIBUTES

- Respect for patients: demands an understanding of patient/client needs and an appreciation of how professionals' behaviours can be interpreted.
- Working with others (teamwork): has become an essential requirement in recent times.
- Social responsibility: through the social contract with society, professionals must be aware and sensitive to the range of views on health issues.

How can these personal attributes be best assessed? This is an area of assessment that continues to challenge assessors of professional health care students. Toohey (2002:533) suggests that the purpose of such assessment is not to certify competence but to 'harness and direct the powerful effects of assessment onto an important aspect of practice and to provide opportunities for students to reflect, self-evaluate and receive feedback'. Toohey's formative assessment of personal attributes used various educational and assessment strategies. Readers are directed to the discussion of assessment methods for suggestions on how to approach the assessment of personal attributes.

As well as considering the approach to this aspect of assessment, it is also important to set criteria to guide students and assessors toward the development and assessment of personal attributes. Using the empirical evidence from the work of Fraser et al (1997) and Hart et al (2001) and the behaviours identified by practice educators as essential behaviours that a student midwife should demonstrate, a tool termed the *professional behaviours inventory* is proposed to facilitate the development and assessment of prespecified behaviours expected of a professional exhibiting the accepted conduct of a midwife. These professional behaviours reflect the professional conduct expected of health care students as laid down by the NMC (2011b) and the HCPC (2008). The professional behaviours consist of highly specified descriptors that are observable and can be readily used by the student, practice educator and other members of the team working with the student. The professional behaviours inventory may be used as one component of the assessment of practice of preregistration health care students. As such, it may serve as both a formative and a summative tool. This assessment tool is shown in Appendix 4.

CONCLUSION

To achieve the aim of preparing health care practitioners who are fit to practise, it is necessary to be clear about what we want to assess in the clinical setting. The NMC and HCPC specify statutory standards for preregistration education. These are to be achieved through the principles of a competency-based model of assessment. Two particular applications of this model have been described in this chapter. First is the NVQ system, which is seen to focus almost exclusively on the performance of discrete tasks and is therefore reductionist in nature. This application of the competency-based model is therefore not entirely appropriate for assessing professional health care education such as nursing and midwifery. Second, the other application of the competency-based model uses the holistic/integrated approach as implemented by the professions in Australia (Gonczi et al 1993) and is now endorsed by the NMC. This approach conceives of competent health care as the capacity of the practitioner to employ a complex interaction of attributes needed for intelligent performance in a range of contexts. Thus a knowledge base and the possession of a repertoire of practical skills will need to mesh with, amongst other things, ethical values and interpersonal skills. Clinically, the assessment can be integrated by using those methods that assess a number of elements and all their performance criteria simultaneously so that evidence toward the achievement of one or several competencies can be generated. The holistic/integrated competency-based approach is recommended for the assessment of students in the health care professions.

All existing methods of clinical assessment are potentially appropriate for use in the holistic/integrated competency-based approach. This is because it is not the methods that are competency based, but the way they are used, the emphasis given to each method and the way in which the results are interpreted that are important. The following chapter examines the range of methods available and how these can be used in competency-based assessment.

KEY POINTS FOR REFLECTION

A competency-based approach to education and training potentially provides a framework for bringing together professional policies for training and employment requirements so that practitioners are both fit to practise and fit for purpose.

A competent professional has the attributes necessary for job performance to the appropriate standards. This encompasses the three key components of attributes, performance and standards:

- **Attributes**: professionals are competent as a result of possession of a set of relevant attributes such as knowledge, understanding, skills, personal traits, attitudes and values. These attributes, which jointly underlie and determine competence, are referred to as competencies. A competency is therefore a combination of attributes underlying some aspect of successful professional performance.
- **Performance** is directly observable, whereas competence is inferred from performance. The notion of competence integrates attributes with successful performance.
- **Standards** specify the skills, knowledge and understanding that underpin performance in the workplace. The judgement of the performance of a role and its associated tasks is either competent or incompetent; competence therefore requires that the performance is judged against prespecified standards.

The NVQ framework represents a very particular application of competency-based assessment. It applies competency-based assessment in a very tightly defined format and embraces the performance philosophy of competency-based systems to the very core. The NVQ model is criticized as being highly reductive, providing atomized lists of tasks and functions. Competence is conceived of in terms of the discrete behaviours associated with the ability to complete individual tasks. There is a danger that this will fragment the learning of care activities by health care professionals.

The holistic/integrated competency-based model is more valid and reliable than current ways of assessing professionals. It enables us to come closer than we have in the past to assessing what we want to assess (i.e., the capacity of the professional to integrate knowledge, values, attitudes, skills and other attributes in the real world of practice). This model requires the components shown in Fig. 3.4 to be considered.

The specification of component skills that contribute to being competent would enable students to develop the essential practical skills required of the competent practitioner. These skills could be in the form of a clinical skills checklist, which, in turn, can be grouped into proficiencies (e.g. assessing needs and planning care). These essential skills should be assessed at prespecified standards commensurate with the stage of the education programme.

The assessment of personal attributes is a challenge. The specification of criteria will guide students and practice educators toward the development and assessment of personal attributes that are essential for effective professional practice.

REFERENCES

Ashworth P, Morrison P. Problems of competence-based nurse education. *Nurse Educ Today*, 1991;11:256–260.

Bedford H, Phillips T, Robinson J. Assessing Competencies in Nursing and Midwifery Education: Final Report. The English National Board for Nursing, Midwifery and Health Visiting, London:1993.

Benner P. Issues in competency-based testing. *Nurs Outlook*, 1982;30:303–309.

Black H, Wolf A. Knowledge and Competence: Current Issues in Training and Education. Employment Department, Sheffield:1990.

Bloom BS, Engelhort MD, Furst EJ. Taxonomy of Educational Objectives, Handbook 1: Cognitive Domains. Longman, London:1956.

Bradshaw A. Defining competency in nursing (part II): an analytical review. *J Clin Nurs*, 1998;7:103–111.

Bradshaw A. Editorial. *J Clin Nurs*, 2000;9:319–320.

Braithwaite DN, Elzubeir M, Stark S. Project 2000 student wastage: a case study. *Nurse Educ Today*, 1994;14:15–21.

Castledine G. New nurse competencies: are they adequate? *Br J Nurs*, 2000;9(5):314–315.

City and Guilds, 3033: Care – NVQ Level 2. City and Guilds of London Institute, London:1992.

Department of Health, Making a Difference. Department of Health, London:1999.

Department of Health. The NHS Knowledge and Skills Framework (NHS KSF) and the Development Review Process. Department of Health, London:2004.

DfES, 2005. NVQ. Available: https://www.gov.uk/government/organisations/department-for-education. Accessed: May 2020.

Department of Education- GOV.UK [online]. Available: https://www.gov.uk/what-different-qualification-levels-mean/list-of-qualification-levels. May 2020./DG_10039029. Accessed: March 2012.

Eraut M. Concepts of competence. *J Interprof Care*, 1998;12(2):127–139.

Farley A, Hendry C. Teaching practical skills: a guide for preceptors. *Nurs Stand*, 1997;11(29):46–48.

Fletcher S. NVQs Standards and Competence. A Practical Guide for Employers, Managers and Trainers. Kogan Page, London:1991.

Fraser D, Murphy R, Worth-Butler M. An Outcome Evaluation of the Effectiveness of Pre-registration Midwifery Programmes of Education. The English National Board for Nursing, Midwifery and Health Visiting, London:1997.

Gerrish K, McManus, M, Ashworth P. Levels of Achievement: A Review of the Assessment of Practice. The English National Board for Nursing, Midwifery and Health Visiting, London:1997.

Gonczi A, Hager P, Athanasou J, The Development of Competency-Based Assessment Strategies for the Professions. National Office of Overseas Skills Recognition, Research Paper No. 8. Australian Government Publishing Service, Canberra:1993.

Hager P, Gonczi A, Edwards R, Hanson, Raggatt P. Professions and competencies. Boundaries of Adult Learning. In: Edwards R, Hanson A, Raggatt P, Boundaries of Adult Learning. Routledge, London:1996, pp. 246–260.

Hart A, Lockley R, Henwood F. Evaluation of the Effectiveness of Midwifery Education in Preparing Midwives to Meet the Needs of Women from Disadvantaged Groups. The English National Board for Nursing, Midwifery and Health Visiting, London:2001.

Health and Care Professions Council. Standards of Conduct, Performance and Ethics. HCPC, London:2008.

Health and Care Professions Council. Guidance on Conduct and Ethics for Students. HCPC, London:2009.

Health and Care Professions Council. Fitness to Practise Annual Report 2010. HCPC, London:2010a.

Health and Care Professions Council. Information for Employers and Managers: The Fitness to Practise Process. HCPC, London:2010b.

Health and Care Professions Council 2011. Standards of Proficiency. Available: https://www.hcpc-uk.org/resources/standards/standards-of-education-and-training/. Accessed: August 2011.

The Health and Care Professions Order, Consolidated text incorporating repeals and amendments made up to 1st April 2010. HCPC, London:2001.

Hilton PA. Record of achievement. In: Hilton PA, Fundamental Nursing Skills. Whurr, London:2004, pp. 306–313.

Hilton SR, Slotnick HB. Proto-professionalism: how professionalisation occurs across the continuum of medical education. *Med Educ*, 2005;39:58–65.

Hutt R. Lasting the course, Part IV: findings and conclusions. *Senior Nurse*, 1988;10(3):4–8.

Jervis A, Tilki M. Why are nurse mentors failing to fail student nurses who do not meet clinical performance standards? *Br J Nurs*, 2011;20(9):582–587.

Jessup G. Outcomes: NVQs and the Emerging Model of Education and Training. The Falmer Press, London:1991.

Le Var R. NVQs in nursing, midwifery and health visiting: a question of assessment and learning? *Nurse Educ Today*, 1996;16:85–93.

Lindop E. Factors associated with student and pupil nurse wastage. *J Adv Nurs*, 1987;12:751–756.

McGaghie WC. Professional competence evaluation. *Educ Res*, 1991;20(1):3.

Manpower Services Commission. Guidance Notes for Two-Year Youth Training Schemes. Manpower Services Commission, Sheffield:1985.

Miller C. Literature review: improving and enhancing performance in the affective domain of nursing students. *Contemp Nurse*, 2010;35(1):2–17.

Moore D. Assuring fitness for practice: a policy review. Nursing and Midwifery Council Task and Finish Group, London:2005.

NCVQ. Guide to National Vocational Qualifications. National Council for Vocational Qualifications, London:1991.

Norris N. The trouble with competence. *Camb J Educ*, 1991; 21(3):331–341.

Novak, 1988 S. Novak, An effective clinical evaluation tool. *J Nurs Educ*, 1988;27(2):83–84.

Nursing and Midwifery Council. The Nursing and Midwifery Order 2001 (SI 2002/253). The Stationery Office, Norwich:2001.

Nursing and Midwifery Council. Consultation on Proposals Arising from a Review of Fitness for Practice at the Point of Registration. NMC, London:2005.

Nursing and Midwifery Council. Essential Skills Clusters for Pre-registration Nursing Programmes. NMC, London:2007.

Nursing and Midwifery Council. The Code: Professional standards of practice and behaviour for nurses, midwives and nursing associates. NMC, London:2018.

Nursing and Midwifery Council. Standards of Pre-registration Midwifery Education. NMC, London:2023.

Nursing and Midwifery Council. Standards of Pre-registration Nursing Education. NMC, London:2023. Available: https://www.nmc.org.uk/globalassets/sitedocuments/standards/2023-pre-reg-standards/new-vi/standards-for-pre-registration-nursing-programmes.pdf.

Nursing and Midwifery Council. Fitness to Practise: How the Process Works. NMC, London:2010b.

Nursing and Midwifery Council. Guidance on professional conduct for nursing and midwifery students. 2nd ed. NMC:2010c.

Nursing and Midwifery Council. Nursing and Midwifery Council: Annual Fitness to Practise Report 2010-2011. NMC, London:2011a.

Nursing and Midwifery Council. Guidance on Professional Conduct for Nursing and Midwifery Students. NMC, London: 2011b.

Papadakis MA, Hodgson CS, Teherani A. Unprofessional behaviour in medical school is associated with subsequent disciplinary action by a state medical board. *Acad Med*, 2004; 79:244–249.

Papadakis MA, Teherani A, Banach MA. Disciplinary action by medical boards and prior behaviour in medical school. *N Engl J Med*, 2005;353:2673–2682.

Percival E, Anderson M, Lawson D. Assessing beginning level competencies: the first step in continuing education. *J Contin Educ Nurs*, 1994;25(3):139–142.

Phillips T, Schostak J, Tyler J. Practice and Assessment in Nursing and Midwifery: Doing it for Real. The English National Board for Nursing, Midwifery and Health Visiting, London:2000.

Roberts D. Editorial: newly qualified nurses – competence or confidence? *Nurse Educ Today*, 2009;29:467–468.

Rutkowski K. Failure to fail: assessing nursing students' competence during practice placements. *Nurs Stand*, 2007;22(13): 35–40.

Skills for Health. Skills for Health, 2005. National Occupational Standards and National Workforce Competences. 2005. Available: http://www.skillsforhealth.org.uk/frameworks.php. Accessed: December 2005.

Skills for Health 2020. Better skills, better jobs and better health. Available: https://skillsforhealth.org.uk/. Accessed: May 2021.

Steinaker N, Bell M. The Experiential Taxonomy: A New Approach to Teaching and Learning. Academic Press, New York:1979.

Storey L, O'Kell S, Day M. Utilising National Occupational Standards as a Complement to Nursing Curricula. Department of Health, London:1995.

Sutton FA, Arbon PA. Australian nursing – moving forward? Competencies and the nursing profession. *Nurse Educ Today*, 1994;14;388–393.

Teherani A, Hodgson CS, Banach M. Domains of unprofessional behaviour during medical school associated with future disciplinary action by a state medical board. *Acad Med*, 2005;80(Suppl.):17–20.

Toohey S. Assessment of students, personal development as part of preparation for professional work – is it desirable and is it feasible? *Assess Eval High Educ*, 2002;27(6):529–538.

Training Agency, Development of Assessable Standards for National Certification. Guidance Note 1: A Code of Practice and a Development Model. Training Agency, Sheffield:1988.

UKCC, Fitness for Practice. United Kingdom Central Council for Nursing, Midwifery and Health Visiting, London:1999.

Watson R, Stimpson A, Topping A, Clinical competence assessment in nursing: a systematic review of the literature. *J Adv Nurs*, 2002;27(5);519–524.

Wolf A. Competence-Based Assessment. Open University Press, Buckingham:1995.

Worth-Butler M, Murphy R, Framer D. Towards an integrated model of competence in midwifery. *Midwifery*, 1994;10: 225–231.

How Do We Assess?

CHAPTER CONTENTS

INTRODUCTION

It is discussed in Chapter 3 that competence is a construct that is not directly observable, but rather, is inferred from performance. Assessing performance will therefore be important to infer clinical competence. Equally important will be the requirement to gather sufficient evidence to justify the inference and, in particular, that a safe inference has been made (Gonczi et al 1993). Clinical competence is a complex entity, and it almost always requires the practitioner to use a combination of attributes simultaneously and adapt practices to different contexts. Thus the assessment of clinical competence is not straightforward, and no one method can hope to assess overall competence. Moreover, some competencies are less easily assessed through performance than others. However, overall, the Standards for Student Supervision and Assessment (NMC 2018b) are outcome focused with a practice assessor making and recording,

objective, evidenced-based assessments on conduct, proficiency and achievement, drawing on student records, direct observations, student self-reflection, and other resources.
NMC (2018b:7.3:9)

These standards make clear that students should learn from a range of people such as registered health and social care registrants, nonregistered staff, service users and other students (Leigh & Roberts 2018). Documented feedback will provide a 'range of forms of evidence' to enable practice assessors to make valid and reliable inferences. An extensive review of the literature on assessment of competence to practice by Redfern et al (2002), concluded that a multimethod approach enhances validity and ensures comprehensive assessment of the complex range of skills required of preregistration nursing and midwifery students. Consequently, it is necessary to use planned combinations of a variety of methods of assessment to obtain the range of evidence to evaluate overall clinical competence so that assessors of clinical practice know with confidence that the student has the necessary knowledge, skills and attributes to ensure public safety and protection.

There is one key similarity between the processes of clinical assessment and research: simplistically, both seek to obtain data or evidence to add to the knowledge base about the subject and/or prove or disprove the case under investigation. In clinical assessment, we seek data by which we obtain clearer perspectives of our learners and evidence to confirm the achievement of competence for safe practice. When conducting clinical assessment, there is much to be learnt from the rigour with which research studies are generally conducted to achieve valid and reliable results. One rigorous research strategy is the use of triangulation.

In this chapter, the importance of using the strategy of triangulation to achieve validity and reliable assessment is explored. In research, the technique of triangulation is used to obtain more valid and reliable research data. The principles guiding the use of this technique will be extrapolated for use in assessment so that assessments can also be conducted with the same degrees of validity and reliability as in research. The uses, merits and limitations of a range of methods that can be used in the competency-based approach for the assessment of clinical practice are also explored and debated. To reflect the principle of integration through the use of the holistic/integrated competency-based model of assessment (see Fig. 3.4), integrated assessment approaches that use a combination of methods are put forward so that a number of competencies and their performance and knowledge outcomes can be assessed simultaneously.

TRIANGULATION

The theoretical perspectives of the term 'triangulation' are drawn from the literature on research, as literature that relates this term to the conduct of assessment is perfunctory and indirect (e.g. see Bedford et al 1993). Triangulation is a term borrowed by the social sciences from surveying and navigation. It refers to the principle of geometry that the third point of a triangle can be plotted using the two known points as the vertices (Fielding & Fielding 1986, in Redfern 1994). This concept of triangulation was first applied to

research methodology by Campbell and Fiske (1959, in Redfern 1994) in psychological research as a metaphor to describe the use of several methods to measure a single construct to confirm a hypothesis. Triangulation in this context then does not mean three. Later researchers such as Denzin (1989) argue that triangulation is more than the use of several methods–it is the combination of 'methodologies' used to investigate the same phenomenon. These methodologies are referred to as *types of triangulation*: four of them are described by Denzin (1989). From the work of Denzin, three types of triangulation are selected for exploration here because these are seen to be relevant and applicable for the conduct of integrated assessments: they are therefore discussed and extrapolated to our discussion on assessment in this chapter. The types of triangulation are:
- method triangulation
- data triangulation
- investigator triangulation.

METHOD TRIANGULATION

There are two kinds of method triangulation: within methods and between methods.

Within-methods triangulation is the application of different types of the same method to measure a phenomenon. An example is that of using different scales to measure pain, such as a visual analogue scale, a Likert-type scale and a semantic differential scale. All these scales are different in the way they assess the amount and/or the quality of pain, but they are all examples of the same kind of method (i.e. scales). As a test of reliability, the issue is whether they come up with the same answer when applied to the same patients at the same time.

When a student is assessed while caring for patients experiencing pain, the student can be observed by the practice supervisor or assessor during clinical. This sentence is incomplete. The sentence should continue to say… practice when caring for these patients arrangements may also be made for the student to be observed by another practice supervisor or assessor, thus generating evidence of performance using the 'testimony of others'. Both assessors are using the same assessment method (i.e. observation). As a test of reliability, the issue is whether they come up with the same or similar answers of what the student can perform.

Between-methods triangulation uses different methods to measure the same phenomenon. The important point about using between-methods triangulation is that it is much more than the mere combination of several methods. Rather, the methods should be selected as a combined strategy so that the strengths of each are maximized and their limitations are minimized. Linking the data in a coherent and systematic way is essential. In the case of the student assessment previously discussed, an example of using between-methods triangulation is to ask questions about care you have observed the student giving. Questioning will establish, for example, whether there is a sound understanding of the needs of the patients who are experiencing the pain, which in turn should influence the care given. It may also reveal the attitudes of the student on this aspect of care or his/her attitudes towards the patients. The strengths and weaknesses of observation in determining performance evidence are complemented by the strengths and weaknesses of questioning in determining knowledge and understanding. As a test of validity, the answers of the student will augment the assessor's observation of performance.

DATA TRIANGULATION

Data triangulation refers to the use of multiple data sources, with each source focused upon the phenomenon of interest (Denzin 1989). These data sources can differ by person, time or place, providing multiple perspectives (Carter et al 2014). For example, data can be collected from different people or during different times or at different locations. The aim is that the data sources provide unique and diverse views about the same topic to contribute to validity and reliability: this enables the researcher to discover the dimensions of a phenomenon that are similar and dissimilar. As shown below, it is appropriate to make use of the three data sources as described by Denzin (1989) for the purposes of clinical assessment:

- Person: assessment evidence is collected from other assessors, supervisors, service users and student self-evaluation.
- Time: assessment evidence is collected on different clinical shifts over a period of time.
- Place: assessment evidence is collected from the different instances of practice provided within the range of context in the learning contract (see Chapter 6).

If we return to the example of assessing the student caring for patients who are experiencing pain, we can see how evidence from the three data sources can provide the practice assessor with diverse views about the student when caring for patients experiencing pain. Evidence provided by the testimony of others will contribute to the validity and reliability of assessments of the student. If all sources agree that the student has achieved the performance and knowledge outcomes and is able to care for this category of patients, the assessment is likely to have validity. Conversely, if there is disagreement, the assessment could lack validity and/or reliability. The use of continuous assessment of practice will help to ensure that evidence collected on different clinical shifts reflects a wide range of conditions. Caring for different patients, working at different times of the day and working with different environmental stresses such as noise and busyness of the ward are factors that may influence how the student practises.

The evidence collected from a range of occasions when the student cared for patients experiencing pain will provide information about the quantity and quality of learning. It will also serve to identify the strengths and weaknesses of the student in this aspect of care. For instance, does the student provide better care for the younger than the older patient? How well does the student cope when caring for these patients? Is the student able to assess the patient's need for pain relief with accuracy? Is the student able to plan care for these patients so that they are as comfortable as possible?

INVESTIGATOR TRIANGULATION

Investigator triangulation occurs when the different knowledge and expertise held by members of the research team are used in the analysis of raw data. When several investigators are involved in a study, this type of triangulation helps reduce the potential bias that occurs when only a single investigator is involved. In clinical assessment, investigator triangulation takes place when the range of evidence contributed by different assessors, supervisors, peers and service users is used in the analysis of student competence. Each person is likely to know the student in slightly different ways and be able to contribute to identification of the range of learning that has taken place, what the strengths and weaknesses of the student are and so on. Investigator triangulation may be particularly valuable when attempting to evaluate the student's attitudes. Several people's views are likely to have been collected after independent assessment of the student, thus reducing biases and adding to the reliability of the assessment (Phillips et al 2000).

So far, then, triangulation is about:

- the use of different assessment methods or ways of collecting assessment evidence
- ensuring that different assessment methods complement each other.

The main aim of using triangulation in clinical assessment is to obtain as complete a picture as possible of the student's achievement of competence in terms of their conduct, proficiency and achievement to ensure that objective, evidence-based assessments are valid and reliable. It is therefore important to remember that triangulation is more than just obtaining multiple sources or types of evidence; the evidence also needs to be linked so that an integrated and comprehensive assessment of the student is made.

ADVANTAGES AND LIMITATIONS OF TRIANGULATION

Practically, triangulation may be quite straightforward to arrange when plans are made for the supervision and assessment of students. Using triangulation to the extent that an integrated and comprehensive assessment of the student is made can prove to be challenging, which may be construed to be a limitation by some. However, the use of triangulation carries many advantages. Advantages and limitations are now considered.

You may wish to try Activity 4.1.

ADVANTAGES

1. It allows confirmation of assessment evidence and increases confidence in the assessment decision made. By combining the types of triangulation; that is, method, data and investigator triangulation–a fuller and more complete picture of the student's achievement or nonachievement is obtained. Different aspects of the student's competence can be identified so that there is a richer and deeper understanding of the student's learning, be it performance or knowledge and understanding or the development of some attitude or a set of values, which confirms our assessment of the student. This therefore increases our confidence when we are making the assessment decision. Consider this scenario: you have a student who is not achieving several competencies. You have come to this decision over several weeks of observing the student in practice and asking them questions about their practice. You wonder whether your decision is influenced by the fact that you do not like the student's visible tattoos! Another assessor provides assessment evidence that confirms your decision. You probably breathe a sigh of relief and say: I'm not biased after all. The testimony provided by another assessor increases your confidence in your assessment decision. Does this enhance the validity, or reliability, or both, of your assessment? (See discussion in Chapter 5.)

2. It guards against a blinkered perspective. The use of triangulation can potentially help to overcome the bias of 'single-method, single-observer' assessments, although the use of several methods and assessors may not compensate for assessor bias (Redfern 1994). It can be difficult to overcome strong likes and dislikes. It can also not compensate for assessor bias caused by other factors such as comparing a student to other students (Yeates et al 2014).

3. It is more likely to portray a 'whole picture' of the student. Rowntree's (1987) book has this question as the title: *Assessing Students: How Shall We Know Them?*

Attempting to know students so that we are fair in our assessments of them requires us to understand a complex and multidimensional being. Furthermore, competencies are generally complex, which requires the student to learn and develop several attributes concurrently (see Chapter 3 for a discussion of the holistic/integrated competency-based model). A range of assessment evidence will provide a richer and deeper understanding of the student's strengths and weaknesses and what has and has not been achieved so that a fuller picture of the student's achievement is obtained. We will then be in a better position to provide the guidance and support that the student requires to learn and achieve their full potential.

4. It allows divergent evidence to enrich explanation. When triangulation is used, we are more likely to obtain or be given unexpected and divergent assessment evidence about the student. Such evidence may explain some aspect of the student's personal circumstances or performance that has been eluding us. For example, a colleague who was working with your student may report to you that your student was observed to have been in tears when caring for a patient with terminal cancer. The student subsequently revealed that a close friend had recently died of cancer. For several weeks, you have been attempting to involve the student in this aspect of care but had been unsuccessful because the student was always reluctant. You were getting concerned that the student is not learning about care of patients with terminal cancer. The evidence from your colleague has served as a source of divergent evidence.

LIMITATIONS

1. It is expensive on resources. When using triangulation, arrangements need to be made for the student to learn and practise over a range of contexts over time. Several assessment methods, including other suitably prepared health and social care registrants, need to be used; more resources, such as time and extra staff, are required. In today's climate of health and social care, where such resources are in short supply, the need for student supervision and assessment competes with the need to deliver care (Leigh & Roberts 2018). It would be tempting, and certainly easier, to ignore the use of triangulation when assessing students! As was practised by the General Nursing Council for England and Wales in the 1970s, the use of one-off assessment when student nurses were assessed on four one-off occasions, for a stated period of time on each occasion, for four aspects of learning, was much more economical on resources. However, the current Nursing and Midwifery Council

(NMC) standards (2018) mean triangulation to generate a diverse evidence base to determine competency and progression cannot be ignored. Practice assessors are required to liaise with practice supervisors in formulating assessments.

2. It cannot compensate for assessor bias. If we cannot overcome our biases, or if we are not aware of them, the use of triangulation will not help us achieve the validity and reliability we desire in our assessment.

3. It may compound sources of error. This point relates to Point 2. If we hold some biases and others that have provided performance feedback also hold some biases that are different from ours, our assessment evidence will not be as objective as we perceive. In fact, the student could be more disadvantaged than if we had not used the evidence from others.

4. Methods selected may be inappropriate. As discussed earlier, the assessment methods selected should complement each other so that a rich range of evidence is provided to allow the development of professional competence to be assessed fully (Fotheringham 2010). This means we must assess the development of knowledge, attitudes, skills and attributes. The selection of methods should allow the assessment of those areas of learning, performance and development equally and not focus on the assessment of one or two domains of learning. For example, if we and other practice supervisors/assessors all use observation to assess the student's performance, we will have assessed the student's abilities to perform a skill, but may not have assessed attributes such as understanding and attitudes well, if at all.

5. Triangulation is no use with the 'wrong' research question. This limitation is equally relevant to assessment. If we are not clear about what we want to assess, then triangulation is not going to enhance the validity and reliability of the assessment. It is therefore important to define, and describe clearly, the competency statement, the knowledge and performance outcomes we wish students to achieve.

You may wish to try Activity 4.2.

Activity 4.2

Debate the following with your colleagues:
The limitations of the different types of triangulation are real and daunting. What can be done to reduce these limitations?

Despite the challenges and difficulties associated with triangulation, the advantages of using this strategy indicate that it can give better opportunities to achieve validity and reliability of assessment. What this means when using the holistic/integrated competency-based approach to assessment is that both the attributes of the learner and the performance of key professional tasks are assessed. The discussion of competence in Chapter 3 stated that the attributes of individuals do not in themselves constitute competence. Nor is competence the mere performance of a series of tasks. Rather, the notion of competence integrates attributes with performance. Also remember that competence is a construct that is not directly observable but is inferred from successful performance. Therefore combinations of assessment methods need to be considered and used so there is a diverse evidence base from which to safely decide upon the competency of a given proficiency.

ASSESSMENT METHODS

This section starts with Activity 4.3.

Activity 4.3

What methods do you frequently use to assess students you work with? Can you give reasons for your selection?

The following methods are the most commonly used by assessors:

- working with the students and observing their practice
- asking questions leading to reflective discussions on contextualized practice
- obtaining the opinion (testimony) of other practice assessors, practice supervisors, student peers and service users
- checking care records made by the students.

Gonczi et al (1993) say that all existing methods of assessment used by a profession are potentially appropriate for use in the competency-based approach to assessment. They go on to explain that it is not the methods themselves that are competency based but the way they are used, the emphasis given to the methods and how results are interpreted that are important in competency-based assessment. The uses, merits and limitations of a range of methods that can be used for the assessment of the different components of professional competence are now explored.

OBSERVATION OF PRACTICE

Observation simply means watching and noting what you see (Stoker 1994). Stoker (1994:iv) says that 'observation is an essential tool in assessment–it is one of the most effective ways of finding out whether learning has taken place'. Furthermore, NMC (2018) explicitly states that practice supervisors 'contribute to the student's record of achievement by periodically recording relevant observations on the conduct, proficiency and achievement of the students they are supervising' (NMC 2018b:4.1:7) and engage with practice assessors and academic assessors to share these observations (NMC 2018b:4.3:7). Likewise, practice assessors '…periodically observe the student across environments to inform decisions for assessment and progression' (NMC 2018b:7.6:9) as well as using the direct observations of others as one of the resources used to inform their assessments on competency.

Learners can be assessed on a number of occasions in their everyday working environment while they are performing in their 'natural' surroundings to give us a picture of their ability to perform a variety of real tasks so that direct evidence of competence can be collected. As the learner is watched in action, direct evidence of behaviours and behavioural patterns is obtained. Far more reliable judgements about professional competence are therefore possible than with assessments conducted over limited time periods in limited ranges of context. Assessments are also more likely to have predictive validity.

There are two ways we can observe the learner's performance: by participant and nonparticipant observation. Working directly with the learner is known as *participant observation*. In research, during participant observation, researchers join the group, often keeping their identities a secret to try to minimize any changes in behaviour that participants may be inclined to make as a result of being observed (Guest et al 2013). In clinical assessment, however, the identity of the assessor cannot be concealed. Therefore, the effects of being observed–the observer effect–may affect the learner's performance. The observer effect is discussed in Chapter 5. Another important point to bear in mind when observing practice is that of observer bias, just as in research, there is researcher bias (Kawulich 2005). Observer bias may affect assessment, which is also discussed in Chapter 5.

Try Activity 4.4.

> ### Activity 4.4
>
> If you were being directly observed, how might your performance be affected?

The fact that someone is looking at us may make us nervous. Our actions may not be as smooth as usual, or we may have lapses of memory. On the other hand, we may exercise more attention to the task than we normally would. Can you recall being observed as part of an assessment and

uncharacteristically fumbling and stumbling? Likewise, can you recall knowing you were going to be assessed and spending days and days meticulously planning and preparing for the task?

In these instances, we are obviously not giving a true picture of the way we practise. Is the validity, or reliability, or both, affected?

Observing the learner from a distance is known as *nonparticipant observation*. In research, the researcher does not interact with the participants; instead they are detached and objectively observe social action and interaction (Caldwell & Atwal 2005). During clinical assessment, we may observe the learner caring for a patient while we are performing another activity such as dispensing medications, talking to someone else and so on. This mirrors the idea that 'the level of supervision can decrease with the student's increasing proficiency and confidence' (NMC 2018b:4). What strategies have you used for observing a learner from a distance?

Nerve-wracking or an opportunity to outshine Fig. 4.1?

USING THE STANDARDS AND PERFORMANCE CRITERIA IN A CHECKLIST

Although the NMC 2018 standards emphasise the importance of students learning in a range of environments with a range of people and being proactive and taking responsibility for their own learning (NMC 2018b:1:5), there remains a requirement for the achievement of proficiencies and programme outcomes to justify progression and eventual registration. The listing of professional body competencies in practice assessment documentation is widely used to demonstrate the student's standard and scope of achievement.

Fletcher (1991:66) stated that in competence-based assessment, 'it is individual performance which is judged – and judged against explicit standards which reflect … the expected outcomes of that individual's competent performance …'. When assessing for the development and achievement of a professional competency, the assessor looks for prespecified behaviours such as the ways a skill is performed, or the ways the learner interacts with a patient, or how care is being given. These criteria are used to determine whether learning has taken place.

In using a competence-based assessment tool, reliability and validity are essential. Wu et al (2015) found that most have face and content validity established through expert consensus and criterion validity because they are mapped to national standards and literature. However, psychometric properties could be better established, as well as their reliability and validity in a variety of settings. Ewan and

White (1996) recommend the use of written checklists because they have a high interobserver agreement. They also have the advantages of ensuring validity, discriminatory power and feasibility (Stoker 1994), concepts that are discussed in Chapter 5.

When using written checklists, the following points may be useful to remember (Ewan & White 1996):

- longer checklists tend to be more reliable than shorter ones
- as checklists require the observer to judge whether certain behaviours have taken place, they are most effective when components of performance are specified in detail
- it is possible to include behaviours that may underpin aspects of attitudes and interpersonal relationships
- have three options for recording (i.e. observed, not observed, not applicable)
- important errors should also be noted
- if any essential component of the performance is omitted, the learner is assessed as not yet competent and is reassessed.

In particular instances, it becomes necessary to assess the process of performance (Gonczi et al 1993). When observing these instances of practice, the ways of performing a task can also be included in a checklist, such as:

- accuracy or lack of error
- speed of performance
- choice of the correct techniques
- the proper sequence of techniques
- adherence to regulatory and policy requirements.

Although the use of checklists has advantages, Ewan and White (1996) warn that if the criteria in the checklist emphasize the performance of a specific skill, then beginning students may become fixated on specifics rather than learning the perspectives of care as a whole. Further disadvantages of checklists or competencies listed in a practice assessment document for a practice assessor were identified by Almalkawi, Jester and Terry (2018) in their iterative review:

- difficulties in the language used to describe competencies
- the challenge of distinguishing between different levels of competence
- lack of transparent and explicit criteria.

They suggested such document limitations could affect the accuracy and fairness of a student's assessment as well as result in impaired feedback on performance to the student. The future may see the introduction of scoring rubrics with clear and understandable competency descriptors to aid accurate assessment.

ALLOW ENOUGH TIME FOR OBSERVATION

Assessments, in general, sample only a fraction of what a learner is expected to know. This is inevitable because it is not feasible or desirable to attempt to assess every aspect of learning; for example, it would be impractical to attempt to assess a pharmacist's knowledge of every drug that could be encountered in everyday practice. Likewise, when assessing the competent clinical practice of students, inference of competence is inevitably based on a sampling of performance.

Fish and Twinn (1997:114) made this important point about observing practice: 'all seeing is selective, and all reporting of what is seen is interpretive; there is no such thing as purely objective factual observation'. Remember that competence is a construct that is not directly observable but is inferred from successful performance. There must therefore be enough evidence so that we are confident it is safe to make the inference that the learner is competent. The practice assessor must therefore allow enough time to observe the learner on a number of occasions so that it is possible for sufficient evidence of conduct, proficiency and achievement can be demonstrated.

How does the practice assessor know when there is enough evidence? Making an assessment decision based on a range of evidence is one of the key principles of competency-based assessment. This important aspect of competency-based assessment is discussed in Chapter 7. It is also a key principle of NMC (2018) standards: '…drawing on student records, direct observations, student self-reflection, and other resources' (Section 7.3) and '…gather and coordinate feedback from practice supervisors, any other practice assessors, and relevant people, to be assured about their decisions for assessment and progression' (Section 7.7).

So far, there has been a consideration of how to use observation as an assessment method, its usefulness or otherwise in ascertaining a true picture of the learner's ability in natural surroundings and some of the difficulties associated with its use. To summarize, effective assessment using observation requires you to:

- use a checklist or assessment tool
- allow enough time for observation
- be aware of observer bias
- be aware of observer effect.

Which components of competence can be assessed with any accuracy using observation? When a learner's performance is observed, only overt behaviours and behavioural patterns exhibited by the learner when care is performed can be seen. Although behavioural patterns may indicate the underlying attitude (Andrusyszyn 1989), inwardly held beliefs, values or feelings cannot be seen (Dawson 1992), nor can knowledge and understanding of the care or task be determined. As an observer, one can only say that the observable performance is mainly a reflection of the possession of skills. Observation is therefore useful only for the assessment of the skills developed that are contributing to effective performance at the time. Gonczi et al (1993), however, claim that observation allows assessment of attitudes and interpersonal skills.

Try Activity 4.5 on the use of observation as an assessment method.

Activity 4.5

Make a list of the uses/merits of observation and another of the limits of observation.

ADVANTAGES OF OBSERVATION OF PRACTICE

- Can provide a high level of integrated assessments. Because the learner is observed performing care and tasks, it is possible to use evidence of performance to assess several competencies and several components of competence simultaneously.
- Allows assessment of attitudes and interpersonal skills. Attitudes can be inferred from behaviours and behavioural patterns. Interpersonal skills can be directly observed.
- Offers realistic evidence of competence. Competence-based assessment uses explicit standards of occupational performance as its foundation. The logical way to assess whether someone is meeting those standards is to watch them working in that occupation (Fletcher 1991).
- Allows evaluation of problem-solving. Because the learner is observed managing a situation, it is possible to assess how well the learner has managed the situation. From this, it can be inferred that the learner has been able to solve the problem.
- Mistakes in performance can be corrected. Direct observation and supervision of practice will enable the supervisor to identify and correct any mistakes at the time or immediately afterwards.

DISADVANTAGES OF OBSERVATION OF PRACTICE

- Circumstances of observation may be too specific. Evidence obtained about the ability to perform in care situations that occur rarely generally cannot be used with any degree of validity towards the assessment of many competencies.

- Requires lengthy and costly assessments for reliability. The learner needs to be observed on more than one occasion to ensure reliability. This means that the period of assessment is longer rather than shorter and is therefore costly in terms of time and effort required.
- Gives indirect evidence of knowledge/understanding only. If a learner can perform the care or task, it can only be inferred that knowledge/understanding underpins that performance.
- Does not assess ability to learn through practice. Even if a learner can perform a task, or care for a patient, it cannot be assumed that the learner can transfer this performance to another situation and perform to the same standards another time.
- Subject to observer bias and observer effect. Polit et al (2010) state that one of the most pervasive problems with observation is the vulnerability of observational data to distortions and biases; human perceptual judgmental errors can pose a serious threat to the validity and accuracy of observational information.

In summary, direct observation of clinical practice is used primarily to obtain evidence of ability to perform when we assess the learning of practical skills and behaviours, which may indicate the underlying attitudes and value systems held by the learner. However, an ability to perform is only one component of competence. Evidence of achievement of the other components of competence needs to be obtained using other assessment methods. Questioning frequently complements observation in that we are obtaining the indirect evidence of competence, which is hidden and not open to observation (Stoker 1994).

EXAMINATION OF PRODUCTS

There are occasions when evidence of ability to perform may be inferred from an examination of the product of the learner's work–items that the learner produced or has worked on (e.g. a made bed and the surrounds, the bandaged stump of a below-knee amputation). The level of achievement is judged by assessing the quality of the piece of work.

QUESTIONING

It is discussed in Chapter 1 that one of the purposes of assessment is to maximize learning. Gipps (1994:15) made the point that 'assessment alone will not develop higher-order skills in the absence of clearly delineated teaching strategies that foster the development of higher-order thinking in pupils'. Asking questions is an integral part of teaching and learning and places students in the role of active learners (De Young 1990). It is one teaching/learning strategy to help students develop higher-level cognitive skills. Questioning can also serve as positive reinforcement for students when we indicate that answers are correct and/or insightful. This gives feedback to the student that material has been understood and higher-level thought processes were used (Activity 4.6).

Activity 4.6

For what purposes have you used questioning?

In clinical assessment, questioning can be used for the following purposes:

- To assess baseline knowledge (e.g. knowledge of the stages of the grieving process).
- To assess ability to form links between previously isolated information (e.g. if a student midwife is learning how to support women in labour, questions could be asked about the support strategies used for the individual woman and how well these worked for that woman; further questioning could then lead the student to explore those common strategies that work, or do not work, for a number of women the student has looked after).
- To assess application of theory to practice (e.g. using the policy on infection control you had previously discussed with the learner, ask your learner to discuss the actions they would take when preparing for the admission of the next patient who requires barrier nursing).
- To assess understanding of care given (e.g. the rationale for using certain communication skills when comforting the dying patient; if the learner understands the why behind the use of these ways of communicating, it indicates that theory underpins practice).
- To assess problem-solving skills (e.g. by posing: What's the real issue here? What other information do you need before you can solve this problem? How else could you … ? Give reasons for …. What would happen if you tried … ? What other options do you have?).
- To assess decision-making skills (e.g. by posing: What action would you take if … ? Give reasons …. What do you intend doing about it?).
- It is possible to obtain an indication of underlying attitudes, values and beliefs (e.g. by posing: What do you think of physician-assisted suicide? What do you think of detaining patients under the Mental Health Act? Do you agree with Jenny's opinions? Why?).
- It is possible to assess verbal communication skills by the ability of the student in verbalizing responses.

From this discussion of the uses of questioning, it can be seen that learning in the cognitive domain and affective domain (Bloom et al 1956)–and thus, several attributes of competence–can be assessed using this assessment method. When we assess learning in the cognitive domain, it is important to assess not only the knowledge base but also higher-level thinking so that the range of cognitive skills is assessed. The kinds of questions asked will stimulate different kinds and levels of thinking, and the learner will then become aware of the kind and level of thinking expected (Perrott 1982). Formulating questions to assess higher-level thinking can be tricky. An understanding of how questions can be classified may assist in the framing of those questions that are necessary to elicit the level of thinking required of the learner.

The most popular classification system is based on Bloom's taxonomy of educational objectives (Bloom et al 1956). Although the taxonomy was developed to classify educational objectives, questions can be related to each level of the taxonomy. Lower-order cognitive skills reside mostly in Bloom's categories of knowledge and comprehension, whereas Bloom's categories of application, analysis, and evaluation require higher-order cognitive skills (Lemons & Lemons 2013). Table 4.1, adapted from De Young (1990), lists the cognitive activity at each level, as well as some sample questions.

With the assistance of the information in Table 4.1, try Activity 4.7.

Activity 4.7

Examine one learning outcome that a learner must achieve. Formulate one question at each level of Bloom's taxonomy so that you can assist your learner to develop the range of higher-level cognitive skills.

The aim is to structure questions so that they define a linking path because these are more valuable in assessing the quality of learning and helping the learner to develop higher-level thinking (Minton 1997). Do not be too concerned if you have had difficulties formulating the questions. Many trained teachers manage only to ask questions predominantly at the lower cognitive levels (De Young 1990). In view of the high-level thinking required of health professionals, however, it is beneficial to assess students at the application through to evaluation levels (see Table 4.1).

Remember that, when questioning is used in clinical assessment, the main aim is to gain evidence about how much learning has taken place (i.e. how much of the competency the student has achieved). As students become more practiced with being asked higher-order questions, to be asked such questions will start to feel routine, and they

TABLE 4.1   Question Classification According to Bloom's Taxonomy

Category	Cognitive Activity Required	Sample Question Words	Examples of Questions
1. Knowledge	*Recall*	What	What is the definition of glaucoma?
Questions, regardless of complexity, can be answered by simple recall of previously learnt material	Identify Define When Describe List Which Who	At what age do infants begin to crawl?	
2. Comprehension	*Understanding*	Compare	What does the nursing process have in common with the scientific method?
Questions can be answered by merely restating and reorganizing material in a rather literal manner to show that there is understanding of the essential meaning	Contrast	Differentiate Explain Extrapolate	Why does intravenous tubing have to be free of air?
3. Application	*Solving*	Apply	Given these arterial blood gas results, what nursing interventions are needed?
Questions involve problem solving in new situations with minimal identification or prompting of the appropriate rules, principles or concepts	Consider How would Checkout	How would you obtain a blood pressure reading on a person with third-degree burns of all extremities?	
4. Analysis	*Exploration of reasoning*	Support your	What is the major premise behind Kubler-Ross's theory of death and dying?
Questions require the student to break an idea into its component parts for logical analysis, facts, opinions, logical conclusions, etc.	What assumptions What reasons	What data would you need to support this nursing diagnosis?	
5. Synthesis	*Creating*	Think of a way	Given all of the data in this case study, what nursing diagnoses can be developed?
Questions require students to combine ideas into a statement, plan, product, etc., that is new for them	Create Propose Plan Suggest	Think of a way that we could research the relationship between those variables.	
6. Evaluation	*Judging*	Judge	Of the two possible nursing interventions in this situation, which would be more appropriate?

TABLE 4.1   Question Classification According to Bloom's Taxonomy—cont'd

Category	Cognitive Activity Required	Sample Question Words	Examples of Questions
Questions require students to make a judgement about something using some criteria or standard by making their judgement, principles, or concepts	Which would Consider Defend What is the most appropriate?		

From Craig JL, Page G. The questioning skills of nursing instructors. *J Nurs Educ*, 1981:20:20. With permission.

will become quicker and easier to answer. However, this is the aim, to enable students to problem solve diverse, complex questions and scenarios to develop high-level cognitive skills (Lemons & Lemons 2013). Questions asked should therefore be related to the competency and be based on the context of the practice event. The following checklist on the use of questioning may be helpful. It builds upon the work of Stoker (1994):

- Are the questions relevant to the learner? Do they relate to things the learner needs to know and should know rather than focusing on unusual aspects of the subject?
- Are the questions appropriate for the stage of the course of the student?
- Is the wording clear? Does it indicate what sort of answer you require?
- Have you provided some sort of feedback at the time? Be especially aware of how you deal with incorrect or incomplete answers. Try not to let your reaction have the effect of demotivating the learner.
- Be careful not to make learners feel that you are trying to catch them out.

The limitations of using questioning for assessing clinical practice are:

- Questions cannot assess attitudes, values and beliefs with accuracy because what the learner says may not be a reflection of inwardly held beliefs.
- The learner may feel threatened. This may affect the responses, and an inaccurate picture is formed of the student's ability.
- Inappropriately framed questions may not elicit the correct responses.
- Questioning can be time consuming.
- It may not have predictive validity. Correct responses to questions may not reflect the ability to perform.

Because the use of questioning in the clinical setting is frequently related directly to the caregiving experiences of the learner, questioning sessions may lead to a discussion

of these instances of practice. It is generally believed that reflection on practice–where the thinking done in one situation is made explicit and built on to be used in another–should be developed through discussion that takes place away from the arena of care activity (Bedford et al 1993). The use of discussions in clinical assessment is now examined.

DISCUSSION AROUND CARE AND CARE ACTIVITIES

De Young (1990) says that topics that are most suitable for discussion are controversial issues, clinical or professional problems and emotionally laden topics such as death and dying. After deciding on which clinical event you wish to explore further with the student through discussion, you need to provide some structure for the discussion. De Young (1990:87) made this important point about the use of discussion: 'Good discussions do not just happen spontaneously; they require careful planning'. She suggests making the following arrangements before you start:

- Be clear about what you want the student to learn—set some objectives.
- Plan the physical environment—use a room where you will not be interrupted; ensure that the seating is adequate.

During the discussion, take on the role of the facilitator (Rogers 1983). As you work with students during discussions, you can assess their development of those attributes desirable of a competent practitioner. Depending on the topic and the skills of the facilitator (De Young 2009, 1990; Ewan & White 1996; Oliver & Endersby 1994), students may have the following learning opportunities:

- To consider and explore the principles, concepts and theories used in that particular practice situation and transfer such learning to new and different situations.
- To clarify information and concepts.

- To develop critical-thinking skills, leading to the development of problem-solving and decision-making skills. Bedford et al (1993) emphasize the importance of postevent discussion in fostering the development of high-quality decision-making and problem-solving skills.
- To develop and evaluate their beliefs, values and attitudes, leading to attitude change. The use of discussion to bring about attitude change is well documented (De Young 1990). Because students are facilitated to give and take during the discussions, they learn whether the stance they take on a particular issue is clear, logical and defensible.

Bedford et al (1993:39) advocate that discussions should be critical and take place before, during and after an activity 'through which the activity is reviewed and analysed'. They say that these critical discussions move the assessment activity from being mere surveys of activities done and skills covered to a collaborative, analytical discussion about practice and divorce criticism from personal attack. Bedford et al (1993:136) emphasized that it is 'assessment discussion' rather than simple discussion that complements observational data in the assessment of competent practice:

Through discussion about a particular event, students can demonstrate the attributes of critical thinking, which von Colln-Appling and Giuliano (2017) determined from a review of the literature, were knowledge acquisition and application, analysis of information, decision making and reflection. The great advantage of assessment dialogue, as opposed to simple discussion, is that it facilitates learning as part of the assessment process.

Assessment discussions can help students to develop 'situational understanding' that will help them live with, and negotiate a way through, the competing and contradictory values they encounter as they perform care (Phillips et al 2000). Among others, Elliott (1991) and Schön (1987) postulated that professional practice is learned and developed through doing and reflection on doing. During the course of assessment discussions then, students are allowed to voice their understanding, views and opinions, disagreements and doubts; their range of cognitive skills and attitudes, values and beliefs can be assessed.

Assessment discussions around practice can thus be held:
- Before an activity when the student is being prepared for taking part in the care. The student's knowledge, understanding and perhaps attitude, values and beliefs can be assessed when questions are asked during discussions.
- During an activity as the student performs, discussions can be held to check understanding. Care has to be taken that there is minimal interruption to the student's attention and concentration on the performance.
- After an activity when care is reviewed and analysed. During the analysis, the range of cognitive skills, such as

knowledge, understanding, problem solving and attitudes, values and beliefs developed or altered as a result of the experience can be discussed. Postactivity discussion should be held as soon as possible after the experience, while events are still fresh in the mind, to allow more accurate recall of details and for any feedback to have more impact.

REFLECTIVE JOURNALING/LEARNING DIARY

The new NMC standards are clear that 'student self-reflection' is part of the portfolio of evidence the practice assessor will use to determine competence (NMC 2018b:7.3). Reflection is therefore part of assessment. Student practice assessment documents provide sections for students to record their reflections that can then frame discussion and critical analysis with their practice supervisor, practice assessor or academic assessor. Reflective journaling in a practice assessment document or learning diary are useful strategies for improving reflective skills, fostering professional growth, and can add another dimension to assessing their learning outcomes (Allan & Driscoll 2014). Reflective journaling will provide an indication of the learning that has occurred and how critical thinking is developing within the student (Wedgeworth et al 2017). Practicing the skill over time can also enhance the student's ability to write reflectively (Epp 2008).

Reflective journaling can offer insight into how students make sense of and feel about their practice. Indeed Lauterbach and Becker (2005) said that journaling 'is a critical nursing education strategy that makes explicit both "knowing" and the process of how nurses "come to know"'. It is possible that students may choose to write only that which they want to be read (Phillips et al 2000). Nevertheless, it provides an evidence base and focus for dialogue (Phillips et al 2000) and gives a starting point from which to begin an assessment discussion with the student.

Facilitating and assessing learning through reflective assessment discussions using the student's diary is not straightforward (Stuart 1997). Flexibility and abilities to deal with the unexpected are required. When working with a student's diary entry, the following framework may assist in carrying out the reflective assessment discussion with intent:

1. Consider the level of detail in the student's account of the incident.
   - Is there any description/discussion of the incident in relationship to personal involvement?
   - Have the actions taken by the student been discussed in terms of the negotiation undertaken within the situation (Phillips et al 2000)?
   - Is there any description/discussion of the incident in relationship to the involvement of others?

- What suggestions would you make so that the quality of the account could be enhanced?
2. Consider the ways in which the student has explored personal behaviours, feelings and thoughts, and those of others involved.
   - Is there a constructive exploration of behaviours and actions, thoughts and feelings?
   - How perceptive is the student?
   - Was there an objective appreciation of how and why self and others behaved, felt and thought as they did?
   - Was there any indication of how these affected the incident?
   - What suggestions would you make to help the student explore these further?
3. Consider the ways in which the student has used or referred to relevant theory and literature.
   - Is relevant underpinning knowledge identified?
   - Is there any indication of application of theory to practice?
   - Has the student critically analysed theory and current literature and their relationship to practice?
   - What broad theoretical areas may be included to explore the incident further?
   - What broad professional issues may be brought into this incident?
4. Consider the amount of learning the student has extracted through the incident.
   - Has the student identified any implications for future practice?
   - Does the student specify how their own practice can develop?
   - Does the student integrate any new learning with previous knowledge to reach different/new perspectives about care?
   - Have any assumptions about current practice been critically appraised?
   - Has the student suggested alternative ways for practice?
   - What influenced the choices made about the way care was provided (Phillips et al 2000)?
   - What constraints affected any decisions made (Phillips et al 2000)?
   - What suggestions would you make to help the student develop the above issues further?

Try Activity 4.8. Do not rush it.

Activity 4.8

Obtain a reflective journal or learning diary entry of a student. Using the discussed framework, work through the entry with a colleague.

Reflective journaling is an effective way of encouraging active reflection on experience, particularly where a review takes place with the assessor at some point in the future (Boud et al 1985). Hwanga et al (2018) found that students welcomed reflective journaling because it provided them with repeat opportunities for self-reflection and self-emancipation. However, the students reported in this study that they wanted opportunities to build on their diary entries to further develop their critical-thinking and reflection skills through face-to-face feedback and group discussions. As the basis for reflective assessment discussion, reflective journaling and diaries will allow the student opportunities to justify personal actions by giving the rationale for choices in different circumstances. The student is likely to feel valued because the incident under discussion has been personally identified as important. To an extent, the student is taking control of personal learning by identifying what is important. By an inclusion of the requirement to record not only behaviours and actions but also feelings and thoughts, the student may indicate attitudes, values and beliefs held about particular situations. Although diaries can be used to assess attitudes, values and beliefs, Dawson (1992) says that any such assessment should be formative because attitude is dynamic and changes over time.

What aspects of learning can be assessed through the reflective assessment discussion of a student's diary? Assessing learning through this process is complex (Boud et al 1985). In using the framework suggested to facilitate the reflective discussion, the following aspects of learning may be assessed:

- the perceptiveness of the student in the situation
- the self-awareness of the student
- communication and interactive skills
- unobserved practical skills
- underpinning knowledge
- ability to apply theory to practice
- higher-level cognitive skills such as problem solving and decision making
- attitudes, values and beliefs.

Every assessment method has disadvantages and limitations! There are several limitations of using the student's learning diary for assessment:

- it does not assess the ability to perform in the practical setting
- it can be time consuming
- it may not have predictive validity
- it may not have reliability because each incident is different
- it may not elicit the appropriate responses if the assessor is unskilled in facilitating reflective assessment discussions.

TESTIMONY OF OTHERS

Harlen (1994:3) observed that 'all forms of assessment are subject to human judgement and thus require some form of moderation'. In the section on triangulation, the use of investigator triangulation was suggested as a means of reducing the potential biases of a single assessor. The potential diversity of views from a range of supervisors and others would also enrich and strengthen the assessment database on the learner. It is also now a fundamental requirement of the assessment process in the NMC 2018 standards. This section will consider the use of testimony of others as an assessment method.

TESTIMONY FROM OTHER PRACTITIONERS

In practice, the NMC (2018) standards require that explicit arrangements are made for the student to be supervised by other health and social care registrants who may contribute to the assessment of and feedback to the student by observing the student's practice. Evidence from observation can be complemented with evidence from other assessment methods. Making arrangements for the student to work with and be assessed by others has the advantage of making the assessment more feasible because the student will have more opportunities to practise. The practice assessor will have a key role and responsibility for coordinating learning and assessment activities so that they are purposeful. The student will then have a fair chance of achieving learning outcomes and competencies. The arrangements made with other practitioners should include:
- briefing them about the learning experiences that the student needs
- the learning outcomes and competencies to be achieved
- the level of performance expected of the student.

The academic assessor, link lecturer and local practice education team can be resources in assisting with this.

Ewan and White (1996) and Bedford et al (1993) caution that we have different standards of practice, which may lead to inconsistent expectations and judgements of our student. These issues may be compounded if practice educators lack confidence in their professional expertise and feel threatened by students with a more theoretical orientation (Jevis & Tilki 2011). The reliability of assessments will be reduced, and validity may be compromised.

An issue that is gaining increasing prominence is 'failing to fail' a student. Duffy (2004) found that one of the reasons that assessors were not failing students was that they had inadequate knowledge of the assessment process of students they were assessing. Later studies, for example, by Jevis and Tilki (2011) and Luhanga et al (2008), found that assessors lacked confidence in making decisions to refer/fail students. Moreover, Elliott (2016) conducted a review and thematic analysis of the literature, identifying reasons why assessors failed to fail poorly performing students. The themes were:
- difficulties in assessing a student's attitude
- the subjective nature of assessment
- 'benefit of the doubt' culture
- perceived lack of support when failing a student
- confidence to decide to fail a student.

In these instances where unsafe students are passed, the reliability and validity of assessment are clearly compromised. Assessors of student healthcare practitioners need moral courage encompassing moral stress, moral integrity and moral residue (Black, Curzio & Terry 2014) in not shying away from failing a student when necessary.

Try Activity 4.9.

Activity 4.9

Make some suggestions to reduce inconsistencies among practice educators and thus increase the validity and reliability of your assessment.

Some suggestions practice assessors and practice supervisors may wish to consider are:
- regular practice educator meetings to confer on criteria for high standards of practice
- regular practice educator meetings to confer on the expected levels of performance in comparison with an ideal standard; having a common standard among practice educators will help to rate a student's performance at the level expected of students for that stage of the training, which has the advantage of ensuring that assessments have discriminatory power (see Chapter 5 for a discussion of this)
- using the proficiencies in the practice assessment document or a checklist for observation
- discussing the criteria in the practice assessment document or checklist with other practice educators to avoid multiple interpretations
- appropriate training and regular updating of practice educators
- openly discussing personal biases with each other to deal with them objectively
- soliciting the assistance of the academic assessor or link lecturer from the higher-education institution.
Testimonies should:
- be specific to the clinical activity
- give a brief description of the background and circumstances of practice

BOX 4.1 Witness Testimony on Student Nurse, Mary

During an afternoon shift, Mary was assisting in the care of clients on the short-term area of the unit. When sitting with a client called Joseph during teatime, Mary observed him having an epileptic seizure. I was away from the area at the time, so Mary immediately called for help. On entering the dining room, I observed that Mary had moved Joseph's food and drink away from him and was supporting his upper body and head while offering reassurance. It was obvious to me that Joseph was experiencing a series of seizures because he appeared to regain consciousness for a short time and then enter into another seizure. Both of us continued to support him until he had fully recovered.

During the discussion that followed this incident, I praised Mary for acting quickly by calling for help and ensuring a safe environment by removing the food and drink, which may have harmed Joseph. Although Mary could not name the specific type of seizure, she was able to describe the client's behaviour, which allowed me to assess the type of seizure. More importantly, Mary had remembered the importance of maintaining the safety of the client by supporting his upper body and head to ensure a clear airway. Mary also reported that she had made a note of the time and duration of the seizure and was able to explain the reasons for recording such information in the client's care file.

Mary acted in a competent and professional manner during this incident and followed the correct procedure when administering first aid.

- identify the aspects of competence demonstrated
- state the standard achieved by the student; that is, how well the student has performed.

Box 4.1 is an example of a witness testimony.

TESTIMONY FROM USERS

Another group of people who could potentially provide testimonies about student performance are service users. Users are patients, clients and carers who are current or recent recipients of a service (Jones et al 2009). There is an increasing impetus to involve users in all aspects of health and social care education (Department of Health 2002, 2009; NMC 2010). In 2005, the NMC explored ways of involving laypeople in the assessment of practice by, for example, directly soliciting feedback from patients/clients and carers on care given by students, or indirectly by contributing to examination boards and moderating panels as members. The involvement of users is now explicitly embedded in the NMC's student assessment expectations as stated in NMC (2018a) Part 1: Standards Framework for Nursing and Midwifery Education: 'a range of people including service users contribute to student assessment' (5.14:12).

As recipients of care given by students, users are a legitimate source of assessment data. Who can say with more accuracy whether the nurse was kind or gentle or explained and reassured before giving an injection, for example? Neary (2001:9) found that patients and clients do assess students informally, as illustrated by this statement from a patient: 'Nurse [name] took me for a bath today. I feel safe with her, the way she encouraged me into the bath, … I was frightened I'd fall … Nurse [name] never left my side, gave me confidence, she did, good lass that she is'. A study by Redfern and Norman (1999a, 1999b) found that the congruence between patients' and nurses' perceptions of quality care was high and significant. There is also evidence from the field of medicine where the high scores given by patients on the performance of medical students correlated well with the scores given by the doctors (Braend et al 2010). This suggests that user assessment of student performance is likely to be valid and reliable. User comments and complaints (following the appropriate investigations) could feed into the assessment of individual students.

However, formalizing and gaining access to this source of assessment evidence can be fraught with difficulties around organizational barriers, professional and academic politics (Repper & Breeze 2007). Moriaty et al (2010) report that the most frequent type of involvement was informal feedback with some service users completing a compliments form and feedback forms where their involvement was formalized. However, to make service user involvement more meaningful in the assessment process and providing student feedback, there are potential problems. Casey and Clark (2014) suggested these might include:

- Service user reluctance to critically evaluate a student
- Poor service user preparation for the role
- A detrimental effect on the service user's health and well-being from the responsibility of the role
- Service user feedback may not be genuine or meaningful
- Service user not understanding the purpose of their feedback
- The illness of the service user affecting their capacity to provide meaningful feedback
- Service user judging the student against the performance of other students
- Tokenistic use of service users in the assessment and feedback process
- Difficult for the service user to complete practice assessment document

- The additional time required for staff to involve a service user in the assessment process

From their work on developing a user testimony tool to assess the clinical practice of preregistration nursing students, Chapman et al (2011) identified that communication, comfort and treating individuals with respect are areas of care that could be assessed by users. Overall, Muir and Laxton (2012) found that service users bring their personal and professional experiences to assessment process and providing they have received suitable preparation for their role, they are a valuable source of feedback for students, practice supervisors and practice assessors.

TESTIMONY FROM THE STUDENT'S PEERS

Another group of possible assessors comprises the student's peers. Peer reviews are becoming an increasingly important feature of professional practice (Lankshear & Nicklin 2000) and may be an additional source of evidence from which a practice assessor draws to make their objective, evidenced-based assessments. There are a range of potential benefits for students either acting as the assessor or the student being assessed. Tornwall (2018) undertook an integrative review of peer assessment and identified from the literature that benefits could include:

- Assessing self in the context of their peers
- Less stressful than being assessed by a professional
- Could enhance critical thinking
- Could improve student motivation, autonomy and workplace preparation
- Could enhance peer support

Furthermore, peer assessment during training provides opportunities for students to learn to rate the work of other students, helping students to develop collaborative skills; it builds on the skills of giving feedback and develops professional responsibility (Papinczak et al 2007), thereby preparing aspiring professionals for evaluating the work of others.

However, Tornwall (2018) also noted a range of potential challenges with peer assessment:

- Could create an anxiety-ridden, competitive and hostile learning environment
- Peers could feel that they lack the expertise and feedback skills to be part of the assessment
- A student might not feel accepting of their peer's judgement or feedback
- A student might feel that it is for the professional to assess them not a peer
- For the teacher or professional, not knowing how to prepare and support students to provide accurate and effective peer feedback, particularly if it was going to be negative feedback.

- Ensuring selected peers had the motivational and cognitive abilities to provide meaningful feedback
- Peers lacking confidence to undertake the task

If students are to be expected to perform peer assessment, training should be provided. Guidelines, criteria and a rubric are all strategies that would help alleviate some of the challenges and concerns of peer assessment (Boehm & Bonnel 2010). Peers frequently work for sustained periods in close proximity; they therefore have the opportunity to make assessments that may be inaccessible to others. Overall, the student's peers have a useful contribution to make in the overall assessment process of both theory and practice. However, it is probably a strategy that needs to be started early in a student's programme so it becomes a routine feature and needs student and supervisor preparation so that the challenges do not outweigh, to the detriment of all concerned, the benefits of peer assessment and feedback.

SIMULATION

In their glossary of terms, the NMC defines simulation as:

an artificial representation of a real-world practice scenario that supports student development and assessment through experiential learning with the opportunity for repetition, feedback, evaluation and reflection. Effective simulation facilitates safety by enhancing knowledge, behaviours and skills.

NMC (2018a:14)

However, with reference to Article 31(5) of Directive 2005/36/EC, the NMC also states that:

'only simulated experiences which involves direct contact with a healthy or sick individual and/or community can be counted as practice hours under the EU directive'.

Although this directive only applies to adult nursing programmes, creative solutions to using simulation within practice learning are being developed.

In directly addressing the question of whether simulation can be used to assess student proficiency of a skill, the NMC state in their online supporting information:

Simulated assessment … should be used in a proportionate way. Most skills should be demonstrated in a practice setting, but if opportunities to demonstrate some skills are limited, then by exception, some procedures may be demonstrated in simulation.

Therefore, the NMC, through their 2018 standards, embraces the use of simulation as a strategy to develop proficiencies and competence in a safe and supportive environment. Simulation can be particularly helpful in assisting students to explore human factors that may impact on clinical decision–making and practice in rapidly changing and unpredictable situations. However, simulation by exception may only be used as a means of summatively assessing a student in a given proficiency; for example, to enable mental health students to develop proficiency in nasogastric intubation or management of intravenous infusions, when opportunities are lacking in clinical placements.

Simulation embraces both technical and operative skills, nontechnical skills (such as communication) and cognitive ability (such as decision making, managing uncertainty) and can be delivered using a variety of modalities. Modalities may include procedural simulation, virtual reality, computer-assisted simulation up to simulated clinical immersion (INACSL 2016). These modalities may incorporate a range of activities including:

- Role-playing
- Simulated patients
- Haptic devices
- Avatars
- Part-task trainers
- Hybrid models
- Full-body manikins
- Complex simulated environments (ASPiH 2016)

Fidelity refers to the creation of a perception of realism for learners (INACSL 2016) and may be broken down into three aspects: physical, conceptual and psychological. Physical fidelity refers to how realistic the simulated environment is compared with the real-life situation in which a situation would occur; for example, simulated ward environment or clinic room. Conceptual fidelity refers to the elements of a scenario and how they relate to each other; that is, is the scenario feasible and realistic? Psychological fidelity maximizes the contextual contexts within a simulated environment; for example, noise and lighting, distractions, other members of the health care team, time pressures and competing priorities (INACSL 2016).

Drawing from the findings of a systematic review by Norman (2012), the potential benefits to students from the use of simulation include knowledge and skills, safety, communication, clinical judgment, satisfaction and confidence. An integrative review by Foronda, Liu and Bauman (2013) found that students felt simulation created greater confidence and self-efficacy, skills and knowledge acquisition, and they gained interdisciplinary experiences. However, they also found simulation could increase feelings of anxiety and stress. Additionally, simulation enables students to identify what issues they felt they needed to improve on, practice as many times as they wanted and learn from their mistakes without harming real patients (McCaughey & Traynor 2010; Ricketts 2011).

The overarching principle to guide which type of simulation is most appropriate should be what are the intended learning outcomes (Tosterud, Hedelin & Hall-Lord 2013; Shin, Park & Kim 2015), and whatever approach is taken should be carefully planned and suitable for the students at whatever stage of their programme they are at (Ricketts 2011).

An activity is now used to illustrate how a simulated exercise of a clinical situation can be carried out (Activity 4.10).

Activity 4.10

You are planning to involve your learner in a simulated exercise to give them practice in explaining aftercare and home visits to a patient following discharge from the ward. How should you plan for and conduct the simulation?

There are several key steps to follow:

1. Thoroughly prepare the scenario, including setting learning outcomes for enacting the simulated clinical situation. In Activity 4.10, you will need to collect information about the patient and any problems the patient may encounter at home, the illness of the patient, the home and surrounding environment, any social support and so on. Creating a simulation as near as possible to the real-life situation that the learner will encounter enhances retention so that the established behaviours can be transferred more easily to the real setting (Quinn 2000).

2. Brief the learner and the person who is playing the part of the patient. The learner and the patient need to be prepared, particularly if they have not been involved in a simulated exercise before. This involves thorough briefing about the roles they will be playing, the intended learning outcomes to be achieved and agreeing on any ground rules. Briefing ensures that the learner is more likely to benefit from the activity.

3. Allow sufficient time to carry out the activity. The learner is expected to behave and react in any way they feel is appropriate, as the simulation is not scripted.

4. Debriefing and processing the learner's responses and behaviours to give feedback is an important final step. Debriefing should be immediate and is the key to successful simulation (Wotton et al 2010). It should facilitate reconstruction of real-time representations of students' interactions and build on existing knowledge

to form mental representations of clinical problems. The following points may be used to guide the debriefing:

- allow the student to self-evaluate
- identify the concepts learned
- relate learning to the outcomes of the exercise
- discuss any problems encountered
- discuss application to clinical practice
- give feedback (e.g. discuss if the student needs to do it differently).

What aspects of learning can be assessed using enactment of a simulated clinical situation?

What can be assessed will depend on the simulated activity. In the example provided, it is possible to assess the following aspects of learning:

- knowledge of how the illness has affected the patient
- knowledge of resources and social and support services for the patient
- knowledge of the arrangements to be made before discharge of a patient
- communication and interpersonal skills
- decision-making and problem-solving skills
- attitude about discharge planning.

If a scenario requires the performance of physical activities (e.g. enacting the drill for an emergency situation, as in a cardiac arrest) responses and reactions during an emergency can be assessed. In these simulated clinical situations, the use of the 'thinking aloud' technique is helpful in developing knowledge and clinical reasoning processes (Corcoran-Perry & Narayan 2000). The 'thinking aloud' technique requires the learner to think aloud while making decisions: this makes the reasoning process of the learner explicit and transparent. In their study, Corcoran-Perry and Narayan tape-recorded the thinking aloud verbalizations for later transcription. Analysis of the transcripts revealed the cues attended to, the inferences generated and the actions proposed.

What aspects of learning can be assessed using analysis of a simulated clinical problem?

To analyse a simulated clinical problem successfully, the student requires prior knowledge and, perhaps, practical experience of similar situations. During the analysis and the subsequent solving of the problem, the student has to exercise higher-level cognitive skills.

In the scenario given in Box 4.2, it is possible to assess the following aspects of learning:

1. Underpinning knowledge, ability to assess the situation and planning the care
   - analysis of the facts presented
   - formulation of an action plan
   - rationale for the choices and strategies in the action plan.

BOX 4.2   Undiagnosed Twin Births

It is fairly busy on the labour ward in a consultant obstetric unit. There are three midwives on duty, including you and two student midwives. One of the student midwives is with you for the shift.

You admit a 30-year-old multigravida woman at 36 weeks of pregnancy in advanced labour. She is accompanied by her husband. A female baby is delivered soon after admission. The baby appears smaller than you would expect for the gestation. On palpation of the mother's abdomen, a second fetus is detected. Fortunately, the oxytocic drug has not been administered.

How would you manage this situation?

---

2. Problem-solving and decision-making skills
   - ability to predict potential problems and/or complications
   - ability to select relevant cues and to discriminate to reach an appropriate decision
   - ability to prioritize actions and the rationale for the decisions
   - ability to delegate care.

Although all types of simulation may have a limited place within the summative assessment of student proficiencies, they have a very valuable and growing place in safely practicing and developing proficiencies and understanding the multidimensional, interdisciplinary nature of health and social care.

OBJECTIVE STRUCTURED CLINICAL EXAMINATIONS

In their literature review on the use of objective structured clinical examinations (OSCEs), Redfern et al (2002) reported that, following its introduction by Harden et al in Scotland in 1975, the OSCE is now widely used in medicine in Canada, the United States, the Netherlands and elsewhere. An OSCE is not an assessment method in the same way as observation or question and answer. It is basically an organization framework comprising multiple testing points called *stations* around which students rotate. Students perform at these stations and are assessed on specific tasks. The OSCE is best suited to the testing of clinical, technical and practical skills and can do so across a broad range, often with a high degree of fidelity (Newble 2004). OSCEs have been used predominantly by teaching staff in university laboratory settings to assess competence in performing psychomotor skills, ability to analyse and interpret data, take a patient's history, identify and solve problems, make clinical decisions and for use of interpersonal and communication skills (e.g. see Meechan et al 2011; Rentschler et al 2007; Govaerts et al 2001; Phillips et al 2000). The assessment evidence of competence from this source can supplement other sources of evidence.

Because students have to be tested at each station in turn, it means that several students can be tested simultaneously during each OSCE. In practice, the number of stations set up will determine the number of students going around during the OSCE. The conventional use of an OSCE is to rotate students through a series of 5- to 10-minute stations where standardized simulated professional tasks are performed under the observation of one or two assessors who score the performance against a checklist on a marking sheet. Questions may be asked during the performance to supplement evidence obtained through observation.

There are alternative ways of conducting an OSCE. For example, stations may be much longer, and examiners may not be present if the simulated patient on whom the task is performed undertakes the marking. Another variant is the inclusion of stations where multiple-choice questions or other forms of written responses are required (Newble 2004).

One key limitation of assessment evidence from OSCEs is that the performance of students under laboratory conditions may not reflect their performance in real clinical settings. Furthermore, ability to perform the specific task or solve the specific problem at one station is a very poor predictor of ability to perform another, even similar, task or problem (Newble 2004). This means that wide sampling across problems is required to obtain an adequate level of reliability and content validity. Another limitation is that students can find it stressful (Phillips et al 2000).

Evidence of the reliability and validity of assessment evidence from OSCEs is conflicting. Nicol and Freeth (1998), Govaerts et al (2001) and Ladyshewsky (1999) report high reliability and validity of this test procedure, whereas Phillips et al (2000) report that as a form of assessment, it is seriously flawed, having neither inter- nor intraassessor reliability. Although acknowledging the value of intense psychometric research since the introduction of OSCEs, Walsh et al (2009) and Hodges (2003) also question the validity and reliability of OSCEs. Hodges stated that an OSCE is a 'social drama' with 'scripts and parts for actors to play', and 'students modify their performance to convey the impressions they believe their audience desires' (Hodges 2003:1134, 1136). The following measures have been reported to increase the validity and reliability of the use of OSCEs:

Reliability is increased when:
- Assessors are carefully trained (Nicol & Freeth 2002; Redfern et al 2002).
- Assessors are experienced (Nicol & Freeth 2002).
- There is more than one assessor (Weinrott & Jones 1984).
- Scoring is standardized (Nicol & Freeth 2002).

With reference to the standardization of scoring, a checklist could be used. Newble (2004), however, warns that the phenomenon of trivialization could occur when using checklists. This is when detailed checklists do produce reliable scores but which do not truly reflect the examinee's performance of the task; only criteria that are easy to define are included at the expense of equally or more important criteria, and appropriate weightings of the criteria are not made. He suggests that, within the framework of structured tasks, the use of global ratings by informed or trained assessors may be as reliable or even more reliable.
- A large number of stations are used to enable wide sampling across problems and learning tasks (Newble 2004).
- A separate written test is added to the requirement to perform at the stations (Redfern et al 2002; Verhoeven et al 2000).
- There is periodic review of assessment procedures to confirm that testing remains unbiased (Humphris & Kaney 2001).

Newble (2004) suggests that validity is increased when:
- Problems that learners need to be competent in dealing with are generated by expert groups or by more formal studies based on observation and analysis of what that group of learners will have to undertake.
- Tasks within the problems or conditions in which the student is expected to be competent are defined. For example, if the problem was 'dyspnoea', tasks might include taking a history from a patient with dyspnoea, performing and interpreting a pulmonary function test, demonstrating competence in assisting a patient into the optimal position for minimal respiratory effort, demonstrating competence in the administration of oxygen using the range of equipment available and educating a patient about the use of medication for the relief of dyspnoea and, if appropriate, health promotion measures to prevent the deterioration of the respiratory illness.
- A blueprint is constructed. This is a way of including the sample of items to be included in the test. The simplest form is a two-dimensional matrix with one axis representing the generic competencies such as history-taking, communication, management and care-planning skills. The other axis represents the problems or conditions on which the competencies will be demonstrated.
- There is wide sampling across the competencies.

Readers are referred to papers by Walsh et al (2009), Brannick et al (2011) and Bobos et al (2021) that provide literature reviews of research on OSCEs. A systematic review and meta-analysis of measurement properties of objective structured clinical examinations used in physical therapy licensure and a structured review of licensure practices in countries with well-developed regulation systems.

The next three methods of assessment to be considered will focus on the use of written evidence of competence. These methods are:
- care records made by the learner
- case study presentation by the learner
- project or assignment compiled by the learner.

CARE RECORDS MADE BY THE LEARNER

This section starts by considering a scenario: try Activity 4.12.

Activity 4.12

You wish to assess your learner's ability to record an accurate history as well as assess, plan and document the care needs of a client admitted to the unit. How can the learner be assessed?

The learner has to demonstrate the ability to obtain the history in the first instance and subsequently to record the history, assessment of the client and plan of care in writing. The most appropriate way to assess this is to observe the student taking the history and then to examine the written records made by the learner. The activity of interviewing a client to obtain a history followed by the formulation and documentation of a care plan is one way of integrating assessment so that several competencies can be assessed concurrently.

WHAT CAN WE FIND OUT ABOUT THE LEARNER?

The observation will tell us how the student attempted to establish rapport and develop a relationship with the patient, how and what type of communication skills were used, the accuracy of the questioning and so on. The care plan and records made by the learner will tell us whether:
- all the relevant information has been obtained
- the student is able to analyse and synthesize the information in a meaningful way, resulting in an accurate assessment of care needs
- the student is able to plan care using the information
- the student has achieved accurate record keeping as required (in NMC. Future Nurse: Standards of Proficiency for Registered Nurses; Platform 1:1.16: 9, 2018d; and Annexe A: 1.8:28 as well as NMC's 2018. NMC The Code was updated and re-published in 2018).

Subsequently, as the learner cares for the client and is able to maintain a continual review of care needs, this should be reflected in the changes made to the care plan.

In this instance, we will be able to assess the learner's ability to:
- evaluate the effectiveness of care given
- solve any problems
- involve the patient/client in planning care
- make decisions about client needs
- manage change
- work as a member of the multiprofessional team because most patient/client needs require input from a range of professionals.

Most of these are higher-level cognitive skills that the beginning student may not have acquired. It would therefore be inappropriate to assign such a task to a junior student. There are other areas of learning that can be assessed through a student obtaining a client history with the subsequent development of a care plan:
- underpinning knowledge of the condition or illness
- knowledge of the history to be taken and effective communication skills to obtain an accurate and comprehensive history; an understanding of the information obtained and the ability to analyse the information to synthesize information meaningfully
- problem-solving and decision-making skills to evaluate and make changes to care as required
- effective written communication skills to maintain standards of record keeping
- the standards of the records may tell us about how important the student views record keeping.

Examination of care records, however, may not tell us about the student's attitudes towards the task.

CASE STUDY PRESENTATION BY THE LEARNER

Case studies provide students with the opportunity to carry out an in-depth study of one particular patient/client in their care over a period of time. In the written format, this method of assessing learning is more frequently used for the assessment of theory. However, the evidence of learning provided by a case study can be used as one source of evidence for the assessment of competence in the clinical setting. This evidence can be examined in the written format or be presented verbally by the student. Some elements guiding the compilation of a case study are:
- an orientation to the patient/client
- the socioeconomic background of the patient/client and the influence of this on the development of the condition/illness
- draw on and integrate theory from a range of subjects to explain the nature and cause of the condition/illness
- the problems/difficulties encountered by the patient/client and the care required

- the rationale for the care, management and treatment
- contributions made by other members of the multidisciplinary team and their importance
- identify services available
- evaluate the effectiveness of care.

WHAT ASPECTS OF COMPETENCE CAN BE ASSESSED USING A CASE STUDY?

These include:
- knowledge base surrounding the case study
- an understanding of that knowledge
- application of theory to practice
- ability to assess, plan, implement appropriate care and evaluate care
- possibly assessment of attitudes and interpersonal skills.

Practical skills cannot be assessed. A difficulty when assessing the case study is that it may reflect idealized standards of care rather than actual care given (Lankshear & Nicklin 2000). This will then reduce the validity and reliability of that assessment.

PROJECT OR ASSIGNMENT COMPILED BY THE LEARNER

It is possible to arrange for the learner to carry out a small-scale project or assignment. On completion of the work, it is usual to provide a written record for assessment. Rowntree (1987) suggests that, if students are allowed to set their own objectives and how to achieve them, we can assess not only the product but also, more importantly, the process of learning. Similar to the case study, a project or assignment is more frequently used for the assessment of theory. The evidence of learning, however, can be used as one source of evidence for the assessment of competence in the clinical setting to give us a more holistic measurement of competence. Through examination of a project or assignment, it is possible to assess the following (Quinn 2000; Rowntree 1987):
- knowledge and understanding of the subject under investigation
- application of theory to practice
- creativity
- independence and resourcefulness
- how the situation was managed (e.g., coming up with solutions to problems will be indicative of problem-solving and decision-making skills).

These qualities and attributes are some of the hallmarks of a competent practitioner and are therefore important for the student to develop. Practical skills and attitudes cannot be assessed with accuracy.

SELECTING AND COMBINING METHODS OF ASSESSMENT

Some methods of assessment are simply inappropriate for the assessment of certain aspects of competence; for example, interpersonal communication skills cannot be assessed using written assessment methods; manual dexterity and psychomotor skills cannot be assessed through verbal assessment methods. Attitudes, the most difficult aspect of competence of all to assess, may elude assessment altogether if special care is not exercised. The careful selection of method is thus required so that the assessment method matches the type of attribute being assessed. An examination of the uses, advantages and limitations of the assessment methods discussed in this chapter will help you consider which combination of methods will be most suitable to assess the particular attributes of competence.

When selecting methods for use in the holistic/integrated competency-based assessment system, Gonczi et al (1993:20) provide two guiding principles:
1. The assessment should be as integrated and holistic as possible (i.e., combinations of attributes should be assessed simultaneously); for example, when a student is observed admitting a patient, attributes such as knowledge of the admission procedure, communication and interpersonal skills, record-keeping skills and so on can be assessed simultaneously.
2. The assessment should be as direct as possible (i.e., as close as possible to the real-work situations in which these combinations of attributes are employed).

The key question arising is this: How well will the methods assess the capacity to function appropriately across the uncertain situations of professional practice? Redfern et al (2002) found that the use of a multimethod approach enhances validity and ensures comprehensive assessment of the complex repertoire of skills required of students in nursing. Although this may be the case, inevitably, not all the professional attributes needed to function in the dynamic world of practice can be assessed holistically and directly. Therefore, combinations of methods need to be considered that will provide the range of evidence on which a judgement of competence can be made. The principles underpinning the use of the strategy of triangulation should also be considered when selecting and combining methods.

Other factors to be considered when selecting methods are:
- The time available to assessors–busy practitioners are generally hard pushed for time to be assessors to learners who end up competing for the practitioner's time (Beskine 2009; Phillips et al 2000).
- The confidential nature of some aspects of work limits the capacity to undertake assessment in the real situation; for example, when learning counselling skills in

the mental health setting, it may not be desirable to learn the skills and be assessed when working directly with these clients. Simulated activities may be required.

- The methods should be acceptable to the learners (e.g. not all learners feel comfortable taking part in enacting simulated clinical situations).

The following combinations of methods are suggested for assessing the components of competence discussed in Chapter 3:

1. To assess higher cognitive skill development:
   a. questioning
   b. assessment discussion
   c. simulation
   d. OSCE
   e. care records
   f. testimony of others
   g. project or assignment
   i. case study
2. To assess technical skills and performance, use:
   a. direct observation of practice
   b. examination of work products
   c. testimony of others
   d. simulation
   e. OSCE
3. To assess reflective practice, use:
   a. questioning
   b. assessment discussion
   c. testimony of others
   d. care records
   e. case study
   f. project or assignment
4. To assess attitudes and ethics of care use:
   a. questioning
   b. assessment discussion
   c. observation
   d. testimony of others
   e. simulation

Assessment of attitudes and ethics of care abound with difficulties (Dawson 1992; Andrusyszyn 1989) and frequently pose a gap in assessment strategies (Fraser 2000). Toohey (2002) warns that what we do not assess sends a particular message to students because they tend to view that only what is assessed deserves their time, attention and effort. It is difficult to assess and measure attitudes, beliefs and values directly. We can, however, observe behaviours and behavioural patterns that may be reflective of their personal attributes (Toohey 2002) and the underlying attitudes and values held by the students (Andrusyszyn 1989). As discussed in Chapter 3, the use of criteria in the format of prespecified behaviours expected of a professional exhibiting the appropriate conduct may assist.

CONCLUSION

In a system of competency-based assessment, any of the assessment methods described in this chapter can be used. From the discussion on the uses and limitations of the range of assessment methods, it can be seen that no one method will enable the assessment of all the components of competence. It is, of course, neither desirable nor economical to use all the assessment methods. It is, however, important to select and combine methods so that their strengths and weaknesses complement each other, and methods are relevant to the nature of the competency being assessed. In choosing the methods to be used, there will always be a need to balance the competing demands of resources and availability of learning opportunities and the necessity to obtain the range of evidence and feedback required for the practice assessor to make objective, evidenced-based assessments on conduct, proficiency and achievement.

In general, a move in the direction of competency-based assessment requires the greater use of more direct methods of assessment that more closely match the kinds of day-to-day tasks undertaken by professionals. This emphasizes the importance of the use of methods that directly assess performance and the other attributes of competence and requires practice assessors and supervisors to make professional judgements in interpreting what the minimum acceptable levels of competence are in respect to professional standards. Assessment methods that are 'subjectively scored', such as observation and simulation of practice, need to be managed to ensure reasonable reliability to accompany greater validity. A high level of professional expertise is required to assess the work of others (Luhanga et al 2008; Phillips et al 2000). Being an expert in a profession is essential but is not enough. It is important to have some level of expertise in the assessment process. The next chapter addresses issues relating to the management of the assessment process, in particular the competency-based assessment system, so that assessments can be made with validity and reliability.

KEY POINTS FOR REFLECTION

Competence is a construct that is not directly observable but is inferred from successful performance. Therefore, combinations of assessment methods need to be considered and used so that a range of evidence of capable performance is provided to enable a safe judgement of competence to be made.

- The strategy of triangulation in clinical assessment is to combine the use of several methods of assessment to obtain as complete a picture as possible of the student's achievement of competence. Methods selected should complement each other so that a rich range of evidence is obtained.

- Triangulation allows confirmation of assessment evidence and increases confidence in the assessment decision made, guards against a blinkered perspective, is more likely to portray a 'whole picture' of the student and allows divergent evidence to enrich explanation.
- However, it is expensive on resources, it cannot compensate for assessor bias, it may compound sources of error and it is of limited use if assessment outcomes are unclear and assessment methods selected are inappropriate.

- In competency-based assessment, it is not the methods themselves that are competency based; rather, it is the way they are used, the emphasis given to the methods and how results are interpreted that are important.
- Assessment methods selected should be most direct and relevant to the nature of the competency being assessed. Combinations of methods need to be able to obtain and provide the range of evidence on which a judgement about conduct, proficiency, achievement and ultimately progression can be made.
- When selecting and combining methods, ask how well the methods will assess the capacity to function appropriately across the uncertain situations of professional practice.

OBSERVATION

- This is an essential tool in assessment. It is one of the most effective ways of finding out whether learning has taken place as direct evidence of competence can be collected.
- Working directly with the learner is known as *participant observation* but beware of observer effect and observer bias.
- Observing the learner from a distance is known as *non-participant observation.*
- Using checklists contributes to validity and reliability of the observation.
- Allowing enough time makes the use of observation more effective.

QUESTIONING

- Asking questions is an integral part of teaching, learning and assessment and places students in the role of active learners, assisting them to develop higher-level cognitive skills.
- Structure questions so that they define a linking path, as these are more valuable in assessing the quality of learning and helping the learner to develop higher-level thinking.
- Questioning is used to assess learning in the cognitive and affective domains, thus assessing several attributes of competence.

DISCUSSION

- The discussion of a particular care event can assess the knowledge, understanding and values that have informed their actions in the clinical area on a given occasion, enabling assessors to test their own observation-based judgements about the quality of those actions.

- During these assessment discussions, students should be facilitated to voice their understanding, views and opinions, disagreements and doubts.
- Assessment discussions can also be conducted using the student's reflective journal or learning diary entries as the basis.

TESTIMONY OF OTHERS

- The feedback of practice supervisors, service users, student peers and others is a central component to assessment in the NMC (2018b) standards.
- All forms of assessment are subject to human judgement and thus require some form of moderation.
- The student's practice assessor needs to take into account the testimonies of others as part of their assessment both commonalities and points of disagreement.
- Testimonies should be specific to the clinical activity, give a brief description of the background and circumstances of practice, identify the aspects of competence demonstrated and state the standard achieved by the student; that is, how well the student has performed.
- It is possible to use testimonies from patients/clients and their carers and the student's peers.

SIMULATION

- A simulation is the reproduction of the essential features of a social or physical reality that corresponds to a real-life situation that a student might encounter. During a simulated experience, learners can be put into a situation where they can experience some aspect of the real situation by becoming involved in activities that are closely related to it.
- Simulated activities cannot take account of the complexities of the real clinical environment. The validity of this testing procedure is questionable as the amount of

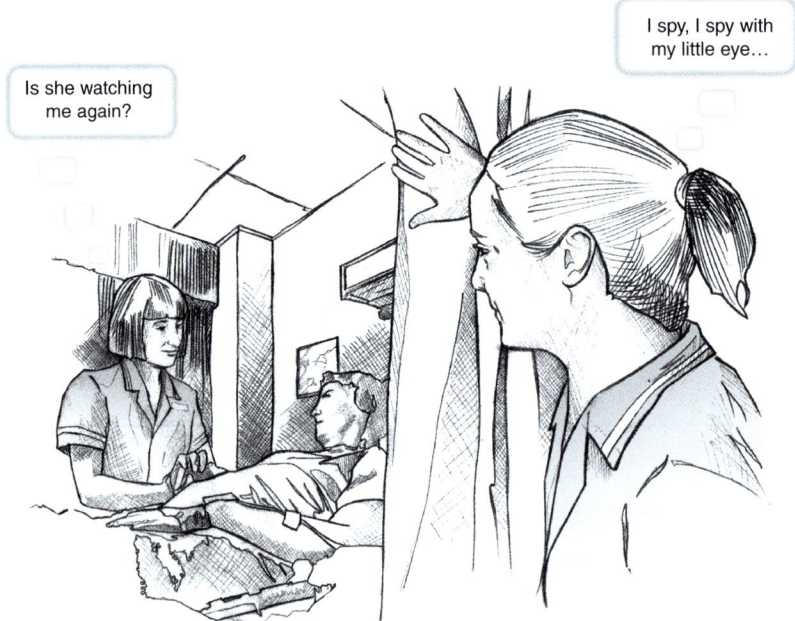

Fig. 4.1 Nerve wracking or an opportunity to outshine?

learning that can be transferred to the real-life setting is debatable.
- Simulations can be delivered through a range of modalities.
- OSCEs can test clinical, practical and technical skills, but may not represent actual performance in the clinical setting.

CARE RECORDS MADE BY THE LEARNER

Formulating, documenting and making changes to a care plan is one way of integrating assessment so that several competencies can be assessed concurrently.

CASE STUDY PRESENTATION BY THE LEARNER

Case studies provide students with the opportunity to carry out an in-depth study of one particular patient/client in their care over a period of time. It is possible to assess attitudes, interpersonal skills, knowledge, understanding and the ability to assess, plan, implement and evaluate care surrounding the case study.

REFERENCES

Allan EG, Driscoll DL. The three-fold benefit of reflective writing: improving program assessment, student learning, and faculty professional development. *Assess Writing*, 2014;21:37–55.

Almalkawi I, Jester R, Terry L. Exploring mentors' interpretation of terminology and levels of competence when assessing nursing students: an integrative review. *Nurs Educ Today*, 2018;69:95–103.

Andrusyszyn MA. Clinical evaluation of the affective domain. *Nurs Educ Today*, 1989;9:75–81.

ASPiH. Simulation-based education in Healthcare. 2016. Available: http://aspih.org.uk/wp-content/uploads/2017/07/standards-framework.pdf. Accessed: 21 May 2018.

Bedford H, Phillips T, Robinson J, et al. Assessment of Competencies in Nursing and Midwifery Education and Training. The English National Board for Nursing, Midwifery and Health Visiting, London:1993.

Black S, Curzio J, Terry L. Failing a student nurse: a new horizon of moral courage. *Nurs Ethics*, 2014;21(2):224–238.

Bloom BS, Engelhart MD, Furst EJ. Taxonomy of Educational Objectives Handbook I: Cognitive Domain. Longman, London:1956.

Boehm H, Bonnel W. The use of peer review in nursing education and clinical practice. *J Nurs Staff Develop*, 2010;26(3):108–115.

Boud D, Keogh R, Walker D. What is reflection in learning? In: Boud D, Keogh R, Walker D, Reflection: Turning Experience into Learning. Kogan Page, London:1985, pp. 7–17.

Braend AM, Gran Frandsen S, Frich JC, et al. Medical students' clinical performance in general practice – triangulating assessments from patients, teachers and students. *Med Teach*, 2010;32:333–339.

Brannick MT, Erol-Korkmaz HT, Prewett M. A systematic review of the reliability of objective structured clinical examination scores. *Med Educ.* 2011;45(12):1181–1189. doi:10.1111/j.1365-2923.2011.04075.x.

Beskine D. Mentoring students: establishing effective working relationships. *Nurs Stan*, 2009;23(30):35–40.

Bobos P, Pouliopoulou DV, Harriss A, Sadi J, Rushton A, MacDermid JC. A systematic review and meta-analysis of measurement properties of objective structured clinical examinations used in physical therapy licensure and a structured review of licensure practices in countries with well-developed regulation systems. *PLoS One*. 2021;16(8):e0255696. doi:10.1371/journal.pone.0255696.

Caldwell K, Atwal A. Non-participant observation: using video tapes to collect data in nursing research. *Nurs Res*, 2005;13(2):42–54.

Campbell DT, Fiske DW. Convergent and discriminant validity by the multi-trait, multi-method matrix. *Psychol Bull*, 1959;56:81–105.

Carter N, Bryant-Lukosius D, DiCenso A, Blythe J, Neville AJ. The use of triangulation in qualitative research. *Oncol Nurs Forum*, 2004;41(5):545–547.

Chapman L, James J, McMahon K. Involving patients in assessment of students. *Nurs Times*, 2011;107–34.

Casey D, Clark L. Involving patients in the assessment of nursing students. *Nurs Stand*, 2014;28(47):37–41.

Corcoran-Perry S, Narayan S. Teaching clinical reasoning in nursing education. In: Higgs J, Jones M, Clinical Reasoning in the Health Professions. Butterworth-Heinemann, Oxford:2000, pp. 249–254.

Craig JL, Page G. The questioning skills of nursing instructors. *J Nurs Educ*, 1981:20:20.

Dawson KP. Attitude and assessment in nurse education. *J Adv Nurs*, 1992;17:473–479.

Department of Health. Requirements for Social Work Training. Department of Health, London:2002.

Department of Health. Education Commissioning for Quality. Department of Health, London:2009.

Denzin N. The Research Act. 3rd ed. McGraw-Hill New York:1989.

De Young S. Teaching Strategies for Nurse Educators. 2nd ed. Prentice Hall, Harlow:2009.

De Young S. Teaching Nursing. Addison-Wesley, Menlo Park, CA:1990.

Duffy K. Failing Students Report. Nursing and Midwifery Council, London:2004.

Elliott J. Action Research for Educational Change. Open University Press, Milton Keynes:1991.

Elliott C. Identifying and managing underperformance in nursing students. *Br J Nurs*, 2016;25(5):250–255.

Epp S. The value of reflective journaling in undergraduate nursing education: a literature review. *Int J Nurs Stud*, 2008;45:1379–1388.

Ewan C, White R. Teaching Nursing: A Self-instructional Handbook. 2nd ed. Chapman & Hall, London:1996.

Fielding NG, Fielding JL. Fielding, Linking Data. Sage, Beverly Hills, CA:1986.

Fish D, Twinn S. Quality Clinical Supervision in the Health Care Professions. Butterworth-Heinemann, Oxford:1997.

Fletcher S. NVQs Standards and Competence. A Practical Guide for Employers, Managers and Trainers. Kogan Page, London:1991.

Foronda C, Liu S, Bauman EB. Evaluation of simulation in undergraduate nurse education: an integrative review. *Clin Sim Nurs*, 2013;9(10):409–416.

Fotheringham D. Triangulation for the assessment of clinical nursing skills: a review of theory, use and methodology. *Int J Nurs Stud*, 2010;47:386–391.

Fraser D. Action research to improve the pre-registration midwifery curriculum. Part 3: can fitness for practice be guaranteed? *Midwifery*, 2000,16:287–294.

Gipps CV. Beyond Testing: Towards a Theory of Educational Assessment. The Falmer Press, London:1994.

Gonczi A, Hager P, Athanasou J. The Development of Competency-Based Assessment Strategies for the Professions. National Office of Overseas Skills Recognition, Research Paper No. 8. Australian Government Publishing Service, Canberra:1993.

Govaerts MJB, Schuwirth LWT, Pin A, et al. Objective assessment is needed to ensure competence. *Br J Midwifery*, 2001;9(3):156–161.

Guest G, Namey EE, Mitchell ML. Collecting Qualitative Data. Sage Publications; London:2013.

Harden R, Stevenson M, Downie WW. Assessment of clinical competence using objective structured examination. *Br Med J*, 1975;1:447–451.

Harlen W (Ed). Enhancing Quality in Assessment. BERA Policy Task Group on Assessment. Paul Chapman Publishers, London:1994.

Hodges B. OSCE! Variations on a theme by Harden. *Med Educ*, 2003;37:1134–1140.

Hovancsek MT. Using simulations in nursing education. In: Jeffries PR, Simulation in Nursing Education: From Conceptualization to Evaluation. National League for Nursing, New York:2007, pp. 1–9.

Humphris GM, Kaney S. Examiner fatigue in communication skills objective structured clinical examinations. *Med Educ*, 2001;35:444–449.

Hwanga B, Choia H, Kima S, Kimb S, Koc H, Kimb J. Facilitating student learning with critical reflective journaling in psychiatric mental health nursing clinical education: a qualitative study. *Nurs Educ Today*, 2018;69:159–164.

INACSL Standards Committee. Standards of Best Practice. *Clin Sim Nurs*, 2016;12(S):S5–S50.

Jevis A, Tilki M. Why are nurse mentors failing to fail student nurses who do not meet clinical performance standards? *Br J Nurs*, 2011;20(9):582–587.

Jones D, Stephens J, Innes W, et al. Service user and carer involvement in physiotherapy practice, education and research: getting involved for a change. *NZ Aust. J. Physiother*, 2009;37(1):29–35.

Kawulich BB. Participant observation as a data collection method. *Qual Soc Res*, 2005;6(2):1–22.

Ladyshewsky R. Simulated patients and assessment. *Med Teach*, 1999;21(3):266–269.

Lankshear A, Nicklin P. Methods of assessment. In: Nicklin P, Kenworthy N, Teaching and Assessing in Nursing Practice. 3rd ed. Baillière Tindall, London:2000, pp. 119–138.

Lauterbach SS, Becker P. Journaling to learn: a strategy in nursing education for developing the nurse as person and person as nurse. *Int J Human Caring*, 2015;9(1):29–35.

Leigh J, Roberts D. Critical exploration of the new NMC standards of proficiency for registered nurses. *Br J Nurs*, 2018;27(18):1068–1072.

Lemons PP, Lemons D. Questions for assessing higher-order cognitive skills: it's not just Bloom'. *CBE—Life Scien Ed*, 2013;12:47–58.

Luhanga F, Yonge OJ, Myrick F. Failure to assign failing grades: issues with grading the unsafe student. *Int J Nurs Ed Scholar*, 2008;5(1):1–14.

McCaughey CS, Traynor MK. The role of simulation in nurse education. *Nurs Educ Today*, 2010;30:827–832.

Meechan R, Jones H, Valler-Jones T. Do medicines OSCEs improve drug administration ability? *Br J Nurs*, 2011;20(12):728–731.

Minton D. Teaching Skills in Further and Adult Education. Revised ed. Macmillan, Basingstoke:1997.

Moriaty J, MacIntyre G, Manthorpe J, et al. My expectations remain the same. The student has to be competent to practise: practice assessor perspectives on the new social work degree qualification in England. *Br J Soc Work*, 2010;40:583–601.

Muir D, Laxton JC. Experts by experience; the views of service user educators providing feedback on medical students' work based assessments. *Nurs Educ Today*, 2012;32:146–150.

Neary M. Responsive assessment: assessing student nurses' clinical competence. *Nurs Educ Today*, 2001;21:3–17.

Newble D. Techniques for measuring clinical competence: objective structured clinical examinations. *Med Educ*, 2004;38:199–203.

Nicol D, Freeth D. Assessment of clinical skills: a new approach to an old problem. *Nurs Educ Today*, 1998;18:601–609.

Norman J. Systematic review of the literature on simulation in nursing education. *ABNF J*, 2012;Spring:24–28.

Nursing and Midwifery Council. Part 1–Standards Framework for Nursing and Midwifery Education. NMC, London:2018a.

Nursing and Midwifery Council. Part 2–Standards for Student Supervision and Assessment. NMC, London:2018b.

Nursing and Midwifery Council. Part 3: Standards for Pre-Registration Nursing Programmes. NMC, London:2018c.

Nursing and Midwifery Council. Future nurse: Standards of Proficiency for Registered Nurses. NMC, London:2018d.

Nursing and Midwifery Council. The Code: Professional Standards of Practice and Behaviour for Nurses and Midwives. 2018. NMC The Code was updated and re-published in 2018. NMC, London:2015.

Nursing and Midwifery Council. Standards for Pre-Registration Nursing Education. NMC, London:2010.

Nursing and Midwifery Council. Consultation on Proposals Arising From a Review of Fitness for Practice at the Point of Registration. NMC, London:2005.

Oliver R, Endersby C. Teaching and Assessing Nurses: A Handbook for Preceptors. Baillière Tindall, London:1994.

Papinczak T, Young L, Groves M, et al. An analysis of peer, self, and tutor assessment in problem-based tutorials. *Med Teach*, 2007;29:e122–e132.

Perrott E. Effective Teaching. Longman, London:1982.

Phillips T, Schostak J, Tyler J. Practice and Assessment in Nursing and Midwifery: Doing it for Real. The English National Board for Nursing, Midwifery and Health Visiting, London:2000.

Polit DF, Beck CT, Hungler BP. Essentials of Nursing Research: Appraising Evidence for Nursing Practice. 7th ed. Lippincott Williams & Wilkins, London:2010.

Quinn FM. The Principles and Practice of Nurse Education. 4th ed. Chapman & Hall, London:2000.

Redfern S, Norman I. Quality of nursing care perceived by patients and their nurses: an application of the critical incident technique. Part I. *J Clin Nurs*, 1999a;8:407–413.

Redfern S, Norman I. Quality of nursing care perceived by patients and their nurses: an application of the critical incident technique. Part II. *J Clin Nurs*, 1999b;8:414–421.

Redfern S, Norman I, Calman L. Assessing competence to practise in nursing: a review of the literature. *Res Papers Educ*, 2002;17(1):51–77.

Redfern SJ. Validity through triangulation. *Nurs Res*, 1994;2(2):41–56.

Rentschler DD, Eaton J, Cappiello J. Evaluation of undergraduate students using objective structured clinical evaluation. *J Nurs Educ*, 2007;46(3):135–139.

Repper J, Breeze J. A review of the literature on user and carer involvement in the training and education of health professionals. *Int J Nurs Stud*, 2007;44:511–519.

Ricketts B. The role of simulation for learning within pre-registration nursing education – a literature review. *Nurs Educ Today*, 2011;31:650–654.

Rogers C. Freedom to Learn for the 80s. Charles E. Merrill, Columbus, OH:1983.

Rowntree D. Rowntree, Assessing Students: How Shall We Know Them? 2nd ed. Kogan Page, London:1987.

Schön D. Educating the Reflective Practitioner. Jossey-Bass, San Francisco:1987.

Shin S, Park J, Kim J. Effectiveness of patient simulation in nursing education: meta-analysis. *Nurs Educ Today*, 2015;35:176–182.

Stoker D. Assessment in learning: (iii) Methods of assessment. *Nurs Times*, 1984;90(13):i–viii.

Stuart CC. Reflective journals as a teaching/learning strategy. *Br J Midwifery*, 1997;5(7):434–438.

Toohey S. Assessment of students' personal development as part of preparation for professional work – is it desirable and is it feasible? *Assess Eval High Educ*, 2002;27(6):529–538.

Tornwall J. Peer assessment practices in nurse education: an integrative review. *Nurs Educ Today*, 2018;71:266–275.

Tosterud R, Hedelin B, Hall-Lord ML. Nursing students' perceptions of high- and low-fidelity simulation used as learning methods. *Nurs Educ Pract*, 2013;13:262 –270.

Verhoeven BH, Hamers JGHC, Schepbier AJJA, et al. The effect on reliability of adding a separate written assessment component to an objective structured clinical examination. *Med Educ*, 2000;34:525–529.

von Colln-Appling C, Giuliano D. A concept analysis of critical thinking: a guide for nurse educators. *Nurs Educ Today*, 2017;49:106–109.

Walsh M, Hill Bailey P, Koren I. Objective structured clinical evaluation of clinical competence: an integrative review. *J Advan Nurs*, 2009;65(8):1584–1595.

Wedgeworth ML, Carter SC, Ford CD. Clinical faculty preceptors and mental health reflections: learning through journaling. *J Nurs Pract*, 2017;13(6):411–417.

Weinrott M, Jones R. Overt versus covert assessment of observer reliability. *Child Dev*, 1984;55(3):125–1137.

Wotton K, Davis J, Button D, et al. Third year undergraduate nursing students' perceptions of high-fidelity simulation. *J Nurs Educ*, 2010;49(11):632–639.

Wu XV, Enskär K, Lee CCS, Wang W. A systematic review of clinical assessment for undergraduate nursing students, *Nurs Educ Today*, 2015;35:347–359.

Yeates P, O'Neill P, Mann K, Byrne G, Eva K. Bias in assessing trainees' clinical competence: the influence of assessors' recent experiences of other performances on present assessment scores. *Lancet*, 2015;383(Suppl 1):113.

5

Conducting Defensible and Fair Assessments

Chris Carter

CHAPTER CONTENTS

INTRODUCTION

Generally, to achieve competency in preregistration education programmes, students spend up to 50% of the course time in clinical practice. Clinical practice provides students with exposure to different health care settings, which allows them to develop the required level of competency to function at the beginning of professional registration (Wu et al 2015). The assessed part of the practice placements provides students with opportunities to prepare and confirm they have the required knowledge, skills, attitudes and competence to meet standards of quality and patient safety (Willis Commission 2012).

A considerable amount of literature has been published attempting to define competency and competence (Brown & Crookes 2017., Hishinuma et al 2016, Nilsson et al 2014, Heaslip & Scammell 2012, Yanhua & Watson 2011, Watson et al 2002 see also Chapter 3). The World Health Organization (2009) defines competence in nursing and midwifery as 'a broad composite statement, derived from nursing and midwifery practice, which describes a framework of skills reflecting knowledge, attitudes, psychosocial and psychomotor elements'. However, each regulatory body has its own interpretation, for example, the UK Nursing and Midwifery

Council (NMC) defines competency as 'the overarching set of knowledge, skills and attitudes required to practice safely and effectively without direct supervision' (Nursing and Midwifery Council 2010). In Australia, competence was defined as 'a combination of skills, knowledge, attitudes, values and abilities that underpin effective and superior performance in a professional/occupational area' (Australian Nursing and Midwifery Council 2006). Furthermore, each approved education provider will interpret how the definition is translated into programmes and assessment processes. Although the concept of competence is not universally agreed, it is recognized as a holistic approach using competency-based assessment tools, which include knowledge, skills, performance, attitudes and values (World Health Organization [WHO] 2019, Gonczi 2013).

The best method of assessment and feedback has not only been the focus of regulatory bodies and education providers, but also students. Students' views towards their assessment has become an integral part of national public surveys used to benchmark universities. For example, in the UK, the National Student Survey allows final-year students to provide feedback on their experiences studying their course. Topics include teaching, learning opportunities, assessment and feedback, organisation and management, learning resources, student voice and overall satisfaction (National Student Survey 2019a). Also, students studying National Health Service–funded courses are asked questions about their placement experiences (National Student Survey 2019b). In consequence, universities and placement providers have invested considerable effort to supporting assessors and students in practice.

Although these are regulatory and academic debates, assessors at the bedside work in the real world and need practical approaches to assessing students. Competency-based assessment in the professions need to be based on realistic, complex workplace problems which generate a range of evidence to make valid and reliable assessments of a student's proficiency (Wu et al 2015). Assessment of students serves three main purposes: formative, summative and evaluative (Harlen 2015). Formative assessments involve students being "assessed for learning" purposes, meaning students use this for ongoing feedback to develop competence, whereas summative assessments involve "assessment of learning" and are formal assessments of the student's performance. Evaluation assessments may be used to assess aspects of the work of the university (Harlen 2015).

RETHINKING THE ROLE OF ASSESSORS IN A CHANGING HEALTH CARE CONTEXT

The Lancet Commission (2010) on Health Education reported 'new infections, environmental and behavioural risks at a time of rapid demographic and epidemiological transitions threaten the health security of all... Professional education has not kept pace with these challenges largely because of fragmented outdated and static curriculums ... mismatch of competencies to patient and population needs; poor teamwork;... narrow technical focus without broader contextual understanding; episodic encounters rather than continuous care; hospital orientation at the expense of primary care'. Although this report approaches health care education in a global context, from both a low- and high-income-country perspective, it highlights the emerging globalisation and changes in health care. The increasing mobility of international nurses and a critical shortage of health care professionals globally have led to increasing numbers of preregistration students requiring clinical placements and assessments (Jones-Berry 2018). In consequence, the role of assessors is changing in response to changing patient need and health care provisions and increasing numbers of preregistration students.

In practice, various terms are used interchangeably to describe the role of the assessor; these have included mentor, preceptor, sign-off mentor, clinical supervisors, faculty and lecturers (Hughes et al 2016). It is widely accepted the role of mentor and assessor are different, and there is

potential role confusion (Donaldson 2019, Bray & Nettleton 2007). As a consequence, the UK nursing regulator took a radical departure from its well-established "mentor" and "sign-off mentor" model to one of "coaching" and assessment (Donaldson 2019, Rosser 2017). The new model replaces the mentorship model with a triad of roles: practice supervisors, practice assessor and academic assessor (Jones-Berry 2018).

The revised NMC (2018) standards will provide greater opportunities for nurses and midwives, as well as other registered health and social care professionals to be involved in student learning. This reflects the long-established position that supervising students is part of every practitioner's role (Department of Health 2000). The role of practice supervisor could be undertaken by any nurse, midwife, associate nurse or registered health and social care professional.

Approved education institutions (AEIs) in partnership with placement providers will be responsible for providing the governance arrangements to prepare and support supervisors. Widening the supervisory role provides opportunities to move away from the current "profession-centric" approach to mentorship to genuine interprofessional learning and teaching opportunities (Leigh & Roberts 2018, Rosser 2017). This approach provides potential harmony with other health care professional models for assessment. The Health and Care Professions Council (2018) has no specific requirements or expectations for the development of its practice-based educators, including the length or content of any training; these are set and managed by education providers.

There are two types of assessor roles, one from practice and another from the AEI. Formalising the assessor roles with requirements from both practice and academic organisations will allow student's achievements across theory and practice to be recognized and assessed (NMC 2018).

What is not clear is the impact of this new approach to coaching and assessing will have on student learning. Concerns have been raised regarding role confusion, heavy and increasing demands of delivering patient care alongside supervisory and assessor roles, a fragmented approach to student learning and a further layer of complexity (Donaldson 2019, Leigh & Roberts 2018, Ferrier 2017, Ramdeen 2017). However, the new model continues to place greater emphasis on teaching and learning in practice and encourages greater collaboration between AEIs and placement providers. Previously, clinical components of courses may have been viewed as separate from the rest of the curriculum, with students left to learn from clinicians with little interaction with university staff. The revised NMC standards encourage greater integration and collaboration between theory and practical aspects of the curriculum (Gonzci 2013). Greater flexibility in the clinical learning environment and opportunity for other professionals to be involved in the supervision of students will prepare students for a changing health care system (Leigh & Roberts 2018).

Critical to implementation and sustainability of the revised NMC standards for preregistration students (NMC 2018) are consistency across the UK, good quality assurance frameworks and strong partnerships between AEIs and placement providers (Jones-Berry 2018). Partnerships between organisations will develop the capacity to support students and develop clinical learning opportunities and knowledge (Gonczi 2013).

Students are exposed to a variety of clinical areas and specialities during their clinical placements, making it difficult to demonstrate competence in all areas (Helminen et al 2016). It is widely accepted that there is a need for longitudinal work or "continuum of time" to track a student's progress throughout their education and during their transition from student to a newly qualified role (Franklin & Melville 2015; Gonczi 2013; Yanjua and Watson 2011). Advances to competency-based assessments include the use of e-portfolios or documents. Green et al (2014) suggested nurse and midwifery education 'is a relatively late adopter' of e-portfolios, which are already used by other health disciplines. Electronic practice documentation will allow greater collaboration between the student, practice supervisor, practice assessor and practice supervisor (Leigh & Roberts 2018), but also reflects the changing demographics of students who are now more familiar with using the internet, social media and technology (Chang et al 2017). This also allows students to collect and select evidence throughout their education and can be summarized as "collect, select, reflect and connect" (Clark & Eynon 2009). Promoting longitudinal approaches to assessment encourages students to recognize their preregistration education is just the first stage in lifelong education (Willis Report 2012).

COMPETENCY-BASED ASSESSMENTS

Providing students with clinical experiences encourages them to take an active role in their learning. The exposure to real-life clinical situations not only helps to prepare them for their future role (Wu et al 2015), but these experiences and situations form the basis of the students' assessment of competence. Assessments are relied upon to make some quite specific, but also far-ranging, judgements about students' future competence as registered practitioners. As the student progresses through their course and knowledge, skills and competence increase, and the supervision and assessment of students should change (Nursing and Midwifery Council 2019).

Competency-based assessment is the favoured approach of several national nursing regulatory organisations (Nursing and Midwifery Council 2019, Australian Nursing and Midwifery Council 2006, Canadian Nurses Association 2010). Determining reliable competency-based assessments, which provide valid, fair and consistent judgements, is a challenge for regulatory organisations, education providers and assessors (Heaslip & Scammell 2012). This can be achieved by the careful selection and combination of methods of assessment that will best assess the particular component of competence (e.g., using observation to assess psychomotor skills and questioning to assess cognitive skills).

It is not possible or desirable to assess everything a person might need to know or be able to do. Therefore, assessment of clinical practice is inevitably based on a sample or snapshot of the student's performance in assessment tasks perceived to be relevant (Wu et al 2015). Nursing requires a complex combination of knowledge, performance, skills and attitudes, but also the hidden aspects of nursing, referred to as the "art" of nursing (Franklin & Melville 2015, Nilson et al 2014, Benner 1984). An inference of competence is then made from the student's performance on the set of arranged tasks. Competence is a construct that is not directly observable; rather, it is inferred from the performance. Most typical assessments involve making inferences (e.g., tests of knowledge usually sample only a fraction of the required knowledge).

These aspects need to be assessed, and there are various methods of assessments used in practice, ranging from pass/fail or a graded system (Heaslip & Scammell 2012). There is no consensus on the best type of assessment strategy to be used (Brown & Crookes 2017). Although core standards exist nationally and regionally, across Europe there remain wide variations in nurse and midwifery education systems and agreement on competency and assessment strategies (Lahtinen et al 2014, Salminen et al 2010).

Grades (numerical, alphabetical or descriptive) can be applied to rate a specific assessment task or the overall performance. Gray and Donaldson (2009) explored the use of grading in practice and found grading can encourage motivation and provide feedback to the student on how they are getting on (rather than a pass or fail) because it also allows a student to be recognized for merit or excellence. Grading can improve the learning experience by providing detailed feedback on the students' performance. It would also provide parity with academic assessments and could be used to influence a student's overall degree classification. Conversely, arguments against grading in practice included that grading was not compatible with the principles of competency-based assessment and can have a negative impact on students' learning and motivation.

There are also risks with grade inflation by assessors, and students may become focused on the grade and not the feedback.

Alternative grading methods include grading the student's expertise using a scale; this may include independent, safe to practice, fitness to practice and dissemination level (Helminen et al 2016, Claman et al 2002). This type of assessment can be traced back to Bondy's (1983) five-point scale, based on an increasing hierarchy of competence to evaluate students' clinical performance.

Pass/fail assessments are commonly used and are associated with competency-based assessments. Challenges with using this system are when assessing those where it is not a clear pass or fail and may be given the benefit of doubt (Duffy 2003). Oermann et al (2009) conducted a national review of assessment and grading strategies used by US schools of nursing and found 83% used pass/fail to assess students in practice rather than a letter of numerical grade. In both the UK and Ireland, educational providers have worked together to develop standardized assessment tools. This has allowed for regional standards to be agreed upon and provide assessors with standardized documentation when dealing with students from different institutions (O'Connor et al 2009).

Given that many educational institutions have developed their grading criteria to meet their needs, this makes comparison of the most effective methods difficult. Regardless of the method of assessment used, evidence obtained may be subjectively scored, resulting in reliability, and perhaps even validity, being compromised. Students may then be assessed unfairly, or incorrect assessment decisions are made—and what could be worse than passing a student who has not achieved the goal of professional health care education, which is to be "fit for purpose" and "fit for practice"?

In deciding whether the assessments are sufficiently robust to enable sound judgements to be made, clear criteria should be used for deciding if the assessments are both defensible and fair. A question to be asked is this: Do our assessments enable us to make such judgements soundly? Deciding whether or not an assessment lives up to this task is not straightforward. There is now an examination of those factors to be considered to make sound judgements in assessments. Measures to attain objective assessments and avoid subjective assessments are suggested.

KEY CONCEPTS OF CONDUCTING ASSESSMENTS

As an assessor, you must make assessment decisions continually, and these decisions about student performance must be just and fair. How can you ensure that this is so?

Furthermore, assessment for certification, so-called *high-stakes* assessment, as in professional health care education, should offer enough reliability and validity for public scrutiny (Hill 2012). This is reflected in the UK nursing and midwifery regulator role in preregistration education programmes to assure programmes prepare and equip students with the skills and knowledge to deliver safe and effective care now and in the future (Nursing and Midwifery Council 2019a). The same applies to standards set by the Health and Care Professions Council for other health disciplines (HCPC 2018). To effectively measure competence, assessment tools must be valid and reliable, which reflect the real world. (Harlen 2015, Franklin & Melville 2015).

VALIDITY

The traditional definition of validity is the extent to which a test measures what it was designed to measure. If it does not measure what it purports to measure, then its use is misleading (Gipps 1994). There are two key issues here that are important to the assessment of clinical practice: how measurements are made and what measurements are made. The use of the strategy of triangulation will help ensure that a complete picture of the student's competence is obtained, thereby enhancing validity. The need for triangulation allows for objectivity because validity in assessments conducted in the clinical learning environment is difficult owing to the complexity in patient care and external factors within the clinical learning environment (Franklin & Melville 2015). Valid assessment in clinical practice depends on methods of assessment used that are appropriate to the attribute of the competence being assessed (e.g., valid assessments of psychomotor skills are unlikely to be provided using questioning). Assessment for accountability purposes, as in health care professions, should aim for high validity because health care professionals must be fit for caring for patients and clients. We therefore must be clear about what we want to measure. When assessing in clinical practice, validity is inferred (Harlem 2015, Gonczi 2013). The way to infer validity is to collect evidence of the different types of validity that matter to us in clinical practice. Types of validity to be discussed here are:

- Face validity involves subjectively judging the validity of the assessment tool to see if it appears to require the use of the intended knowledge or skill to be assessed.
- Content validity involves analysis of what content is covered in the assessment and checked that it reflects the content intended to be assessed. For example, has the assessed sample adequately met the required standards for a particular proficiency?

- Construct validity relates to the full range of knowledge, skills and attitudes being assessed.
- Predictive validity is the extent to which the assessment accurately predicts a future event, for example, completion of a module or overall course.
- Interrater reliability is when one or more assessor assesses a student on a particular proficiency.
- Test-retest reliability asks if the assessment were administered on another occasion, that the outcome for each student would be the same.

  (Harlem 2015, Thompson et al 2012:159).

RELIABILITY

Reliability is a measure of consistency (Adamson et al 2012). Reliability relates to the interreliability of the assessment tool; meaning can the results be reproduced by the same assessor (Harlem 2015). A challenge in practice is, are the same results replicable by another assessor? (Franklin & Melville 2015, Girazadas et al 2007). Validity and reliability may interact and may involve a trade-off; for example, to reduce error, an increase in the range of content to be assessed for each proficiency may be needed, but this would increase the number of items and length of the test. This may then lead to other forms of error, for example, student fatigue, and more items per proficiency would mean fewer could be assessed (Harlem 2015).

FACTORS AFFECTING ASSESSMENT

It is difficult to measure validity because of many factors that can detract from it; this includes the type of assessment used, and the competence can be influenced by student, environmental or situational and assessor factors (Yanhua & Watson 2011). Each set of factors is now considered in turn.

STUDENT FACTORS

As stated, to achieve reliability, student performance must be consistent. Can students perform with consistency all the time? Obviously not—there are human factors that mitigate against being the "perfect all-singing, all-dancing" student. Those physical and emotional factors that may affect performance could be poor health, fatigue, lack of interest in the placement and therefore motivation to learn, anxiety and lack of confidence about giving patient care and personal problems affecting concentration at work. Physical disabilities such as hearing problems or specific learning difficulty may affect learning. The presence of other students in the clinical area may be supportive and positive for each other, thereby enhancing learning, or it may detract from learning if students are negative.

Another group of factors that students have no control over, such as their gender or racial background, may also affect the way they are assessed. Pitt et al (2012) identified four potential themes impacting on student performance; these included demographic background, academic, cognitive and personality/behavioural factors. Now try Activity 5.1.

> **Activity 5.1**
>
> Make a list of those student factors that you have encountered, either personally or from a colleague's experience, that have affected assessments either positively or negatively.

A group of practice educators came up with the following list of factors that they thought might have affected the way they view the students and potentially their assessment of students:

- Physical appearance, such as dress code, body piercing, tattoos and dyed hair.
- Age of the student in relation to themselves—the younger practice educator may feel threatened by the older student, and the mature practice educator may wish to 'mother' a younger student.
- The social class of the student—more may be expected of the student from a higher socioeconomic background because these students are "associated with higher intelligence". Conversely, less may be expected from the student from a lower socioeconomic background.
- The accent of the student—students speaking with the "Queen's English" accent are accorded a higher intelligence and assessed accordingly.

Changes in preregistration funding of courses have resulted in many students needing to undertake additional paid work around their courses. Many students undertake paid health care work, and although this may increase the student's confidence, it may also impact on students' learning. Kajander-Unkuri et al (2013) found that approximately 80% of bachelor-level students worked paid jobs in addition to studying. Several studies have shown full-time students who work extra jobs are likely to have an impact on their academic performance (Pitt et al 2012, Dante et al 2013).

ENVIRONMENTAL/SITUATIONAL FACTORS

There are particular problems that are direct consequences of assessing students in the clinical learning environment.

These problems will contribute to assessments being unreliable if they are not recognized and managed:

- There is inherently high variability in the context of clinical assessment; patients/clients or situations cannot be standardized and therefore cannot produce identical situations in which students can be assessed, for example, a non-English-speaking patient or a patient who continues to deteriorate despite appropriate treatment. The conditions for learning and practice can be highly inconsistent, which will impact directly on the consistency of performance of the student and the assessment.
- The work environment is often very busy. Leigh and Roberts (2018) estimated that with the revised NMC standards, a detailed assessment will take approximately 2 hours per assessment per student. Over the year, this would be equivalent to 1 day of assessment per student per year. The workload of practice educators has increased, while resources and support have not (Beskine 2009). There is therefore insufficient time for reliable evidence collection.
- There are many distractions that may interfere with the student's and the practice educator's concentration. A preoccupation with something that has happened, concern with jobs still to be done and the busyness and noise on a ward are examples of distractions that will affect learning and assessment activities.
- The learning climate of the working environment should also be considered. The pressure for placements and the high turnover of staff can affect the timing of the assessment and/or quality of the assessment (Helminen et al 2015, Heaslip & Scammell 2012). This may limit the support and encouragement given to learners gaining confidence and enabling them to participate more effectively in patient care and their learning.
- The workload of assessors may also influence the student experience. A difference between the UK model of assessment and other countries is that the assessor is a clinical nurse first who is not employed by the university, and supervision and assessment of students is part of their professional role (Heaslip & Scammell 2012). This places considerable pressure on the balance of their clinical and education roles.

ASSESSOR FACTORS

As with factors attributed to the student and the environment, there are many factors attributed to the assessor that can detract from the reliability of assessment. Assessment of proficiency is subjective and difficult to measure due to the diverse nature of health care and involves a relationship between the student and assessor (Franklin & Melville 2015). Hughes and Fraser (2011) found that for students, the relationship with supervisors and assessors was fundamental in developing their competence. Furthermore, Hishinuma et al (2016) found the qualities and skill of the assessor will influence the student's quality of clinical learning and characteristics the students will have in the future as registered professional. Concerns over the competency of assessors have also been raised; for example, Hennerby and Joyce (2011) found 18% of agency staff were below the expected competency. This poses significant concerns regarding the quality of learning, assessment and patient safety in practice.

Helminen et al (2016) suggested assessors felt they were expected to be more knowledgeable about assessing students, causing increased pressure. Changes in supervision and assessment of preregistration students and increasing diversity in supervisors and assessors without formal training may result in the differing interpretation of expectations and understanding of the assessment process. (Franklin & Melville 2015). Also, the impact of 12-hour shifts (long days) on the quality of student experience and learning has yet to be evaluated. However, heavy workloads and the reduction in handover time have all been identified as having a negative impact on assessment (Franklin & Melville 2015, Butler et al 2011).

Assessors need to understand students have different learning styles resulting in different learning needs and preferences. Henderson et al (2012) found students evaluated that their individual learning needs and views were not taken into account in the clinical learning environment. As a consequence, assessors need to invite questions from students and respond to their comments in an open and positive manner. Supervisors and assessors need to be aware of the various resources available and of any reasonable adjustments to appropriately support students. This should be a team approach. However, with students working with multiple staff on placements, the importance of the student–supervisor–assessor role is vital.

Try Activity 5.2. This activity is to help you consider those factors in your work environment that may contribute to unreliable assessments. Remember to ask the following questions about reliability:

- Would I interpret the student's performance of a skill in the same way if I saw it again?
- Would I interpret another student's performance of the same skill in the same way? What quality assurance measures are in place to confirm consistency?
- Would other assessors agree with my interpretations of the student's performance? What quality control measures are in place to check the outcomes are judged comparable?

- How consistent is the student's performance?
- Has there been an adequate sample across the range of context?

Competency-based assessments not only integrate the knowledge and skills with practical application, but they also allow for evidence to be gathered on several occasions, across a variety of contexts (Franklin & Melville 2015). Students may focus their learning on the aspects that will be assessed and experience a dichotomy between what is taught and what occurs in the real world (Helminen et al 2016).

Student performances vary, and assessment relies on assessors' perception of events and the accuracy of their perception (Davis et al 2013). In a university setting, assessments may be filmed or moderated by another marker. In practice, this is not ethical or feasible owing to resources and may lead to conflicting views of events. Indeed, assessors have been found to be inconsistent and focus on different aspects of performance (Dory et al 2018). Assessors may consult other health care professionals who have worked with the student to:

- Limit assessment bias.
- Understand how the student has coped in different clinical and professional situations.
- Obtain several viewpoints for objectivity.
- Confirm the student has demonstrated professional norms and behaviours (Price 2012).

Assessors may want the clinical practice to be a positive experience for students, which may result in assessors passing students or avoiding providing feedback on difficult areas (Wells & McLoughlin 2014, Miller 2010). Failure to fail is a term used to describe situations where assessors pass students who should have failed. The UK nursing and midwifery regulator commissioned a study of this phenomenon (Duffy 2003). Duffy (2003) found where it is not clear if a student should pass or fail, they may have been given the benefit of the doubt and passed. Since then, the concept of failing to fail has been identified in the literature in North America, Australia and the UK (Hughes et al 2019, Hughes et al 2018, Doherty & Dieckmann 2015). Themes which influence an assessor's decision may include: it's too difficult, the emotional process involved, lack of university

support, lack of confidence or unsafe characteristics (Hughes et al 2016). Students may also manipulate the situation and try to influence their assessment, for example, Hunt et al (2016) identified that a small proportion of students could use coercive and manipulative behaviour to elicit a successful outcome to their practice learning assessments. For UK assessors, balancing and deciding the priorities of managing a clinical workload and finding time to fail a student is a challenge; solutions include creating a positive culture in which assessors can raise concerns, coupled with strong leadership and appropriate support from within the placement organisation and university (Woodcock 2009).

FEASIBILITY

Feasibility changes over time and is determined by the time, culture, innovation and funding available (Davis et al 2013). With changing social values, patient expectations and changes in health care delivery, assessment of health care students will need to evolve. If we were given a task to do but had not been given the time or resources to complete the task, we would say that it is unfair because it had not been feasible to complete the task. Likewise, in assessment, it is only a fair assessment if it is feasible in terms of:

- Allowing sufficient time for students to practise and demonstrate competence.
- If there are sufficient resources in terms of opportunities for students to learn and demonstrate that they have developed their abilities and skills.
- If assessors have enough time and opportunities to work with and assess students.

Try Activity 5.3

As outlined, time constraint is likely to be a major restriction to mentoring, due to the length of placement, your workload or differing shifts with your student. All these factors could result in students not having enough time to practice or you not being able to spend enough time with students to perform a fair assessment.

Generally, a student's length of placement in a clinical area cannot be altered because these periods have already been determined in the curriculum. Prior planning of clinical experiences (e.g., agreeing a learning contact/action plan with the student) will maximize the potential of clinical time. The use of alternative assessment methods and strategies other than observing the student in practice yourself can make the assessment fairer, for example, the use of Objective Structured Clinical Examination or high-fidelity simulations (Davis et al 2013).

Remember to ask the following questions about feasibility:

- Has the student been given enough time to practice?
- Has the student been given enough learning opportunities?
- Has enough time been spent assessing the student, either by you or another assessor?

CONCLUSION

All assessments must balance rigour (validity and reliability) against feasibility. Validity is traditionally considered to be more important than reliability. Conducting fair assessments is complex. The biggest challenge to fairness faced by assessors and students during clinical practice is the context: we cannot assume identical clinical experiences for all. Health care is rapidly changing, and educational programmes need to be responsive and keep pace with these changes. Assessors play an important role in preregistration health programmes, as they assess student competence. Assessors' ability to judge a student's fitness to practice is essential in safeguarding the profession and public safety.

REFERENCES

Adamson KA, Gubrud P, Sideras S, Lasater K. Assessing the reliability, validity, and use of the Lasater clinical judgment rubric: Three approaches. *J Nurs Educ*, 2012;51(2):66–73

Australian Nursing and Midwifery Council. National Competency Standards for the Registered Nurse. 2006. Australian Nursing and Midwifery Council. Australia.

Bray L, Nettleton P. Assessor or mentor? Role confusion in professional education. *Nurs EducToday*, 2007;27:848-855.

Benner P. From novice to expert excellence in power in clinical nursing practice. California, United States of America: Addison-Wesley Publishing Company Inc:1984.

Beskine D. Mentoring students: establishing effective working relationships. *Nurs Stand*, 2009; 23(30):35-40.

Brown RA, Crookes PA. How do expert clinicians assess student nurse's competency during workplace experience? A modified nominal group approach to devising a guidance package. *Collegian*, 2017;24:219-225.

Butler MP, Cassidy I, Quillinan B, Fahy A, Bradshaw C, Tuohy D et al. Competency assessment methods – tools and processes:

a survey of nurse preceptors in Ireland. Nursing Education in Practice. 2011;11:298-303.

Bondy KN. Criterion-referenced definitions for rating scales in clinical evaluation. *J Nurs Educ*. 1983;22(9):376-382.

Canadian Nurses Association. Canadian Registered Nurse Examination: competency framework.2010. http://www.cno.org/globalassets/for/rnec/pdf/competencyframework_en.pdf

Chang CP, Lee TT, Mills ME. Clinical nurse preceptors' perception of e-portfolio use for undergraduate students. *J Profess Nurs*, 2017;33:276-281.

Clark JE, Eynon B. E-portfolios at 2.0. Surveying the field. *Peer Rev*, 2009;11(1):18-23.

Claman L, Watson R, Norman I, Redfern S, Murrells T. Assessing practice of student nurses: methods, preparation of assessors and student views. *J Adv Nurs*, 2002;38(5):516-523.

Dante A, Petrucci C, Lancia L. European nursing student's academic success or failure: a post-Bologna Declaration systematic review. *Nurs Educ Today*, 2013;33(1):46-52.

Davis M, McKimms J, Forrest K. Chapter 2: Principles of assessment. In: How to assess doctors and healthcare professionals. John Wiley & Sons Inc, UK:2013.

Department of Health. Meeting the challenge: a strategy for allied health professionals. London:2000.

Doherty A, Dieckmann N. Is there evidence of failing to fail in our schools of nursing? *Nurs Educ Perspec*, 2015;36(4):226-231.

Donaldson E. From mentor to supervisor and assessor: changes in pre-registration programmes. *Br J Nurs*, 2019;28(1):64

Dory V, Gomez-Garibello C, Cruess R, Cruess S, Cummings BA, Young M. The challenges of detecting progress in generic competences in the clinical setting. *Med Educ*, 2018;52:1259-1270.

Duffy K. Failing students: a qualitative study of factors that influence the decisions regarding the assessment of students' competence in practice. Nursing and Midwifery Council (formally The United Kingdom Central Council for Nursing, Midwifery and Health Visiting, 2003.

Ferrier L. Should mentors be replaced by supervisors and assessors? *Nurs Stand*, 2017;31(43):33.

Franklin M, Melville R. Competency assessment tools: an exploration of the pedagogical issues facing competency assessment for nurses in the clinical environment. *Collegian*, 2015;22:25-31.

Gipps in Gipps CV. (1994) Beyond Testing: Towards a Theory of Educational Assessment. The Falmer Press, London:1994.

Girazadas DV, Clay L, Caris J, Rzechula K, Harwood R. High fidelity simulation can discriminate between novice and experienced residents when assessing competency in patient care. *Med Teach*, 2007;26:472-476.

Gonczi A. Competency-based approaches: linking theory and practice in professional education with particular reference to health education. *Educ Philos Theory*, 2013;45(12)1290–1306.

Gray M, Donaldson J. National approach to practice assessment for nurses and midwives: exploring issues in the use of grading in practice – literature review. Edinburgh Napier University, Scotland:2009.

Green J, Wyllie A, Jackson D. Electronic portfolios in nursing education: a review of the literature. *Nurs Educ Prac*, 2014;14:4-6.

Harlen W. Chapter 43: Assessment and the curriculum. In: Wyse D. Hayward L. Pandya J. (Eds). (2015). SAGE handbook of curriculum, pedagogy and assessment. 2 vol set. SAGE Publications, UK:2015.

Health and Care Professions Council. Standards of Education and Training. 2018. https://www.hcpc-uk.org/resources/standards/standards-of-education-and-training/

Heaslip V, Scammell JME. Failing underperforming students: the role of grading in practice assessment. *Nurs Educ Prac*, 2012;12:95-100.

Helminen K, Coco K, Johnson M, Turunen H, Tossavainen K. Summative assessment of clinical practice of student nurses: a review of the literature. *Int J Nurs Stud*, 2016;53:308-319.

Henderson A, Cooke M, Creedy DK, Walker R. Nursing students' perceptions of learning in practice environments: a review. *Nurs Educ Today*, 2012;32(3):299-302.

Hennerby C, Joyce P. Implementation of a competency assessment tool for agency nurses working in an acute paediatric setting. *J Nurs Manage*, 2011;19:237 –245.

Hill TL. The portfolio as a summative assessment for the nursing student. *Teach Learn Nurs*, 2012;7:140-145.

Hishinuma Y, Horiuchi S, Yanai H. Development and assessment of the validity and reliability of a scale for measuring the mentoring competencies of Japanese clinical midwives: an exploratory quantitative research study. *Nurs Educ Today*, 2016;41:60–66

Hughes LJ, Mitchell ML, Johnston ANB. Just how bad does it have to be? Industry and academic assessors' experiences of failing to fail – a descriptive study. *Nurs Edu Today*, 2019; 76: 206–215.

Hughes LJ, Johnston ANB, Mitchell M. Human influences impacting assessors experiences of marginal group performances in clinical courses. *Collegian*, 2018;25:541-547.

Hughes LJ, Mitchell M, Johnston AN. 'Failure to fail' in nursing' – a catch phrase or a real issues? A systematic integrative literature review. *Nurs Educ Prac*, 2016;20:54-63.

Hughes AJ, Fraser DM. There are guiding hands and there are controlling hands: student midwives experience of mentorship in the UK. *Midwifery*. 2011;27(4):477-483.

Hunt LA, McGee P, Gutteridge R, Hughes M. Manipulating mentor's assessment decisions: do underperforming student nurses use coercive strategies to influence mentors' practical assessment decisions? *Nurs Educ Prac*, 2016;20:154-162.

Jones-Berry S. Nurse leaders warn that a growth in career routes will add to staff burden. *Nurs Stand*, 2018;33(6):35-37.

Kajander-Unkuri S, Salminen L, Saarikoshki M, Suhonen R, Leino-Kilpi H. Competency areas of nursing students in Europe. *Nurs Educ Today*, 32013;3(6):625-632.

Lancet Commission. Medical education in the 21st century. 2010. https://www.thelancet.com/commissions/education-of-health-professionals

Lahtinen P, Leino-Kilpi H, Salminen L. Nursing education in the European higher education area — variations in implementation. *Nurs Educ Today*, 2014;34(6):1040-1047.

Leigh J, Roberts D. Critical exploration of the new NMC standards of proficiency for registered nurses. *Br J Nurs*, 2018;27(8):1068-1072.

Miller C. Improving and enhancing performance in the affective domain of nursing students: insights from the literature for clinical educators. *Contemp Nurs*. 2010;35(1):12-17.

National Student Survey. Q&As for students. 2019a. https://www.thestudentsurvey.com/students.php

National Student Survey About the NSS. 2019b. https://www.thestudentsurvey.com/about.php

Nilsson J, Johansson E, Egmar AC, Florin J, Leksell J, Lepp M, et al. Development and validation of a new tool measuring nurses self-reported professional competence – the nurse professional competence (NPC) scale. *Nurs Educ Today*, 2014;34:574-580.

Nursing and Midwifery Council. Our role in education. 2019. https://www.nmc.org.uk/education/our-role-in-education/

Nursing and Midwifery Council. Future Standards of Proficiency for Registered Nurses. 2018. Nursing and Midwifery Council. UK

Nursing and Midwifery Council. Standards for Pre-Registration Nursing Education. 2010. Nursing and Midwifery Council. UK

OConnor T, Fealy GM, Kelly M. Guinness AMM, Timmins F. An evaluation of a collaborative approach to assessment of competency among nursing students of three universities in Ireland. *Nurs Educ Today*, 2009;29(5):493-499.

Oermann MH, Yarbrough SS, Saewert N,. Ard N, Charasika M. Clinical evaluation and grading practices in schools of nursing: national survey of findings Part II. *Nurs Educ Perspec*, 2009;30(6):352-357.

Pitt V, Powis D, Levett-Jones T, Hunter S. Factors influencing nursing students' academic and clinical performance and attrition: an integrative literature review. *Nurs EducToday*, 2012;32(8):903-913.

Price B. Key principles in assessing students practice based learning. Nursing Standard. 26. 2012;49:49-55.

Ramdeen B. Should mentors be replaced with supervisors and assessors? *Nurs Stand*, 2017;31(47):33.

Rosser E. Consultation on the new roles of supervisor and assessor. *Br J Nurs*, 2017;26(15):892.

Salminen L, Stolt M, Saarikoski M, Suikkala A, Vaartio H, Leino-Kilpi H. Future challenges for nursing education – a European perspective. *Nurs EducToday*, 2010;30(3):233-238.

Thompson J, Kenward L, Wilson A. Chapter 6: The mentor as an assessor. In: Kilgallon K. Thompson J. Mentoring in nursing healthcare: a practical approach. John Wiley Sons & Incorporated, UK:2012.

Watson R, Stimpson A, Topping A, Porock D. Clinical competence assessment in nursing: a systematic review of the literature. *J Advan Nurs*, 2002;65(8):1584-1595.

Wells L, McLoughlin M. Fitness to practice and feedback to students: a literature review. *Nurs Educ Pract*, 2014;14(2):137-141.

Willis Report. Quality with Compassion: the future of nursing education. Health Education England, London:2012.

Woodcock J. Supporting students who fail. *Emerg Nurs*, 2009;16(9)18–21.

World Health Organization. Developing a global competency framework for universal health coverage. 2019. https://www.

who.int/hrh/news/2018/developing-global-competency-framework-universal-health-coverage/en/

World Health Organization. Global standards for the initial education of professional nurses and midwives. 2009. https://www.who.int/hrh/nursing_midwifery/hrh_global_standards_education.pdf

Wu XV, Enshar J, Lee CCS, Wang W. A systematic review of clinical assessment for undergraduate nursing students. *Nurs Educ Today*, 2015;35:347-359.

Yanhua C, Watson R. A review of clinical competence assessment in nursing. *Nurs Educ Today,* 2011;31:832-836.

6

Assessment as a Process to Support Learning

Kathy Wilson and Caroline Ogier

CHAPTER CONTENTS

INTRODUCTION

It is discussed in Chapters 2 and 4 that assessors of students on health care courses have both professional responsibility and accountability to ensure that students they assess achieve safe and competent standards of clinical practice. A carefully planned and managed assessment strategy is required so that the goal of professional education, which is to achieve fitness for purpose and practice, is fulfilled through the assessment processes. It would perhaps be a truism to say that students do not just achieve this "fitness"; rather, their learning requires facilitation as they work alongside practitioners during clinical placements.

Price and colleagues (2014) discuss the importance of being assessment literate and define this concept of "assessment literacy" as involving an appreciation of the purposes and processes of assessment, and this applies equally to students and staff involved in the assessment process in practice. It is therefore necessary to effectively plan and manage clinical assessment so that the powerful effects of assessment can be harnessed and directed positively into learning about professional practice.

The continuous assessment process will be explored as the key assessment strategy to facilitate assessment as a learning process. Integral to the continuous assessment of clinical practice are the strategies of using the learning contract, with its concomitant assessment and learning plan, formative assessment and summative assessment. These are examined with respect to the successful management of the continuous assessment of practice to realize the positive impact of assessment on student learning.

CONTINUOUS ASSESSMENT OF CLINICAL PRACTICE

This section starts with an activity reflecting a student experience (Activity 6.1). The assumption made here is that many experiences of being assessed do not necessarily reflect the definition of a "fair" assessment as proposed by the Nursing and Midwifery Council (NMC). The NMC defines a fair assessment as one which is transparent and evidenced based, supported by clear and reliable documentation and includes a variety of viewpoints (NMC 2018a)

Activity 6.1
Recall an occasion as a learner when you felt you were assessed unfairly. What were the circumstances surrounding that assessment?
You may have experienced the following:
• You agreed your learning objectives with your practice educator and agreed a plan of how these may be achieved.
• You worked with several different staff members, achieving a range of skills, receiving some verbal feedback but limited written feedback.
• You had feedback recorded in your assessment document from your identified practice educator at the midpoint of the placement, although you did not have the opportunity to discuss this or undertake your own self-assessment.
• You did meet with your assessor again at the end of the placement to complete your documentation in which you received positive feedback on your performance and achievement, which you were happy to receive.

This activity requires reflection and analysis on the part of the student and those supporting learning and assessment in practice regarding whether this was indeed a fair and evidence-based assessment. As you work through the chapter and review the sections on formative assessment and feedback, you will be encouraged to critically review the process of assessment that was undertaken in this activity and its potential impact on student learning. Students need to be enabled to view assessment not only as an outcome in terms of gaining a pass or specific grade, but as a

process of development (Parker 2010). This will only occur if they can see it as a process that they participate in, rather than just something being done to them at the end of a placement experience.

The Quality Assurance Agency for Higher Education (QAA) definition of assessment is 'any processes that can appraise an individual's knowledge, understanding, abilities or skills' (QAA 2018:2). Nicklin and Kenworthy (2000) and Rowntree (1987) assert that assessments give students opportunities to demonstrate the learning that has taken place, although, as Price et al (2014) indicate, they should equally be about the giving the required level of support and promotion of student learning.

Establishing effective assessment approaches in health care programmes to determine competency has been debated and received significant attention in the literature over a period of many years (Heaslip & Scammell 2011). This remains a complex issue because of the nature of what needs to be learned and assessed in professional programmes and the fact that practical assessments of a student's learning are context bound (Cassidy 2008). Each patient or client cared for has different health care needs, which means that the student must learn different aspects of care and different ways of responding constantly. An "accurate estimate" of total learning can be made only over a period of time, after a student has had continuous supervision and sufficient learning opportunities to experience the range of clinical situations required to develop competence. In the UK, the impetus for the use of continuous assessment of theory and practice in nursing and midwifery education can be directly attributed to the perceived injustices of the final "one-off" assessment, where factors such as anxiety and ill health may adversely affect the competence demonstrated on the day of the assessment. The result may not be representative of the overall abilities demonstrated by the student.

The assessment of learning of theory and practice is a continuous process culminating in a judgement of achievement. Formative processes guide student learning, and summative assessment measures integration of subject disciplines and the application of theories in practice.

The use of continuous assessment allows the quality and quantity of information about the student to be increased; it provides a measure of how a student is developing the professional competencies required of them and checks their progress in achieving the required programme standards, and their performance should be monitored continuously (RCN 2017). In the case of preregistration nursing and midwifery education, the requirement for students to spend a minimum of 40% of their time with their mentors (NMC 2008) is no longer stipulated in the

2018 standards. With the separation of assessment and supervision roles in the standards for student supervision and assessment for nurses and midwives that previously were seen as part of the mentor role, the nominated practice assessor must periodically observe the student to make an objective decision but, more importantly, must seek and review the feedback from practice supervisors to support that evidence-based decision (NMC 2018b)

The collection of a more comprehensive range of assessment evidence will support us in knowing a student's abilities and, hence, the more likely it is that our assessment will be accurate, and because of the nature of care delivered by all health care professionals, it seems more logical to look at a broad range of knowledge, performance and abilities across a range of contexts. Subjectivity is inherent in all assessment activity but probably more so when assessing performance, despite the practice of developing extensive assessment criteria and multiple assessment methods. Cassidy (2008) proposes the need for a legitimate audit trail to support effective decision making. Practitioners need to ensure that their decisions are informed and supported by the feedback received from other registered health care practitioners in a range of care contexts, including the student's own voice in this learning and assessment process. A dialogue with the student involving their self-assessment and feedback adds to the rigor of assessment (Cassidy 2008).

Continuous assessment of clinical practice has the following advantages:

- Practitioners who are responsible for student learning can assess progress as it takes place.
- The context-bound nature of practical assessments is reduced as the learner is assessed over the varied circumstances of different patients/clients cared for.
- The learner receives continual and accurate feedback on performance and can identify areas where improvement is required. The assessor's personal knowledge of the learner and understanding of the context of the performance are significant advantages in providing valid feedback.
- Areas for development and improvement can be planned jointly by the practice assessor and the student.
- The student is likely to feel supported and encouraged because any learning and achievement will be contributing to the summative assessment. Rowntree (1987) reports that students in higher education who have experienced continuous assessment believe it to be less stressful than the "all-or-nothing" final assessment. However, students could equally feel they are under scrutiny at all times and need to be on their best behaviour. If formative assessment is well managed and integral to the student experience, students can feel more confident in the assessment process.

FORMATIVE ASSESSMENT

Measuring performance, summing up what each individual achieves and providing information in a way that is suitable for use beyond the programme, such as access to further stages of education or to employment, remains an important goal of summative assessment (Price et al 2012), although the purpose of assessment goes beyond this. Using assessment to motivate students and steer their approach to learning is regularly defined as formative assessment (Boud & Falchokov 2007).

Formative assessment uses evaluations of what students know and can do in planning future learning activities and to help students improve. Normally, formative assessment informs students about outcomes and provides them with feedback so that they can understand the qualities of their current achievements and how they need to develop further. The QAA defines formative assessment as a developmental process (QAA 2018).

Both formative and summative assessments strongly influence learning (Boud 2000) and more crucially 'affect people's lives' (Boud &Falchokov 2007:3). What underpins assessment for learning is the principle that all assessment, within the overall package, should contribute to helping students to learn and to succeed (Sambell & Mc Dowell 2013).

Summative assessment provides an 'authoritative statement of …what counts and …directs students attention to those matters' (Boud 2000:155). It tells students what to learn. The influence of formative assessment is no less profound. It provides the fine-tuning mechanism for what is learnt and how it is learnt. It should guide students in how to learn what they need to learn. It should also tell them the progress they are making. With health care students spending so much time in clinical practice, these are essential and important messages.

In clinical practice, formative assessment should be used to guide the student to what it is they need to achieve, helping them identify their strengths and recognize areas that they may need to develop through a continuous and well-thought-through process. Formative assessment aims to support student development and provide a systematic appraisal of their learning and is largely diagnostic in nature (Mulholland & Turnock 2007). Students need to be helped to understand the purpose of formative assessment and their role within the process, and this will only occur with regular feedback to feedforward as part of a sustainable model of assessment (Boud 2000)

STUDENT SELF-ASSESSMENT IN FORMATIVE ASSESSMENT

Boud and Falchikov (2007) support the commonly held view that students should be active participants in the process, reflecting, self-assessing and engaging in this two-way communication process; that is, interactive rather than passive partners in their learning (Gibbs et al 2004).

It is important to allow students to assess their own learning and allow them to voice their perceptions of their achievements, ability and level of competency so that learning can start from, and build on, what the student already knows and can already do. From educational psychology, Ausubel (1968:163) stated strongly that:

'If I had to reduce all educational psychology to one principle, it would be this: the most important single factor influencing learning is what the student already knows. Ascertain this and teach him [sic] accordingly.'

With the introduction of apprenticeships and several postgraduate routes into health care programmes, students representing a wide demographic and a diverse range of backgrounds bring a wealth of knowledge and skills to their placement experience, and this needs to be uncovered and built on.

Rowntree (1987:65) highlights the benefits of fully exploring previous knowledge and claims that a 'pupil does not really know what he [sic] has learned until he has organized it and explained it to someone else'. Self-assessment facilitates this process. Students may need to be facilitated to be realistic so that they do not over- or underestimate their ability and capabilities.

Students have an important role to play in planning their own learning and assessment. If they are to become competent assessors of their own work, they need sustained experience in ways of questioning and improving the quality of their work and supported experience in assessing their work. The ability to self-assess one's competence and achievements accurately is not a natural gift but a skill that can be learned and improved upon with practice (Mattheos et al 2004). Feedback is crucial in helping students develop accurate self-assessment skills.

Authors such as Yorke (2003) and Boud (2000) stated that assessors should focus on the quality of feedback given, which, in turn, will enable students to develop and strengthen their skills of self-assessment. There is a discussion later on how to manage feedback constructively.

Students are often well placed to assess their own learning and to regulate their own work appropriately. They will thus be able to indicate the amount and nature of clinical experiences they have had and recognize what clinical experiences they need to achieve competence.

Tan (2007) highlights that the ability for students to self-assess their own learning is strongly linked to enabling them to be lifelong learners because it encourages them to participate in and to self-direct their learning, to work independently and to continuously review their own performance and progress, which Boud refers to as sustainable assessment (Boud 2000).

One key aim of self-assessment should be to shift the student's focus from "how good am I?" to "how can I get better?" (Mattheos et al 2004:385). This ability will help students develop awareness of their own standards of practice. By listening to students, the assessor will learn what students consider their own learning needs to be. The practice educator should respond to the student's expressed learning needs. It may be necessary to probe more deeply so that the self-assessment helps students monitor their own learning to help them become independent learners.

Opportunities and time should be made available to engage in the essential process of formative assessment with learners to provide them with targeted and evidence-based feedback so that action plans for further learning and development of competence can be made. Adequate documentation of progress can thus be made. Duffy (2004) warns that the omission of formative assessment with opportunities for student self-assessment leads to inadequate documentation of progress and is a potential cause for the student's inability to achieve the required level of competence. Good feedback practice can support the development of self-assessment and reflection, including peer feedback, and should involve the student in self-regulating their own work or in this case their performance. This level of feedback is what Carless refers to as sustainable feedback, which is paramount in facilitating students in the development of these important skills needed for lifelong learning (Carless et al 2011).

In clinical practice, how does the formative assessment process discussed fit into the teaching/learning and working cycles of the practice educator and the learner? These issues will be explored in subsequent sections.

FEEDBACK IN ASSESSMENT

Boud and Molloy (2013) highlight the fact that feedback is the one aspect of assessment that creates most dissatisfaction amongst students, and this is clearly evidenced in the scoring of the National Student Survey.

Students need to be part of the feedback process; we need to move away from the transmission of feedback through a one-way process from educator to student to a more enriched dialogue exchange in which the student is fully engaged (Carless et al 2011), and this can be achieved in part by communicating the purposes of feedback and their central role in this process (Carless 2011). Feedback that involves simply telling the student what the practice educator thinks and hoping the student will do what they have been told to achieve a successful outcome is not helpful or appropriate to extending their learning. The key message from all the assessment literature is the importance of involving the student in that process.

Providing feedback is a vital component of student support in clinical practice (Walsh 2010). Duffy (2013) emphasizes the value of constructive verbal and written situational feedback, that is, feedback directly related to the situation in practice. Students often report finding it difficult to get constructive feedback from staff supporting their learning and getting the right amount of feedback, and the type and timing is often inconsistent. Students want and need feedback, whether positive or negative, to support their development (Duffy 2103). The more immediate this feedback and reflection, the greater the potential learning and the greater the possibility that the student will gain in confidence and increase personal autonomy (Neary 2000).

The frequency of formal written feedback is determined by the local university and informed by their assessment processes but is usually structured to occur midway through a placement and at the end of the placement, as a minimum.

However, if a student's feedback is limited to these two occasions, it will not contribute effectively to support their learning and is likely to take the form of a summing up rather than being developmental in nature and hence reflective of poor assessment processes. Many practitioners may claim that they give regular verbal feedback to students, which is indeed an important component of promoting learning; however, students may not always recognize they are receiving feedback. Students may need clarification of the function and nature of feedback and how this will be received during their placement. Understanding the purpose of feedback and their role in feedback will enable students to use this feedback more effectively.

In busy clinical practice environments, it is not always possible to give immediate feedback to students, so practice educators do need to identify strategies for managing this. A student, for example, could be asked to make their own notes after an event and reflect on their learning before spending time with their practice educator to discuss the experience, explore the student's perspective and learning and provide the student with more constructive feedback.

Students need to be supported to develop the commitment to their own learning, and by being active learners, they seek to understand more about what is required of them to succeed and that they proactively seek and act on feedback as active learners in this whole learning process (Boud 2009). Students need to drive their own learning and engage in the process of feedback, seeking knowledge for improvement (Boud and Molloy 2013), be supported to self-assess and reflect on their learning, providing opportunities for service users and carers to input where appropriate (RCN 2017). With the introduction of the 2018 standards for student supervision and assessment in nursing and midwifery programmes, there is significant emphasis on the importance of students receiving ongoing feedback throughout the programme from a range of health care professionals, service users and carers to promote and encourage reflective learning and support the assessor in making a final judgement (NMC 2018b) .

Specific and detailed feedback, with descriptions of what occurred, is required on a myriad of activities and situations that the student will have taken part in. Examples from the student's practice should be used to illustrate points being made in the feedback. This should be clear to the student and offered in terms of specific standards achieved or not achieved.

Formative assessment processes, then, require quality feedback of the kind and detail that not only provides students with insights into their performance and achievement but also tells them what to do to improve; such quality feedback is more effective because students know explicitly and reliably what they are expected to do. What students need to make any improvement is to have knowledge of the desired standard or goal, to be able to compare their own performance with the desired performance and, subsequently, to explore options for improving practice and take part in the appropriate activities to close the gaps—they need to know in some detail what to do and what they can do to improve. Feedback will then help the student to grow, boost confidence and increase motivation and self-esteem (Clynes & Raftery 2008). There is detailed discussion of how to manage constructive feedback sessions in Chapter 7.

SUMMATIVE ASSESSMENT

Summative assessment provides an authoritative statement of "what counts" and directs student attention to those matters. It tells us what to learn. Unfortunately, it does not communicate directly or unambiguously—it uses a form of code that only the most effective learners can decipher. Summative assessment focuses on the whole and is used to provide information about how much students have learned and to what extent learning outcomes have been met. There is a judgement of achievement. In the event of negative outcomes, nothing can now be done to remedy the situation. Whereas formative assessments take place throughout the student's clinical placement, summative assessments usually take place at the end of the placement, where the aggregate of learning is represented.

The influence of formative assessment is subtler in that it provides the fine-tuning mechanism for what and how we learn. Formative assessment guides us in how to learn what we wish to learn, and it tells us how well we are progressing to get there (Boud 2000) and increases the chances of a positive outcome for students. Ironically, summative assessment drives out learning at the same time it seeks to measure it. It does this by taking responsibility for judgements about learning away from the only person who can learn (the student) and placing it unilaterally in the hands of others. It gives the message that assessment is not an act of the learner but an act performed on the learner. How do we replace this misleading image with one that locates assessment in the hands of learners while acknowledging the legitimate role of certification by others?

The specified competencies (in the UK, these are referred to as standards of proficiency for nursing and midwifery professions or standards of competence for preregistration health care courses regulated by the Health and Care Professions Council [HCPC]) for each clinical placement must be achieved at the summative assessment to progress in the programme. Students who are not yet competent at progression points (HCPC 2011, NMC 2018c) are generally not allowed to progress further in their training until they have successfully achieved competence.

Two positions are taken with formative assessment in this discussion: first, it is a facilitative process that aims to guide and maximize learning; secondly, it serves to provide a series of assessments so that a summative assessment can be compiled from them. Rowntree (1987) suggests that final "end-of-the-placement" assessments may be dispensed with altogether if a satisfactory summative assessment can be compiled from the series of formative assessments, although these remain engrained in end point assessments embedded within apprenticeship programmes. Having examined formative and summative assessments, and the continuous assessment process in general, the next section will examine how to engage in and use the process of continuous assessment.

ENGAGING IN THE PROCESS OF CONTINUOUS ASSESSMENT

The three little words "assessment takes time" were probably written with much feeling and understanding by Phillips et al (2000:150) after their intensive investigation of the assessment of clinical practice in preregistration nursing and midwifery education. Assessment does indeed take time, and good assessment takes even more time. Time has to be allocated for "assessment-only" activity to enable assessors to engage in the process of continuous assessment so that assessments serve the intended purposes. The assessment activities to be undertaken within the continuous assessment process are represented in Fig. 6.1.

It can be seen from Fig. 6.1 that one of the central assessment activities is that of student–practice assessor meetings. These meetings are important to facilitate self-assessment, provide feedback, reinforce achievements and progress and discuss areas for development (RCN 2017).

Negotiating how often and planning for these review meetings is important, not least because of the need to meet the assessment requirements and complete the required documentation to support student progression.

Setting specific time out from the day-to-day work in advance and sticking to it is important (Mulholland & Turnock 2007, RCN 2017). Protected, that is timetabled, time should be prioritized and allocated for assessment-only activities (NMC 2008, Phillips et al 2000).

Professional responsibility and accountability for learners require us to ensure that learning takes place, and allocating and spending time with learners is part of that contract we enter into with learners under our supervision. If students are struggling to have these meetings and feel that they pose an additional burden in a busy clinical area, the quality and quantity of learning is extremely negatively affected (Phillips et al 2000).

Readers are directed to Chapter 8 in the section 'Staff commitment to teaching and learning' for some suggestions on how to support student learning and assessment activities.

THE FIRST MEETING/INTERVIEW

This first formalized meeting/interview is important for students; they will be feeling anxious in a new place of work (Phillips et al 2000) and unsure about what to expect from their practice educator they may be meeting for the first time. When asked about their first day on clinical placement, most students in Phillips et al's study (2000:72) provided, as their first word descriptor, "scary", "frightening", "terrified" and "anxious". Students undertake a wide range of learning opportunities across health and social care in both the National Health Service (NHS) and private, voluntary and independent sector areas and will undoubtedly also be feeling uncertain about how the practice area functions, whether they will fit in and be accepted and what they are going to learn, particularly if the student has never worked in that area of practice. The student will thus be looking for support and guidance from the practice educator. The first meeting/interview gives the practice educator an ideal opportunity to start forming a facilitative relationship with the student and introducing the student to, for example, the clinical area, its routine, the learning opportunities available and the members of staff in an effort to reduce anxiety.

Levett-Jones and Lathlean (2007) found anxiety as a barrier to learning. Students in their study who do not feel welcomed reported a diminished sense of belonging, leading to apprehension and anxiety about their clinical experience. Students reported that feeling comfortable and accepted meant they would ask more questions. The sense of belonging impacted on their capacity for learning and motivation to learn, building confidence and self-directedness. Positive

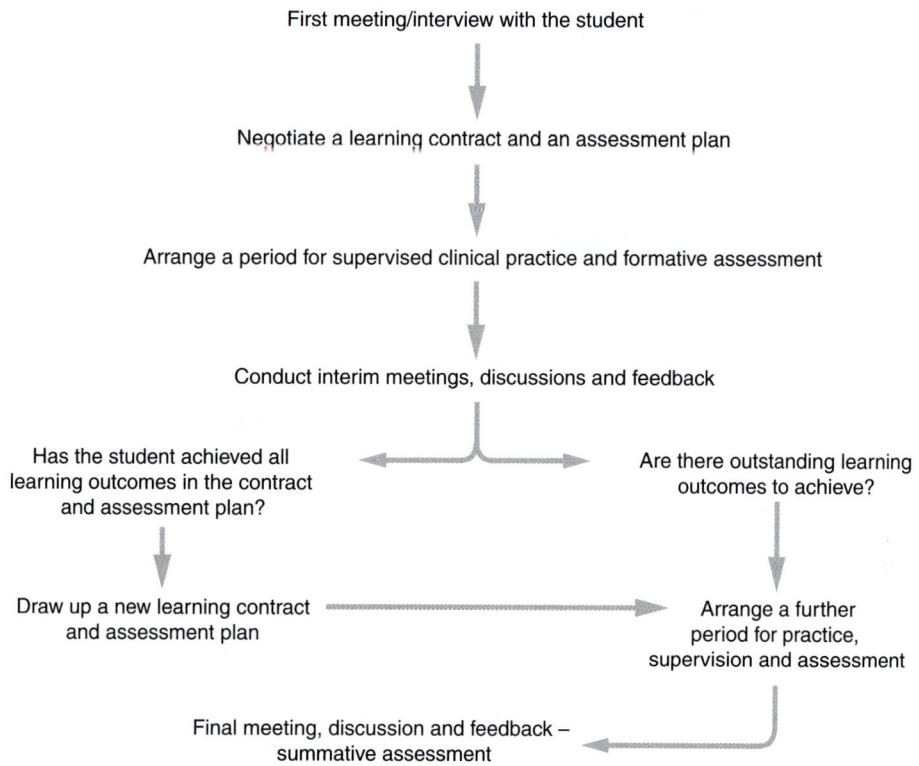

First meeting/interview with the student

Negotiate a learning contract and an assessment plan

Arrange a period for supervised clinical practice and formative assessment

Conduct interim meetings, discussions and feedback

Has the student achieved all learning outcomes in the contract and assessment plan?

Are there outstanding learning outcomes to achieve?

Draw up a new learning contract and assessment plan

Arrange a further period for practice, supervision and assessment

Final meeting, discussion and feedback – summative assessment

Fig. 6.1 The process of continuous assessment of clinical practice.

and productive learning experiences meant that students assumed more responsibility for their learning; they felt empowered and were able to negotiate their learning as partners. Cassidy (2008) also purports that validity of assessment is enhanced if there is investment in the relationship with trust and commitment from both parties.

Vygotsky (1930, in Spouse 1998) introduced the concept of "zone of proximal development" (ZPD) to describe the range of activities in which learners are capable of engaging. The ZPD comprizes a two-stage theory of development whereby a learner who is intellectually ready to move to the next stage could be assisted to reach this potential through support and guidance from a more experienced other. Having an accurate assessment of a learner's level of capability is crucial in assisting a learner to develop a higher level of competence.

By matching the learning tasks to the student's level, the learning contract/assessment plan is individualized, and the emphasis on assessment is placed on the student's progress and learning.

The first meeting/interview with the student should be held as soon as possible—preferably within the first 2 days of the commencement of the placement. This is important to

enable the practice educator and the student to draw up a learning contract that contains an assessment plan. This plan for learning and assessment should use the information from the student self-assessment to contribute to the identification of learning needs. It should also consider the student's ZPD to maximize learning and professional development.

This initial meeting is vital and should provide the space to discuss the student's learning needs and, as Duffy and Hardcore (2007) identify, to also discuss any specific learning difficulties.

As soon as the learning contract and assessment plan are negotiated and agreed upon, the direction that both the practice educator and student require for the teaching/learning and assessment processes to commence is provided.

In Chapter 2, it was discussed that one of your responsibilities as an assessor is to be familiar with the structure, organization and content of the programme of study of students you are assessing. This will allow you to have cognizance of the learning outcomes that your students will be required to achieve during the placement. The first meeting/interview allows you to evaluate what prior learning has taken place to inform and guide subsequent plans for learning. Phillips et al (2000) found that students on new placements often had to endure being treated as though they knew nothing—previous learning and accomplishments were ignored. Apart from this being disabling and demotivating, it can lead the practice educator to shape learning experiences inappropriately. Phillips et al (2000) contend that all students know something, and some know a great deal.

Activity 6.2

Make a list of the points you would discuss with your student during the first meeting/interview. Why have you included these points?

The points to discuss with the student should include the following:

- explore and attempt to allay any anxieties
- confirm the student's stage of training and current module of study to ascertain programme learning outcomes
- discuss any personal learning outcomes the student may have planned
- jointly examine and discuss the student's portfolio of learning to ascertain prior learning and progress
- ask about any written assignments or projects that have to be prepared
- discuss the learning opportunities the placement can provide to generate assessment evidence to enable achievement of competencies and learning outcomes
- discuss arrangements to supervize and support the student in your absence
- discuss the ward's routine and care philosophy.

One specific requirement of the standards for student supervision and assessment for nurses and midwives is that there is a nominated person for each practice setting to actively support students and address student concerns. This could be the area manager or an identified member of the team whose act is a supporting role for student learning, such as a student coordinator (NMC 2018b). The outcomes to aim for after the first meeting/interview are represented in Fig. 6.2. This meeting/interview should culminate in the mutual drawing up of the learning contract and assessment plan. The next section examines the learning contract, which also contains the assessment plan.

THE LEARNING CONTRACT AND THE ASSESSMENT PLAN

The use of learning contracts can be made integral to the continuous assessment process because both the formative and summative assessment components of this process can be fulfilled. As discussed, the intention of formative and summative assessment processes is to guide learning. Careful negotiation and planning of a learning contract will result in a framework to guide the teaching, learning and assessment requirements of the student. This framework will also provide the direction for teaching and assessing activities, including the management of feedback for the practice assessor and practice supervisors. This framework should not be seen as something that fixes students to a certain course of action. It should be a statement of intent that gives structure to learning activities to facilitate the fulfilment of educational learning outcomes and the development of professional competence.

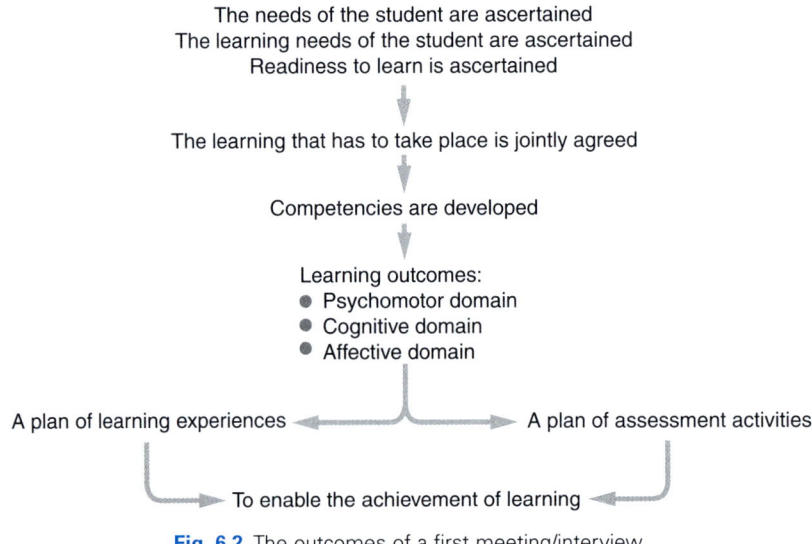

Fig. 6.2 The outcomes of a first meeting/interview.

In the clinical setting, the learning contract approach involves an individual student negotiating with, and entering into an agreement with, a practice assessor to pursue certain goals of a course of training. Commonly, in a preregistration programme, these goals are to achieve the competencies of the training programme. Postregistered practitioners may enter into contracts with their preceptors or managers to develop further their competence, roles and expertise. Because the purpose of these kinds of learning is to develop and/or improve one's competence to perform as a professional, the needs and expectations of the profession must be considered. How the learning is to be assessed is usually determined by the necessity to produce practitioners who have the knowledge and skills to meet the proficiencies of their profession (NMC 2018). Learners may have limited choice in what they have to learn and how they are assessed owing to the constraints of the programme of learning. Furthermore, in the clinical setting, although there are many resources for learning, these are not unlimited. Constraints may also be imposed by timing of the availability of some resources. For example, certain clinical experiences, such as rarely occurring clinical events, do not manifest to order so that the student can learn and be assessed.

These imposed structures on learning and assessment frequently conflict with an adult learner's need to be self-directing and having the "freedom to learn" (Rogers 1983). They may also stifle a learner's creativity and motivation to learn and, according to Knowles et al (2015), may induce resistance, apathy or withdrawal. The use of learning contracts could be one way of reconciling the requirements imposed by the discussed structures and the learner's internal need of having freedom to learn. Chan and Chien (2000) and Sajadi et al (2017) found this reconciliation possible within the constraints of the curriculum; they used learning contracts in the clinical setting, which increased self-directed learning. Interactions for planning and feedback activities between the clinical instructor and the student also improved—this finding confirmed Knowles et al's (2015) belief that learning contracts provide the means through which the planning of learning experiences can become a mutual undertaking between the student and the practice assessor. In the health and social care literature, Chan and Chien (2000), Bailey and Tuohy (2009) and Boitel and Fromm (2014), for example, report other benefits of using the learning contract in the clinical setting. Knowles et al (2015) reported the disadvantages and benefits of contracting based on the experiences of several teachers in higher education. It is not the intention here to enter into a debate of the advantages and disadvantages of using learning contracts, and the reader is therefore directed to the work of these authors for further information.

THE ELEMENTS OF A LEARNING CONTRACT

The core that underpins any learning contract is made up of learning objectives, learning activities to be completed, strategies and resources for learning and both learner and practice assessor evaluation of outcomes. Specific elements can be developed from this core to suit individual and institutional practices as well as fulfil the learning needs of students in a complex area, rich with learning opportunities, such as the clinical setting. For the purposes of competency-based assessment in the clinical setting, the elements given in Box 6.1 are suggested as the framework for the development of a learning contract. A discussion of these elements and how to develop them now follows.

PLANNING A LEARNING CONTRACT

An understanding of the format of the learning contract and this approach to learning is important for the successful implementation and their use. Students must be well prepared for this form of learning to succeed; preparation is crucial and should not be omitted (Knowles et al, 2015). Personal discussion with students and practice assessors tells us that the planning, developing and writing of a learning contract is not a straightforward affair. Authors, such as Boitel and Fromm (2014) and Sajadi et al (2017), report that learners and practice educators require support in their use.

Using the elements of a contract as shown in Box 6.1 as the basis for planning, the sequence of steps given in Box 6.2 is proposed for planning and developing a learning contract/assessment plan for competence-based assessment in the clinical setting.

BOX 6.1 Framework for Developing Learning Contracts

The elements of a learning contract for competency-based assessment
1. Clear statements of the aim and learning outcomes
2. State the level of performance to be achieved
3. Define the range of context for clinical practice to enable the achievement of the aim and learning outcomes
4. Specify the resources and learning activities
5. Develop an assessment plan
6. Identify the roles and responsibilities of both the learner and the practice educator
7. Decide a time frame—set review date(s) and a target date
8. Signatures

BOX 6.2　Steps for Construction of a Learning Contract

The steps to the construction of a learning contract/assessment plan

Step 1

At the initial interview/meeting:

- Facilitate student self-assessment.
- Identify prior learning and clinical experiences the student had engaged in.
- Examine student portfolio.

Step 2

- Identify and jointly agree learning needs and competencies to be achieved.
- For each competency, identify the knowledge outcomes, performance outcomes and attitudes and values to be developed.

Step 3

- Identify the range and context of practice for each competency.
- Identify resources and learning activities such as clinical experiences that are required to enable the student to achieve each competency.

Step 4

- Consider how evidence of learning can be generated and evaluated.
- Decide most appropriate assessment methods to assess learning.
- Map methods against clinical activities and other learning activities.

Step 5

- Agree on the roles and responsibilities of both to achieve the leaning contract/assessment. plan

Step 6

- Set and agree review and target dates.

There is now a discussion of the rationale underpinning each element of the contract and how each element can be developed and used for learning and assessment activities.

1. STATEMENTS OF THE AIM AND LEARNING OUTCOMES

Once the learning needs and expectations are outlined from the perspective of the student, the practice educator will be in a position to both define and describe what needs to be achieved. These require being developed into statements that can provide the direction for learning and assessment strategies. The statements can then act as the criteria against which student progress can be measured.

In a preregistration programme, the learning, of necessity, needs to be related to the achievement of the statutory professional competencies. In the case of midwifery and nursing students and students in professions regulated by the HCPC in the UK, these proficiencies are laid down by the NMC (2018c) and HCPC (2017) respectively. In terms of statements of the aim and learning outcomes for competency-based assessment, the following aspects should be addressed:

- Define the element of competency to be achieved.
- Define the attributes that underlie the successful performance of the competency.

For the purposes of this discussion, the example is used of a student nurse or student midwife who has identified the need to learn about caring for clients and others at times of loss and death. Elements of competence are the tasks within the wider function described by a "unit of competence", which represents a wide work function. This element of competency may be written thus: "to be able to deliver compassionate end of life care to clients and others at times of imminent death, death and loss". Professionals are competent as a result of the possession of a set of relevant attributes such as knowledge, understanding, skills, personal traits, attitudes and values. The attributes that underlie the successful performance of the element of competency to be able to care for clients and others at times of imminent death, death and loss need specifying so that they serve as the criteria for the assessment of successful performance of this element of competency. These criteria are the standards in competency-based assessment. Performance is judged against these prespecified standards. It is suggested here that these standards are specified under the three domains of learning:

- the cognitive domain—knowledge outcomes
- the psychomotor domain—performance outcomes
- the affective domain—attitudes and values to be developed.

Thus the standards, which are not intended to be an exhaustive list, for this element of competency may be grouped under these headings, as follows.

KNOWLEDGE OUTCOMES

- Discuss the stages of the grieving process and the individual's needs during each stage.
- Describe the policies and guidelines relating to care of clients and others at times of loss and death.
- Discuss recent research in this area and recommendations for practice.

PERFORMANCE OUTCOMES

- Support clients, significant others and friends of clients during their initial adjustment to knowledge of the client's condition.
- Support clients during the critical period before death.
- Comfort and support significant others and friends of clients who have suffered loss.
- Comfort and support significant others and friends of clients who have died.
- Debrief and support colleagues as necessary.
- Use the appropriate verbal and nonverbal communication skills.
- Perform the necessary care of the dead person.

ATTITUDES AND VALUES

- Be empathetic towards grieving clients, significant others and friends of clients.
- Be empathetic towards colleagues.
- Possess the appropriate respect for clients from diverse cultural and religious backgrounds.
- Show the appropriate respect for the dead person.

Zasadny and Bull (2015) found that incorporating these domains promotes reflective discussion of practice and integrates theory with practice. This research team also found that defining and documenting the competency statement, knowledge and performance outcomes and the attitudes and values enabled the practice assessor to use them as measures of the complexities of clinical practice and later analysis of student achievement of competence. This is perhaps the most persuasive argument for using standards in the assessment of clinical practice. Standards define what are meant by quality care practices and quality practitioners. When standards and other requirements of good performance (see section 2) are made clear before tasks are attempted, misdirected efforts and undue anxiety can be avoided.

2. STATE THE LEVEL OF PERFORMANCE TO BE ACHIEVED

A statement of the level of performance tries to make clear the degree of proficiency expected of the learner. The specified level of performance required is an important component of any learning contract because it is the measure used for the summative assessment of the element of competence. The specified level of performance also guides the development of the learner. Generally, in a 3-year preregistration programme, there are three levels of performance to be achieved: level 1, performance to be achieved by first-year students; level 2, performance to be achieved by second-year students; and level 3, performance to be achieved by third-year students.

Specifying the criteria for a level of performance is a thorny issue (Phillips et al 2000, Gerrish et al 1997). The most commonly used conceptual frameworks to support assessment in practice in a nursing context have been the work of Patricia Benner, *Novice to Expert* (Benner 1984), and the work of Kathleen Bondy *Rating Scales in Clinical Evaluation* (Bondy 1983). Both frameworks have often been adapted to represent the development of practitioners from a position of dependence to independence, reflecting and indicating the level of assistance being required at each level. The NMC indicates that the level of supervision required should be based on the professional judgement of their supervisors, 'taking into account any associated risks and the students' knowledge, proficiency and confidence' (NMC 2018:18b) The reader is directed to a discussion of this issue in Chapter 3. One possible way around this problem is to specify the level of performance and then match this with the amount of supervision/support needed, the level of practice that can be expected of the student and the conditions of competent practice for the specified performance level.

This eclectic framework to assess clinical practice is shown in Table 6.1. The reader is referred to Chapter 7, where there is a discussion of the theoretical basis of this format, and how to monitor and assess the progress of students using this framework.

3. DEFINE THE RANGE OF CONTEXT FOR CLINICAL PRACTICE TO ENABLE EFFECTIVE PERFORMANCE OF THE ELEMENT OF COMPETENCE

The range of context for clinical practice identifies the various caregiving situations that the student is expected to be able to carry out to achieve the element of competence in a specified clinical setting. Students deliver care in many different contexts; NHS England's (2014) *Five Year Forward View* proposed further changes to health care delivery, and these present an important context for nurses, midwives and allied health professionals. Some of the proposals have focused on reducing traditional barriers between physical and mental health, and health and social care, with more integrated models developed. These new care models require staff who work interprofessionally and flexibly across public health, community and hospital settings. These different caregiving experiences will provide the student with the opportunities to achieve the knowledge and performance outcomes and develop the appropriate attitudes and values specified in the learning contract, although the lack of familiarity with different care settings can also lead

TABLE 6.1 Matching the Levels of Performance to Levels of Supervision and Practice and Conditions of Competent Practice

Level of Performance	Level of Supervision/ Support	Level of Practice	Conditions of Practice for the Achievement of Clinical Competencies	
Competence Achieved	Competence not Achieved			
Level 1	Direct to close supervision	Observes, participates, assists in	Performs with few prompts	Requires detailed and explicit instructions
Can explain the rationale underpinning practice	Cannot explain the rationale underpinning practice			
Level 2	Close to minimal supervision	Active participation Planning most activities and leading some	Performance is smooth and complete	Performance lacks completeness
Does not require prompting in practised activities	Requires prompting in practised activities			
Can explain the rationale underpinning practice and discuss pertinent research	Cannot explain the rationale underpinning practice			
Level 3	Minimal to indirect supervision	Active participation Planning all activities and leading most	Does not require prompting	Requires prompting
Is organized and efficient	Unable to organize care			
Critiques evidence-based practice and its implementation	Does not consider evidence-based practice			

to anxiety and apprehension. Students need support to develop their objectives and to negotiate new learning if they have already achieved those that are available. Here, there is room for negotiation and the exercise of autonomy by the student. If the student has already had clinical experiences that fulfil the requirements of any of the range statements (see Chapter 3), then further similar clinical experiences may not be a priority in some instances. However, this does provide the student with the opportunity to consolidate their knowledge and skills and apply their learning in a different context.

An example of the range statements for the element of competence—to be able to deliver compassionate end-of-life

care to clients and others at times of imminent death, death and loss—is given later. The following range statements could mean the setting is that of a hospital ward, a care home or a patient's own home:

- the imminent death of patients who have suffered a long and difficult illness
- the imminent death of patients with a sudden acute illness
- the imminent death of patients with different diverse cultural and religious needs
- the imminent death of patients
- patients who have died

The range of statements serves to indicate the range of clinical situations to which the element of competence applies. It ensures that the element of competence has been learned and can be demonstrated in a range of contexts.

Notwithstanding the possible disadvantage of specifying the range, there are sound educational reasons for doing so. What is now known of cognitive processes indicates that there is a close connection between skills and knowledge and the context in which they are learned and practised. Eraut (2004) suggest that we cannot teach a skill component in one setting and expect it to be applied automatically in another. This means, in turn, that a competence cannot be assessed with validity in a context very different from the context in which it has been taught and practiced previously. The inter- and intrarater reliability of assessment tools remains a challenge, with intrarater reliability described as when the results are able to be reproduced by the same assessor, interrater reliability being when the same results are able to be reproduced by another assessor (Franklin & Melville 2013).

The specification of a range of contexts will enable this important guiding principle to be put in place. Assessments will then have more validity, as discussed in Chapter 5.

4. SPECIFY THE RESOURCES, LEARNING ACTIVITIES AND LEARNING OPPORTUNITIES

Resources required may be both material and human. These need to be identified and their use planned. Material resources, which should be available, up to date and directly relevant to the desired learning outcomes, could include equipment and caregiving aids, online resources on the organisation's intranet or via the internet, podcasts and videos, textbooks and journal articles. There should be a discussion of how these resources can be best used to contribute to the achievement of learning outcomes. Learning activities around material resources may include simulated learning activities, listening to a podcast, reviewing policies and protocols, undertaking online activities or learning to use a specific piece of equipment. The practice supervisor/educator should arrange to provide the necessary instructions.

When identifying human resources, the name, designation, availability and contact details of other members of the team that would be valuable to the student learning experience should be clear. There should be a discussion of how the person can contribute to the learning so that the student is better prepared to use the expertise of that person. Learning activities here may include observing and working with the person, followed by discussions, or simply asking questions and talking to the person. In the example of the element of competence used so far (to be able to deliver compassionate end-of-life care to clients and others at times of imminent death, death and loss) human

resources and learning activities could include working alongside and observing the palliative care team and observing and working with the bereavement counsellor, hospital chaplain and so on.

Some learning opportunities, such as direct participation in certain clinical experiences, may not be identified ahead of time. It should, however, be made clear to students those specific types of clients/patients whose care they need to participate in. The student will then be in a better position to negotiate with other team members they need to work with when they are looking after such clients/patients.

The reader is directed to the discussion on identifying and using resources and learning opportunities in the clinical environment in Chapter 8.

5. DEVELOP A LEARNING AND ASSESSMENT PLAN

There should be a clear plan of how the learning and assessment of the element of competence are to proceed over a specified period. Both the student and practice educator should agree on the following:

1. How learning and assessment will be managed, for example, making firm arrangements:
   a. to look after certain clients/patients and their family/carers
   b. to work together on specified shifts
   c. to spend time together to review progress on specified occasions.
   d. to gather feedback from others in the team
2. What evidence of learning should be collected.
3. How the evidence will be generated and collected.
4. What will be accepted as evidence that learning outcomes are achieved.

Students should be allowed to exercise choice and autonomy, where feasible, when decisions are made about how evidence is to be generated and provided. The student may negotiate to do a presentation to colleagues/peers, present information verbally to others and to support the achievement of specific learning outcomes, in particular the knowledge outcomes. If an oral presentation is to be given, the student must know how long the presentation will last and how it will be evaluated so that further anxiety is not created.

Evidence of having taken part in care may be collected in a written format in an evidence log or portfolio that may contain feedback from a range of staff that the student has worked with, from service users, carers and peers. Some assessment documents may include sections for students to complete and record their evidence. It is suggested that the student is responsible for maintaining this log/portfolio and records details of clinical activities undertaken that will act as evidence of achievement of learning outcomes in the learning contract. Questioning and reflective discussions of these records will provide evidence of the underpinning knowledge and understanding of care delivered. The reader is directed to the section on recording evidence in Chapter 7 for a further discussion of the use of evidence logs.

Within a scheme of the continuous assessment of clinical practice, the student will generally work alongside the practice supervisor so that the practice supervisor/assessor facilitates learning at the same time as assessing learning and progress. The practice assessor will be gathering evidence of learning that should be discussed with the student during feedback sessions. In the absence of the allocated practice assessor, firm arrangements should be made for the student to work with another practitioner. As indicated previously, the role of the practice supervisor and practice assessor in nursing and midwifery programmes must be made clear to the student, as well as the ways in which these individuals communicate and collaborate to support effective practice learning and assessment (NMC 2018b). The learning contract should be explained to others involved in supporting student learning so that continuity of supervision and support is maintained and the validity and reliability of the assessment is enhanced.

6. IDENTIFY THE ROLES AND RESPONSIBILITIES OF BOTH THE LEARNER AND THE PRACTICE EDUCATOR

A written learning contract signals a commitment from both the student and the practice assessor in which the student and practice assessor work together to achieve the specified outcomes.

A key aim of using learning contracts is to promote student autonomy and responsibility by encouraging self-directed learning, although Chan and Chien (2000) discussed the uncertainties and anxieties students felt when the use of learning contracts was an unfamiliar learning strategy, and development of these skills needs to begin before the student begins their placement. The practice assessor needs to assess the level of readiness and ability of the student to deal with the demands of using learning contracts as advanced learning skills are required. These advanced learning skills include self-direction, critical self-appraisal, the ability to participate actively in the learning activities provided and in the management of their learning and to seek help, guidance and feedback when appropriate (Refshauge & Higgs 2000).

In the case of the practice educator in the clinical setting, it is suggested here that the role shifts from someone who has the responsibility for making sure that learning experiences take place, and indeed controls the clinical experiences that students have, to that of someone whom students approach to negotiate the types of clinical and other learning experiences they require to achieve the outcomes in the contract. Neary (1998) suggests that what students want to learn can be developed only if the practice educator, through facilitation, directs and gives clear guidelines on expected outcomes of learning. Vygotsky's (1930, in Spouse 1998) theory of the ZPD states that the potential of a learner to progress to the second stage of development could be capitalized upon if support and guidance from a more experienced other is available.

Stenhouse (1975, in Mazhindu 1990) made the contentious point that the quality of the facilitator is either the main weakness or the greatest strength of the learning contract. There is no doubt that the success of this learning approach depends not only on the student's own enthusiasm and commitment to the agreement but also on the enthusiasm, commitment and ability of the practice educator as facilitator. The practice educator needs to assist the student with making a successful transition to this form of learning, if required, and also to help the student sustain the interest and commitment to the contract. One key strategy in maintaining student motivation in their learning is to provide opportunities for success and to give regular immediate formative and summative feedback (Neary 1998).

Students must also make a shift in their perceptions of their roles as learners. A traditional learner role is that of dependency. Students are perceived, and perceive themselves to be, dependent on the teacher for planning and evaluating their learning and are more or less dependent and passive recipients of transmitted content. Some roles and responsibilities of the practice supervisor/assessor could be to:

- act as a resource and share ideas and recommend learning resources
- identify and negotiate learning opportunities for the student
- support and encourage the student
- assess and evaluate the student's work, giving regular constructive feedback
- provide stimulating learning experiences.

Some roles and responsibilities of the student could be to:

- seek out and make use of learning opportunities and resources
- make a study of relevant literature and evidence base to increase underpinning knowledge and understanding
- take the initiative to seek guidance and feedback regularly

- participate in assessment and evaluation through self-evaluation.

7. AGREEMENT ON A TIME FRAME—SET REVIEW DATE(S) AND A TARGET DATE

Setting a target date allows the student and practice assessor to pace the learning and provides the student with goals to achieve. It is important to meet at specified intervals to determine progress, make changes to the contract and provide help if needed. The student should be left with the responsibility of seeking guidance and feedback outside of these scheduled times if required. The frequency varies with the type of contract, the level of the student and the ability of the student for self-direction and discipline. The highly motivated, self-directing and self-disciplined student may require little help and therefore fewer occasions for formal review and feedback. The student who is less motivated or has difficulty in maintaining self-discipline will require more frequent meetings to verify understanding, check progress and to provide encouragement and motivation.

It is useful to identify some specific outcomes from the learning contract to work towards during a specified period so that these can be evaluated at each review meeting. This will provide the direction and the goals for learning for that period. Learning is then divided into chunks and is likely to be more manageable and achievable. Opportunities for success are provided; these will act as extrinsic motivators to encourage the student to set sights that are progressively higher (Neary 1998). At these review meetings, the student should participate actively through self-assessment and by the seeking of feedback about performance and learning. The following points may be useful for the review of progress:

- Review the learning contract. Discuss how far the activities that the student has participated in have contributed to the achievement of the learning outcomes and the range.
- Discuss any difficulties that the student may be experiencing.
- Discuss and plan future learning activities.
- Amend the learning contract if necessary—few learning contracts ever go to plan.

If the learning outcomes and the range have been achieved before the target date, a new learning contract should be drawn up. If the actual clinical experience cannot be provided towards the end of the contracted period, plans should be made to use simulation in the place of naturalistic observation as the alternative method of assessment.

8. SIGNATURES

It is suggested that both the student and practice assessor sign the contract because this strengthens the commitment of both participants.

The following checklist of questions may be helpful when you are reviewing the completed contract that has been drawn up:

- Are the identified learning opportunities relevant to the needs of the learner?
- Do the selected learning opportunities use a range of common and less common clinical events?
- Have arrangements been made to use continuous assessment to monitor progress?
- Has the learner been involved in discussing and agreeing the contract?
- Does the contract specify the level of performance, knowledge and performance outcomes?
- Do knowledge and performance outcomes illustrate a link between theory and practice?
- Do knowledge and performance outcomes reflect evidence-based practice?
- Are the roles and responsibilities of you and the learner clearly identified?

PERIOD OF SUPERVIZED CLINICAL PRACTICE AND FORMATIVE ASSESSMENT

The learning contract and assessment plan formulated will provide the practice educator and the student with the framework for teaching, learning and assessment. The period of supervised clinical practice and formative assessment can now proceed more meaningfully and with the intent that is required to help the student achieve the learning during the precious time spent on clinical placements. During this period, the student is learning under supervision and working towards achieving the competencies that the training requires. This learning may occur as a result of interacting with patients/clients, giving patient/client care and being taught by yourself and other staff members. With reference to the learning outcomes and range of context identified in the contract discussed, it is clear what types and nature of learning experiences are required. Arrangements should be made so that the student and the practice educator work together and with other members of the team as necessary to enable the student to engage in the necessary clinical experiences. Working with other team members will also provide assessment evidence that can be attributed as "testimony of others".

During the formative assessment period, assessment activities are informal; you may observe activities, evaluate care given, give feedback, pose questions or discuss care given in a planned systematic or ad hoc way. The information obtained may be partial or fragmentary in the early days and will not allow you to make a firm evaluation of the student's competence. But repeated assessments of this sort, over a period of time and in a range of contexts, will allow you to build up a solid and broadly based assessment of your student's attainment. This will increase the validity and reliability of assessment.

Phillips et al (2000) found that where practice assessors can work with students for only short intermittent and ad hoc stretches, they are not able to collect reliable assessment evidence. This in turn reduces the validity of the assessment. They recommend that there should be a minimum time prioritized for assessment-only activities involving working and observing alongside the learner as part of a specified minimum overall learner entitlement. It has previously been a NMC (2008) requirement that a mentor supports the student for at least 40% of the student's placement learning time, and with the removal of this requirement the continuity of support, quality of feedback from practice supervisors and the amount of time the practice assessor spends observing the student and to make an evidence-based decision needs careful consideration to ensure a robust assessment (NMC 2018b).

The formative assessments that take place as you work with the learner and give feedback on performance are generally ad hoc and informal; however, it is recommended that these formative assessment sessions be documented to enable you and the student to review and reflect on experiences, identify learning that has taken place and plan further experiences. Remember that the aim of formative assessments is to motivate your student and maximize learning.

The number of formal meeting/discussion sessions you hold altogether during the student's placement would be dependent on the length of the placement and the progress the student is making. As a guide, try to hold a formal meeting/discussion session at least every 2 weeks so that you can formally review with your student the progress that is made and identify any difficulties at an earlier, rather than a later, stage of the placement. Formalized sessions should be planned and dates specified in the learning contract.

At the end of each interim meeting/discussion session, you and your student should jointly decide to what extent the competencies and learning outcomes in the learning contract/assessment plan have been achieved. As indicated in Fig. 6.1, if all learning outcomes in the learning contract/assessment plan have been achieved, a new learning contract/assessment plan will be drawn up and a further period for practice and assessment arranged. Likewise, if the

student requires more clinical experience to enable the outstanding learning outcomes to be achieved in the existing assessment plan and contract, a further period for practice and assessment will also need to be arranged. It is important to record in writing the discussion that has taken place because this record should be filed in the student's portfolio for future reference. The student's assessment of practice record is completed as required (e.g., signing those competencies that have been achieved). This will serve to motivate the student. If concerns are raised, then a discussion with a university representative should be initiated to support both yourself and the student in clearly identified specific actions that might be needed to support development, and the development of an action plan can provide a clear outline of specific learning objectives and how the student can be supported to achieve these (Duffy 2013).

THE FINAL MEETING/DISCUSSION SESSION AND SUMMATIVE ASSESSMENT

The final meeting/discussion session to perform the summative assessment is held at the end of the placement. As a guide, this meeting should occur during the last week of the student's placement, preferably on the last day. During this final meeting/discussion session, additional time should be allocated to review and analyse fully the evidence of competence. It is important to record the discussion and complete the student's assessment of practice record to be filed in the student's portfolio so that it can be available to the student for future reference and to other practice educators in subsequent placements. Time should also be spent in preparing the student for future placements. As the supervising practice assessor, you can see any changes in the student that provide specific information for fostering future development. Through your guidance, learning can be influenced. Assessment must be looked at not only in terms of outcomes measurement but also in terms of the learning process.

Suggestions on how you might conduct these meeting/discussion sessions and the summative assessment meeting, analyse assessment evidence and give feedback more effectively are made in Chapter 7.

CONCLUSION

It is acknowledged that outcome measurement in the health care professions is important to achieve fitness for practice and fitness for purpose. This chapter has considered that assessment must be an integral part of the learning process and should never be looked at just in terms of outcome measurement. One of the oldest and most robust findings of educational research is that assessment is the major influence on what gets learned (Eraut 2004). Assessment supports students' learning; it is designed to enable students to learn through preparing for and undertaking the assessment and from feedback on their performance in the assessment (QAA 2018). Assessment should be, and can be, facilitative and constructive and should never be used as a punitive tool. It should be used to identify what students have learned, what they have not learned and where they are having difficulty. Assessment can be used to support the development of lifelong learning skills in students because they themselves will use the knowledge and skills gained through the assessment process in their future everyday practice (Boud 2000). In this way, it supports the teaching–learning process; this form of assessment is known as formative assessment. Assessment in the caring professions also needs to be used for accountability purposes to confer competence and certify students; this form of assessment is known as summative assessment.

The continuous assessment of practice allows the practice supervisor and assessor to work closely with, supervize and assess the student in the everyday working environment. Assessments that take place in these natural surroundings are more likely to reflect the real abilities of the student. There has been much emphasis that assessments should be of this nature so that they are "authentic", with emphasis on the realistic value of the task and the context (Havnes & Mc Dowell 2008). It is important to plan assessments carefully so that these time-consuming assessment activities result in high-quality assessment.

If we could work with students all the time they are in clinical practice, we would be in a very good position to support their development as competent practitioners and judge their performance. This is particularly the case with assessments in professional education that confer professional qualifications; for example, a nursing, midwifery or physiotherapy qualification is taken to guarantee safe and competent practice for the public that these professions serve.

KEY POINTS FOR REFLECTION

Assessment should be a cumulative process, relating to learner progress as well as achievement, and be more closely integrated with learning (rather than separated from it) and with development of the individual student. One of the oldest and most robust findings of educational research is that assessment is the major influence on what gets learned (Eraut 2004).

Formative assessment processes guide and maximize student learning and take place throughout the placement. Both the practice educator and learner collaborate actively to produce a best performance where "feedback'" and "feed forward" take place. This also requires students to engage in self-assessment.

Feedback is an essential learning activity. The need to move away from the transmission of feedback through a one-way process from educator to students to a more enriched dialogue exchange in which the student fully engaged can be achieved in part by communicating the purposes of feedback and their central role in this process (Carless 2011). Unless students are able to use feedback to produce improved work (e.g., to improve upon a similar/same aspect of care), neither they nor those giving feedback will know that it has been effective.

Summative assessment measures achievement at the end of the placement. It focuses on the whole and is used to provide information about how much students have learned and the extent to which learning outcomes have been met.

The assessment of clinical practice should be a continuous process that culminates in a judgement of achievement. In summary, the stages of the continuous assessment process are as follows:

1. Arrange and conduct the first meeting/interview. Be clear about what you want to include in the learning contract and the assessment plan.
2. Arrange clinical experiences to enable your student to practise and achieve the assessment plan and the learning outcomes in the contract. During this period, arrange to work with and assess your student in practice.
3. Arrange and conduct interim meeting/discussion sessions — formalized formative assessments —throughout the placement. Facilitate self-evaluation by the student. Gather evidence and feedback from a range of sources and explore written feedback from a range of other practitioners, service users and carers with the student. Complete assessment documentation.
4. Arrange and conduct the final meeting/discussion session —summative assessment, again through a process of dialogue with the student. Complete assessment documentation.

The use of learning contracts can be made integral to the continuous assessment process. Careful negotiation and planning of a learning contract will result in a framework to guide the teaching, learning and assessment requirements of the student. This framework will also provide the direction for teaching and assessing activities for the practice educator.

REFERENCES

Ausubel, 1968 D.P. Ausubel, Educational Psychology: A Cognitive View. Holt, Rinehart & Winston, New York1968.

Benner et al., 1996 P. Benner, C.A. Tanner, C.A. Chesla, Expertise in Nursing Practice. Springer, New York1996.

Billings et al., 2010 D.M. Billings, K. Kowalski, M.L. Cleary, Giving feedback to learners in clinical and academic settings: practical considerations. J. Contin. Educ. Nurs. 41 (4) (2010) 153–154.

Boitel C, Fromm R. Defining signature pedagogy in social work education: learning theory and the learning contract. *J Soc Work Educ*, 2014;50:608-622.

Boud D. Sustainable assessment: rethinking assessment for the learning society. *Stud Continuing Educ*, 2000;22(2):151-167.

Bradbury-Jones C, Irvine F, Sambrook S. Empowerment of nursing students in clinical practice: spheres of influence. *J Adv Nurs*, 2010;66(9):2061-2070.

Cassidy S. Subjectivity and the valid assessment of pre-registration student nurse clinical learning outcomes: implications for mentors. *Nurse Educ Today*, 2008;29:33-39.

Carless D, Salter D, Yang M, Lam J. Developing sustainable feedback practices. *Stud High Educ*, 2011;36(4):395-407.

Chan SW, Chien W. Implementing contract learning in a clinical context: report on a study. *J Adv Nurs*, 2000;31(2):298-305.

Clynes MP, Raftery SEC. Feedback: an essential element of student learning in clinical practice. *Nurse Educ Pract*, 2009;8:405-411.

Crooks TJ. The impact of classroom evaluation practices on students. *Rev Educ Res*, 1998;58(4):438-481.

Duffy K. Failing Students Report. Nursing and Midwifery Council, London

Duffy K. Providing constructive feedback to students during mentoring. *Nurs Stand*, 2013;27(31):50-56.

English National Board. English National Board, Guidelines to Preparing Continuous Assessment. The English National Board for Nursing, Midwifery and Health Visiting, London:1986.

Eraut M. A wider perspective on assessment. *Med Educ*, 2004;38:800-804.

Franklin N, Melville P. Competency assessment tools: an exploration of the pedagogical issues facing competency assessment for nurses in the clinical environment. *Collegian* 2015;22(1):25-31.

Fraser D, Murphy R, Worth-Butler M. An Outcome Evaluation of the Effectiveness of Pre-registration Midwifery Programmes of Education. The English National Board for Nursing, Midwifery and Health Visiting, London:1997.

Gerrish K, McManus M. Ashworth P. Levels of Achievement: A Review of the Assessment of Practice. The English National Board for Nursing, Midwifery and Health Visiting, London:1997.

Govaerts MJB, Schuwirth LWT, Pin A. Objective assessment is needed to ensure competence. *Br J Midwifery*, 2001;9(3):156-161.

Havnes A, McDowell L (eds). Balancing Dilemmas in Assessment and Learning in Contemporary Education. Routledge, New York, United States:2008.

Health Care Professional Council. Standards of Education and Training. 2017. Available: https://www.hcpc-uk.org/globalassets/resources/standards/standards-of-education-and-training.pdf (Accessed February 2019)

Knowles M. The Adult Learner: A Neglected Species 4th edition. Gulf, Houston:1990.

Kowles MS, Holton EF, Swanson RA. The Adult Learner. 8th edition. Routledge, Oxon:2015.

Koretz D, Linn R, Dunbar S. The effects of high stakes testing on achievement: preliminary findings about generalization across tests. 1991. Paper presented to the AERA/NCME, April, Chicago.

Levett-Jones T, Lathlean J. Belongingness: a prerequisite for nursing students' clinical learning. *Nurs Educ Pract*, 2008;8:103-111.

Mattheos NMC, Nattestad A, Falk-Nilsson E. The interactive examination: assessing students' self-assessment ability. *Med Educ*, 2004;38(4):378-389.

Mazhindu GN. Contract learning reconsidered: a critical examination of implications for application in nurse education. *J Adv Nurs*, 1990;15:101-109.

Mulholland J, Turnock, C, Learning in the Workplace: A Toolkit for Facilitating Learning and Assessment in Health and Social Care Settings. 2nd edition. Routledge, London:2007.

Neary M. Contract assignments and change in teaching, learning and assessment strategies. *Educ Pract Theory*, 1998;20(1):43-58.

Nicklin PJ, Kenworthy N. Teaching and Assessing in Clinical Practice. 2nd ed. Baillière Tindall, London:2000.

Nursing and Midwifery Council. Nursing and Midwifery Council, Standards to Support Learning and Assessment in Practice. 2nd ed. \NMC, London:2008. Online. Available: <http://www.nmc-uk.org/Publications/Standards> (Accessed August 2011).

NHS England. NHS England, Five Year Forward View. 2014. Available: https://www.england.nhs.uk/wp-content/uploads/2014/10/5yfv-web.pdf (Accessed 2 February 2019)

Nursing and Midwifery Council. Nursing and Midwifery Council, Standards of Pre-registration Midwifery Education. NMC, London:2009.

Nursing and Midwifery Council. Nursing and Midwifery Council, Standards of Pre-registration Nursing Education. NMC, London:2010.

Nursing and Midwifery Council. Nursing and Midwifery Council, Standards Framework for Nursing and Midwifery Education. 2018a. https://www.nmc.org.uk/standards-for-education-and-training/standards-framework-for-nursing-and-midwifery-education/ (accessed 20 February19).

Nursing and Midwifery Council. Nursing and Midwifery Council, Standards for Student Supervision and Assessment. 2018b. https://www.nmc.org.uk/standards-for-education-and-training/standards-for-student-supervision-and-assessment/ (accessed 20 February 2019).

Nursing and Midwifery Council. Nursing and Midwifery Council, Future Nurse: Standards of Proficiency for Registered Nurses. 2018c. Available: https://www.nmc.org.uk/globalassets/sitedocuments/education-standards/future-nurse-proficiencies.pdf (accessed 20 February 2019)

Parker J. Effective Practice Learning in Social Work. 2nd ed. Learning Matters Ltd., Exeter:2010.

Phillips T, Schostak J, Tyler J. Practice and Assessment in Nursing and Midwifery: Doing it for Real. The English National Board for Nursing, Midwifery and Health Visiting, London:2000.

Price M, Rust C, O'Donovan B, Handley K, Bryant R. Assessment Literacy: The Foundation for Improving Student Learning. Oxford Brooks University, Oxford:2014.

Refshauge K, Higgs J, Jones M. Teaching clinical reasoning. In:J. Higgs, M. Jones, Clinical Reasoning in the Health Care Professions. Butterworth-Heinemann, Oxford:2000, 141–147.

Rogers C. Freedom to Learn for the 80s. Charles E. Merrill, Columbus, Ohio:1983.

Rowntree D. Assessing Students: How Shall We Know Them. 2nd ed. Kogan Page, London:1987.

QAA. UK Quality Code, Advice and Guidance: Assessment. 2018. https://www.qaa.ac.uk/quality-code/advice-and-guidance/assessment (accessed February 2019).

RCN. RCN Guidance for Mentors of Nursing and Midwifery Students, Royal College of Nursing, London:2017.

Sajadi M, Fayazi N, Fournier A, Abedi AR. The impact of the learning contract on self-directed learning and satisfaction in nursing students in a clinical setting. *Med J. Islam Repub Iran*, 2017;31:72.

Spouse J. Scaffolding student learning in clinical practice. *Nurs Educ Today*, 1998;18:259-266.

Stenhouse L. An Introduction to Curriculum Research and Development. Heinemann, London:1975.

Torrance H, Pryor J. Investigating Formative Assessment. Open University Press, Buckingham:1998.

Walsh D. The Nurse Mentor's Handbook; Supporting Students in Clinical Practice. Open University Press, Maidenhead:2010.

Williams S, Rutter L. The Practice Educator's Handbook. Sage and Learning Matters, London:2015.

Yorke, 2003 M. Yorke, Formative assessment in higher education: moves toward theory and the enhancement of pedagogic practice. High. Educ. 45 (4) (2003) 477–501.

7

Monitoring Progress, Managing Feedback and Making Assessment Decisions

Daniel Soto-Prieto and Nigel Davies

CHAPTER CONTENTS

INTRODUCTION

Giving feedback to students in clinical practice is closely related to managing their progress and making assessment decisions, and all are part of continuous assessment of practice. These activities are central to and essential in facilitating student learning to develop their proficiency in clinical practice. Feedback can and should occur on multiple occasions during a shift and throughout a placement.

This may be informally while the student learns alongside a mentor or practice supervisor or formally from a practice assessor at planned times during a placement. For most students, the aim is for assessment to be continuous and reflect the student's ability and progress over time and for assessment not based on individual set points. In some cases, for example, the end-point assessment for those on apprenticeship programmes, a formal assessment is needed. Likewise, achievement of some nursing proficiencies will require specific assessment, as will assessment of clinical competence assessed through objective structured clinical examinations, and feedback may be linked to debriefing exercises. Formal feedback to support learning in this way is discussed further in Chapter 6.

Mentors and practice supervisors are in a unique position to provide precise feedback to individual students on all aspects of practical professional development. As a mentor or supervisor 'you have the unique opportunity to role model the professional values and behaviours and to instill professional integrity. This includes professional socialization and the promotion of positive values, attitudes behaviours, cultural variances and inclusivity (Royal College of Nursing 2017).

If assessment is to be a true learning process, then the student needs to be an equal partner with progress monitored jointly against expectations that are clear and where there is full transparency about the assessment decision. Self-assessment by the student is, therefore, also needed as part of the process, and it is important that these activities occur not only to maintain the integrity of the assessment process itself, but also to meet the rights of the student as a student (Earl 2013).

This chapter considers the roles, functions and responsibilities of both informal mentors, recognized practice supervisors and formal practice assessors in giving feedback, monitoring progress and how they can use colleagues from within clinical teams and from practice educators and link lecturers to manage assessment issues and make assessment decisions.

MANAGING FEEDBACK

"Managing feedback" is used in this chapter to describe the activity of holding constructive discussions with the student about clinical experiences in which the student and the supervisor have been involved. Feedback can take place informally as the supervisor works alongside the student, more formally during prearranged feedback sessions at set times (e.g., midplacement) or, for those on apprenticeship programmes, as part of formal tripartite reviews. Walsh (2014) considers that feedback is a vitally important aspect of supporting a student and that this vital aspect is not always well sustained—feedback is either not done well or as frequently as needed or, worse still, not given at all (Fig. 7.1) (Neary 2001, Clynes & Raftery, 2008). Fitzgerald and colleagues found that there

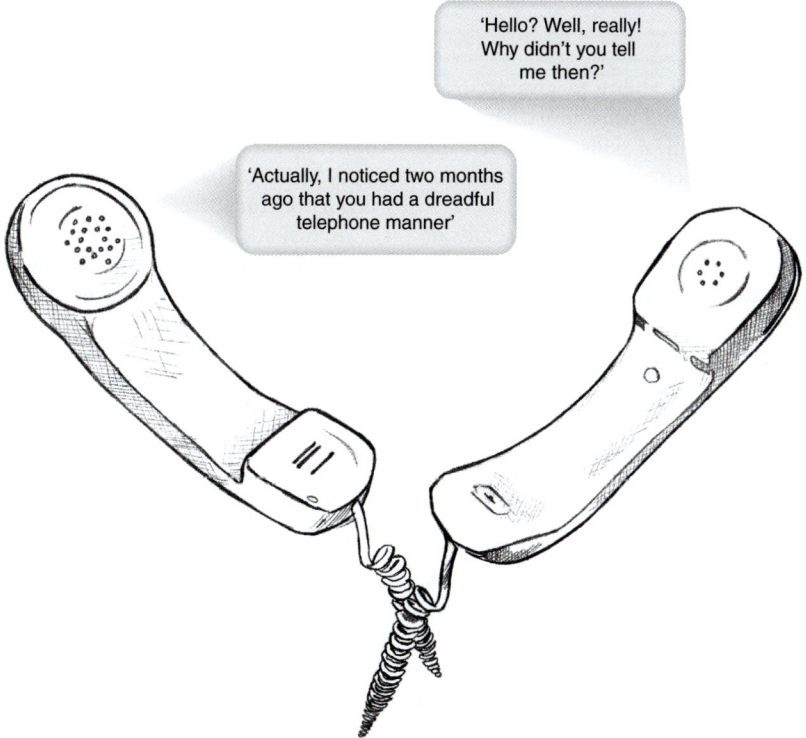

Fig. 7.1 Often, feedback is not done well or as frequently as needed, or not at all.

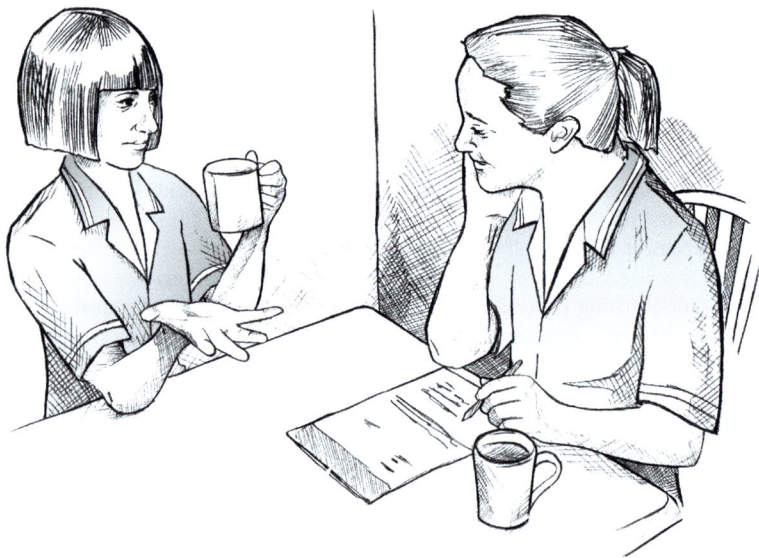

SMILE, LISTEN,
COMMUNICATE,
CLARIFY, COMMIT

Fig. 7.2 Smile, make eye contact and listen to the student.

was 'inconsistency and a lack of ability to give accurate feedback on professional values and behaviours. This is in contrast to the feedback on clinical skills - in which the mentors appeared to be in agreement, with written comments' (Fitzgerald, Gibson & Gunn, 2010:158).

As noted in Chapter 6, it is knowledge of the results of performance provided by detailed factual constructive feedback that enables students to monitor their strengths and weaknesses in performance so that aspects associated with success or good quality care can be recognized and reinforced and unsatisfactory aspects can be changed or improved. Feedback therefore contributes directly to learning through the process of formative assessment.

Constructive feedback has an impact on the teaching and learning process. It also gives messages to students about how their contribution to care is respected, their effectiveness and their worth or self-esteem. Self-esteem is a complex phenomenon which involves both the individual's belief about their competence and feelings, attitudes and beliefs about their worth and, importantly, how these both relate to each other (Mruk 2013).

'Self-esteem has two interrelated aspects: it entails a sense of personal efficacy and a sense of personal worth. It is the integrated sum of self-confidence and self-respect. It is the conviction that one is competent to live and worthy of living' (Branden 1966:110 in Mruk 2013)

Achieving a balance between these crucial components is essential for successful learning.

A major determinant of self-esteem is feedback from significant others. Consequently, students look to and indeed expect and welcome, constructive feedback from their teachers and assessors (Neary 2001, Embo et al 2010) and also from their peers (Rohatinsky, Harding & Carriere,2017, Vandal et al 2018) and look to friends and family for support (Royal College of Nursing 2008). What we know about the effects of assessment on motivation tells us that students give up trying if they do not see themselves as capable of success. If they feel relatively worthless and ineffectual, they will reduce their effort or give up altogether when work is difficult. On the other hand, people who hold positive self-perceptions usually try harder and persist longer when faced with difficult or challenging tasks (Valizadeh et al 2016).

There are therefore many challenges for the assessor or supervisor with regard to how to manage feedback so that it has a positive impact on the self-esteem of the student and importantly their learning.

Managing Feedback Sessions

The following factors are suggested when proposing and setting up feedback sessions:

- Timing of the feedback session;
- Format of the session;
- The student's self-assessment;
- Who should be involved;
- Feedback and the need for "feed forward"

Timing

Feedback will have maximal motivational impact on learning if it takes place while the topic or activity is still recent and therefore still relevant; points and issues raised are therefore more meaningful and alive (Duffy 2013), and the event and its details are fresh and accessible to memory and not distorted with time. In the clinical setting, if appropriate, this could take place as a running commentary while the student is performing the task or as soon as possible after the event. Thus feedback can be offered on aspects of practice that are observed by the supervisor. This opportunistic feedback will, in this way, be situation specific, which ensures that important elements are included. In addition, this can prompt discussion and demonstrations as to how theory is related to practice.

Prompt and timely feedback gives the student the opportunity to act upon feedback as soon as possible to improve future performance. A quote from a first-year student nurse in Neary's study illustrates this point:

'I was nervous because [supervisor] worked with me all week and right away she told me where I was going wrong. She responded quickly by helping me to understand what I needed to learn. [Supervisor] did not waste any time in telling me how and what to do. I like that, I know where I need to improve … I can respond to this level of feedback. I feel more confident now; I can get on with the job.' (Neary 2001:8)

The supervisor who works alongside the student should take advantage of this unique position in being able to offer accurate and timely feedback on all aspects of learning; opportunistic feedback is a vital element of the clinical learning experience.

Feedback sessions after the event will be more beneficial if the supervisor takes responsibility for making time available and arranging a suitable venue. It will not be conducive for engaging in constructive feedback if either the supervisor or the student is still preoccupied with activities in the clinical area. The session may then prove to be counterproductive. Remember that feedback must be timely to give the student enough time and opportunities to improve.

Format

The format can be oral or written or both. Students usually look for both; however, there is little evidence about how students use written feedback and how effective it is for their learning (Glies, Gilbert & McNeill 2013). Written notes are essential in providing continuity in the monitoring of progress and are usually provided in a standardized form as part of the students' practice assessment document (PAD). When written notes are kept, valuable details of the situation are not forgotten, which increases the potential for learning. With the continuous assessment process, which governs the management of preregistration health care students, written records of sessions reviewing progress are required. Constructive feedback sessions may be used to review progress formally and written records kept to monitor and demonstrate progress.

Student Self-Assessment

The importance of asking for the student's self-assessment before giving feedback cannot be underestimated because it provides the supervisor or educators with valuable insights into the student's own perceptions of performance and learning (Earl 2013). Self-assessment by the student will be linked to opportunities to reflect on practice (Bulman & Schutz, 2013). The process of delivering constructive feedback is considerably easier when personal practice limitations are identified by the student. There is more detailed discussion on student self-assessment in the sections on formative assessment in Chapter 6 and the section 'Discussion with the student' later.

Who Should be Involved?

A number of different people are likely to be involved in student supervision, both in a formal and informal manner. It is therefore likely that students will receive feedback from members of their own profession but also from others in the multidisciplinary team. Equally, formal arrangements, such as in nursing, where there is a separation of practice supervision, practice assessment and academic assessment, mean that feedback will be from different people. It is important for students that feedback is consistent and that it is based on observation of proficiencies and skills. The Nursing and Midwifery Council's (NMC) standards state that:

'there are sufficient opportunities for the practice assessor to gather and coordinate feedback from practice supervisors, any other practice assessors, and relevant people, to be assured about their decisions for assessment and progression' (NMC 2018:7.7:9)

BOX 7.1 Suggestions for Effective Feedback

Characteristics of Effective Feedback	Suggested Applications
Create an accepting environment	Use nonjudgemental language and normalise mistakes as a normal part of learning.
	Make feedback an expected part of learning and day-to-day working.
Focus on behaviours	Emphasise personal, direct observations of the student's practice.
	Limit to behaviours amenable to change.
Be specific	Relate to learning goals (goal oriented).
	Focus on performance of proficiencies and skills (task specific).
Compare with a standard	Inform the learner of basic competency requirements related to their stage of learning and placement requirements.
	Provide the anticipated trajectory toward achieving the competency or skills.
Be timely	Give feedback immediately after clinical interactions.
Give the appropriate amount	Limit to clearly defined learning targets.
	Don't overwhelm the student.
Encourage self-directed learning	Involve the student in setting goals.
	Provide time for learner self-reflection.
	Encourage interests to help motivate the student.

Gather feedback from your students Attempt to improve your own skill in providing feedback.
(Modified from Lara RF, Mogensen KM, Markuns JF. Effective feedback in the education of health professionals, Support Line, 2016;38(2):3–8.)

Feed Forward

Feedback should be specific (Duffy 2013) and based on behaviours. There is also a need to feed forward, placing the feedback in the context of what the student should aim for and setting clear expectations for ongoing learning.

> 'Feed forward is equally important to learners' progress. Although feedback focuses on current performance (and may simply justify the grade awarded), feed forward looks ahead to the next assignment. Feed forward offers constructive guidance on how to improve. A combination of feedback and feed forward ensures that assessment has an effective developmental impact on learning.' (Ferrell & Gray 2013)

It is essential that constructive feedback is managed systematically. Box 7.1 contains suggestions for effective feedback, which summarize this section.

MONITORING PROGRESS

Monitoring the progress of students is an essential part of the continuous assessment process. Progress can be monitored more accurately if there is continuity of supervision by the same practice supervisor and assessor. The NMC has grappled with the practicality of this concept in developing the current standards for nursing education (NMC 2018c). During the consultation stage, it was suggested that the same practice assessor should oversee a whole "part" of the student's programme (in reality, often a year of the course). However, during the consultation, it became apparent that with different practice placements and high turnover of staff in some clinical areas, this might be difficult to achieve. Likewise, with allied health students, continuity is often maintained through close liaison between practice and university. In some instances, continuity of practice assessor can be achieved with "hub-and-spoke" placements where the practice assessor in the student's main placement retains an overview of progress when the students completes alternative or complementary practice placements. This is particularly the case for students following an apprenticeship route where they retain a link with their main workplace throughout the programme.

The advantage is that the same practice assessor is able to keep abreast of the clinical activities the student has had exposure to, how these relate to current experience and then looking forward the interrelationships with complementary or alternative upcoming placements. This enables a better assessment of how the student is developing and thus their progress.

Clinical practice placements provide a dynamic situation in which learning can be achieved. Monitoring of progress needs to be seen in this learning context and not as "policing", so students see that learning is paramount. For this to happen, it is important that practice assessors keep track of whether the student is developing competence and achieving the competencies, proficiencies and skills set out by the professional regulators (Health and Care Professions Council [HCPC] 2017a, NMC 2018a). Practice assessors should consider carefully what the student is learning, the clinical activities the student has participated in and how further learning can be facilitated. When monitoring progress it is important to consider:

- Prior clinical experiences of the student;
- The learning outcomes and competencies, proficiencies or clinical skills the student needs to achieve; and
- The stage of the programme the student is at.

Examples of ways in which a practice assessor can ensure they address these key factors are shown in Fig. 7.3.

Developing Levels of Competence

Chapter 4 includes a detailed discussion of how observation may be used as a method of assessment to obtain direct evidence of the ability to perform health care activities. When monitoring the progress of students during observation in the clinical environment mentors or practice, supervisors need to gather evidence of:

- continuing safe and accurate performance of practice;
- increasing speed and dexterity in clinical procedures;
- increasing confidence gained through ever greater clinical experience;
- the development of proficiency during the placement.

Well-established research in education, nursing and health care fields clearly shows that there are recognized characteristics that differentiate the performance of expert practitioners from novices or beginners (Benner 1984, Glaser 1990, Benner, Tanner & Chesla 1996), and this is also true in the development of preregistration students throughout the 3 or 4 years of their respective programmes.

From Novice to Expert

Drawing on Dreyfus' model, Benner's (1984) work has become well known in nursing and provides an authoritative framework to consider progress against. It has also been used in other health care fields. The Dreyfus model (in Benner 1984) considers that a student passes through five levels of proficiency: novice, advanced beginner, competent, proficient and expert. As a student passes through these levels, there are corresponding changes in three general aspects of performance. First, there is a move away from reliance on rules and principles to the use of past experience to guide practice. Secondly, the student begins to see a situation less and less as a combination of equally relevant elements and more and more as a complete whole in which only certain parts are relevant. Thirdly, the student becomes an involved performer and engages in the situation.

Relating this to student development and as a framework for feedback the first three levels become pertinent as the student develops from novice through advanced beginner to competent (Fig. 7.4).

The Novice

- Students enter a new clinical area as novices with no experience of the situations in which they are expected to perform.
- They must be given rules and explicit detailed instructions to guide their performance, for example, procedural lists.
- They focus on getting individual tasks done; novices generally do not see beyond the task at hand and may not recognize any of the underlying problems exhibited by the patient.

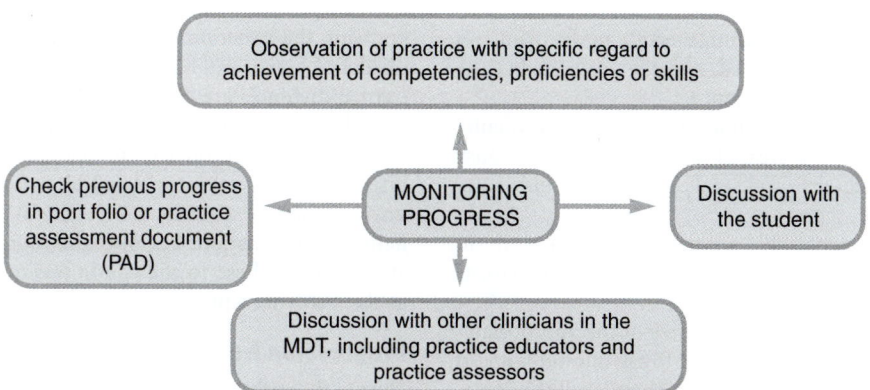

Fig. 7.3 Key assessment activities to monitor progress.

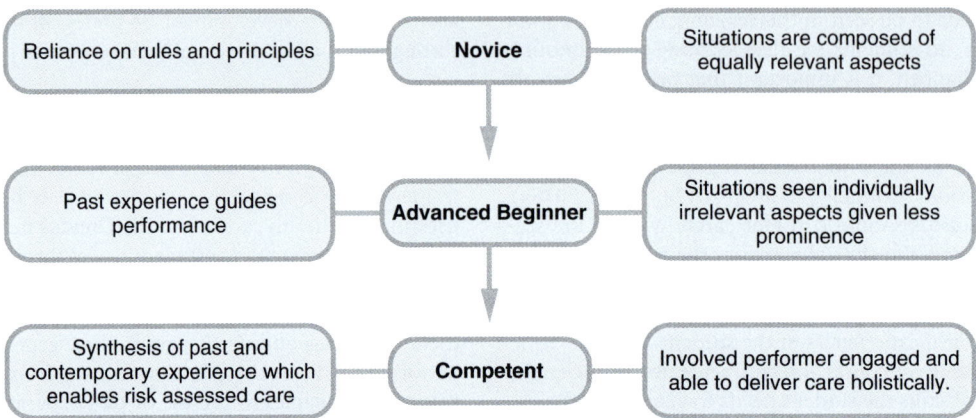

Fig. 7.4 Student development based on Benner's concepts.

- They have little understanding of how to use classroom-acquired theory to guide practice.

The Advanced Beginner
- The advanced beginner can demonstrate marginally acceptable performance.
- As a result of prior experiences, they are able to identify the recurring components of situations but are unable yet to sort out what is most important.
- They cannot order information into a meaningful whole.
- Their concern for good care is almost exclusively related to physical and technological support and to completing all the ordered treatment and procedures.

Competent
- Competent students have increased clinical understanding and are able to focus on the clinical condition and management of the 'whole' client/patient and less on getting tasks done.
- They have increased technical skill; performance is more fluid and coordinated, and they can predict the outcomes of their performance.
- They also have more accuracy at judging the difficulty of a task, with increased ability to handle busy complex situations and make decisions and solve problems.
- Time management skills are developed sufficiently to organize their workload, prioritize care and manage care for several patients.
- They will have increased awareness of the appropriateness of their actions and are able to ask questions about what they have to do to improve their level of competence.

Knowledge Base
Glaser (1990) notes that, as competence in a domain grows, the person displays a knowledge base that is increasingly coherent and useful. The characteristics underpinning these descriptors are described briefly here.

The Coherence of Knowledge
The beginner's knowledge demonstrates superficial understanding: only fragments of information can be accessed for use. Knowledge consists of isolated definitions and superficial understandings.

As competence develops, elements of knowledge are integrated with past organizations of knowledge so that information becomes increasingly interconnected and structured: knowledge gets retrieved in larger units from memory. Proficient individuals are able to access "chunks" rather than fragments of information from memory.

Usable Knowledge
Novices generally possess theoretical knowledge without knowing the situations where that knowledge can be applied and how it can be used most effectively. More proficient individuals are able to understand the relevance of their knowledge and thus access relevant knowledge to inform practice. Proficient individuals are able to make inferences based on interrelated information. Experts and novices may be equally competent at recalling specific items of information, but only the more experienced are able to relate these to the conditions of practice and the goals of solving a problem.

Progression from Novice to Competent Practice
During the early stages of an undergraduate programme, a student who is new to a clinical area is likely to start

practice at the novice level but may achieve competent practice in some aspects of care by the end of the placement. The rate of progression is dependent on many factors, such as opportunities for practice, debriefing and reflection with the supervisor and prior experience of the student. In each new clinical area, the less experienced student may perform at novice level for a longer period before advancing. The more experienced student, who may have been to similar clinical areas, however, would be able to, and indeed would be expected to, move more rapidly to advanced beginner and competent level practice. Remember that the change from the novice level to competent level is incremental (Benner, Tanner & Chesla 1996) and on a continuum.

It is a requirement of preregistration education to prepare students to be able to apply knowledge, understanding and skills to meet the standards for registration (and for employment) at the end of the programme with practice that is safe and effective. It is suggested here that the ability to perform at the competent level is the appropriate level to enable the student to achieve the requirements of the professional body–expected education, and to enable them to make the transition to registered practitioner. The criteria for assessing competent level practice should thus be used when monitoring the progress and assessing the practice of students who are at the stage of being prepared for professional practice. This period of practice will assist the student to start to make the transition from student to registered practitioner.

Levels of Supervision and Support

When monitoring the progress and assessing the practice of students, consider the amount and level of supervision/support required by the student as well as the amount and level of participation in care you expect of the student. When students are at the novice level, they should initially observe care followed by participating and assisting in giving care. When giving care, they should be supervised closely and be supported. Students at the novice level, as discussed earlier, will require detailed and explicit instructions initially and may not be able to explain the rationale underpinning practice. As they learn and progress in their practice, less prompting is required for practised activities, and they should be able to explain the rationale underpinning their actions.

As students progress, encourage them to participate more actively, which includes joint planning of activities. They should also be allowed to lead those activities they are confident in performing. The transition from novice-level practice to advanced beginner level is on a continuum. The amount of supervision required starts to decrease, and supervisors may be able to 'let go' as they learn to trust the performance of the students. From performance that requires to be prompted because it lacks completeness, performance starts to become smooth and complete as students start to internalize the activities. Prompting is generally not required, and the rationale underpinning practice is understood.

As students move from advanced beginner level to competent-level practice, the amount of supervision required becomes minimal, with indirect supervision only required toward the end of the education programme. By this time, students will be taking an active role in giving care. They will be able to plan all practised activities and be leading most of them. They become organized and efficient and can carry out their own workload without having to be reminded about what to do.

Discussion with the Student

Talking, questioning and listening are crucial to monitoring progress and student assessment, and both informal and formal conversations can be used for ongoing review of the student's progress. There is a discussion of how questioning can be used to facilitate and assess student learning during clinical practice in Chapter 4. As the supervisor and student work together, inviting the student to suggest how best to carry out care in clinical situations in which the student has been involved previously will give the supervisor opportunities to consider what the student has learnt from similar past caregiving experiences. It will also provide the supervisor with information about the student's ongoing achievement. Whenever you spend time with your student in care activities, use every opportunity for discussions, with what is going on as the focus. What the student is able to articulate will indicate the amount of progress made. Subsequent discussion and questioning to explore further the quantity and quality of learning, and any difficulties the student may be having with performing particular care activities, will add to this source of evidence of student progression. Through discussion about a particular event, students can demonstrate the knowledge, understanding and values that have informed their actions in the clinical area on a given occasion. Sanzero-Eller et al found that open communication and accessibility was one of the key components of effective mentorship (Lucille Sanzero-Eller, Leva & Feure 2014). This enables the supervisor to ascertain the understanding and the values held by the student about the care given. Activity 1a refers you to a You-Tube talk by Celeste Headlee based on her research, which is also available in a book (Headlee 2017). In this short talk (10 mins), 10 suggestions are made to improve conversations based on social science research, which are pertinent to feedback conversations you may have with students. There is further discussion of using dialogue as a vehicle for preactivity discussion and postevent reflection in Chapter 9.

Activity 7.1   10 Ways to Have Better Feedback Conversations With Students

Celeste Headlee (Headlee 2015) makes the following 10 suggestions for ways to have better conversations. Access and listen to her present these in a You-tube TEDx talk available online.

1. Don't multitask—be present in the conversation and not distracted.
2. Don't pontificate—assume you have something to learn from the student, not just them from you.
3. Use open-ended questions—Who? What? Why? When? How?
4. Go with the flow—consider what is important for the student and how they respond.
5. If you don't know, then say so.
6. Don't equate your experience with theirs – it is never the same; all experiences are individual;
7. Try not to repeat yourself—do not make the same point over and over again.
8. "Stay out of the weeds" —emphasise your main points, but don't stray into giving every minute detail, which can distract from your main message.
9. Listen—pay attention and listen to understand, not just to reply.
10. Be brief.
    - Throughout the talk, consider how each of the 10 points relate to the conversations you have with students as a practice supervisor or assessor.
    - Think about how these are pertinent to the way you give feedback to your students.

https://www.ted.com/talks/celeste_headlee_10_ways_to_have_a_better_conversation?language=en (accessed 21 June 2019)

Progress reviews should also include student self-assessment and constructive feedback from the supervisor. When engaging in self-assessment, students may need help in looking at themselves because they are to judge realistically what they could become while, at the same time, helping them to hold in mind the vision of how they would like to be, perhaps modelled on observations of more experienced practitioners. One aim of self-assessment should be to shift the focus from "how good am I?" to "how can I get better? (Nikos Mattheos et al 2004).

Supervisors should not assume that students are able to self-assess independently, and they should facilitate students' self-assessment of their competency and skills. On the other hand, students are generally aware of the standards against which to measure themselves, for example, by reference to the requirements of PADs based on required professional standards. These documents can be of great value because they appear to prompt students to apply ideas to their own practice and reflect on their learning. If assessments documents are lengthy, then it may be appropriate for mentors or supervisors to point students to specific parts of the document to help facilitate self-assessment about specific proficiencies or skills. This could be done before clinical activities and meeting sessions to discuss progress. Students can then use them to assess their own performance immediately after the clinical activity.

The crucial role of constructive feedback for learning is discussed at some length in Chapter 6. Feedback sessions can be designed to help students grow in their clinical skills and professional competence. Beginning-level students have been found to be anxious about their ability to perform basic clinical skills. They often fail to focus on the patient/client because they have to concentrate their attention on developing clinical skills, and so, feedback for these students should be designed to prompt them to think of the client holistically and to build self-confidence to enable the shift of focus to the patient/client. Advanced-level students, on the other hand, may feel confident about their clinical skills but anxious about becoming a fully-fledged professional in the near future. These students would benefit from feedback designed to promote the growth of professionalism and confidence in their professional personae to enable them to make the transition to registered practitioner.

Checking the Student's Practice Achievement Record

Records need to be kept and documentation made of students' achievements in practice. The terminology used for this document may vary between institutions, but commonly it is known as a practice assessment document and is often referred to in its abbreviated form as the students' PAD. This becomes part of the student's portfolio of learning, providing evidence of practice undertaken and demonstrating a student's fitness for practice. This ongoing achievement record should include comments from supervisors and practice assessors the student has worked with and must be passed from one placement to the next to enable judgements to be made on the student's progress.

Whatever document is used, the following principles will be evident to guide the student's learning and evidence achievement.

1. Ongoing information about the student's achievement of outcomes and learning through reflection, demonstrating the interrelationship of theory and practice

2. Cumulative information about the outcomes of assessment of practice

3. Evidence of rational decision-making and clinical judgement

4. A record of issues raised in discussion, including causes for concern between the supervisor, the student and the personal/ named lecturer as part of the formative process of development

5. A collection of the action plans or learning contracts agreed between supervisors, the student and the personal/ named lecturer

6. Information on key issues from the student's experience which will inform the preparation for subsequent clinical experience. These key issues should stem from student self-assessment and constructive feedback from the supervisor.

Recording Evidence

The use of different methods of assessment to gain a comprehensive picture of the skills, knowledge, attributes and attitudes (see Chapter 4) will clearly produce a comprehensive range of different kinds of evidence. If several methods are used on a day-to-day basis, it may become difficult to keep track of all the evidence that is produced. Even over a week, there will be more evidence than either the student or supervisor can remember, and memory is by its very nature selective. Different documents, as mentioned previously, may be used, but there are increasing calls for consistency and standardization, both for the benefit of students and for the mentors and supervisors recording evidence. In nursing, an initiative first adopted across London to have a universal PAD (Baillie et al 2016) has now spread across much of the UK. The document continues to meet the NMC standards (NMC 2018a), having first been validated in 2012 and subsequently updated in 2019. Now try Activity 7.2.

Some students, particularly those undertaking apprenticeships or support workers undertaking vocational qualifications, are encouraged to record details of achievement in an evidence log. This typically contains details of activities and achievement. Fig. 7.5 is an example of the evidence log of a student learning to undertake blood glucose measurements on a ward. This example of an evidence log compiled by a student indicates the occasions and types of medications administered and the aspects learned. It also shows the progress the student made. These evidence logs are usually filed with other documented evidence of learning in a portfolio. The maintenance of evidence of learning in this format will enable sufficient information of a student's ongoing achievement in practice to be available to supervisors, but importantly also for practice assessors, and for reviews involving students, practice and university educators (for example, tripartite reviews for apprentices).

The supervisor or cosupervisor may also provide written evidence logs of learning. Fig. 7.6 is an example of the evidence log kept by a supervisor in the operating theatre for an ODP (operating department practitioner) student. This evidence log shows the areas of difficulties experienced by the student and the facilitation of further learning, which led to progress and subsequent achievement of learning outcomes. It is, of course, not possible or feasible to compile evidence logs of every learning task, but crucial aspects of learning can be identified in each clinical area so that such logs of learning can be compiled. There should, however, be an accumulation of sufficient evidence for a valid assessment to be made on whether a student is competent at the point of registration (HCPC 2017a, NMC 2018a).

Discussions Between Practice Supervisors and Assessors

It is not always possible for the named supervisor to work with the student on every shift, and at times, it is advantageous for the student to work alongside other members of the multiprofessional team. However, feedback from supervisors and assessment decisions (e.g., in nursing by a different practice assessor) require enough of those involved to have observed the student's practice on sufficient occasions to monitor the progress of the student with validity and reliability. It is important and only fair to the student that both supervisors and assessors seek the views of other practitioners who have worked with the student and are consistent in their feedback. This needs to be managed within the real-world busyness of clinical practice. Myall et al (2008) reported that although most students were able to work with their supervisors for the majority of their clinical placement, others were spending less than the recommended amount of time with them (Myall, Levett-Jones & Lathlean 2008). Assessment should be a team effort to obtain a stronger and wider evidence base on which formative and summative assessments may be made. Good assessment practice would include the following actions:

• assessment should include discussion that occurs as part of the working day;

• evidence and issues should be contributed, where possible, by all members of the team, including the student;

• routine meetings such as handovers, case conferences or some other ward or team event should be used.

When discussing the performance and ongoing achievement of students as part of the process of monitoring

16.12.18 – 11.30 hours

Today I was asked to perform a blood glucose recording, on a 72-year-old gentleman; we chatted away, while I explained the procedure to him. He was quite *au fait* with what was happening, having been diabetic for some years. Between us we chose the finger which I would be pricking. I gathered the equipment I needed, washed my hands and put on some gloves. I carried out the procedure as I have been taught. I chatted to this gentleman throughout the procedure giving reassurance. I discarded all the used equipment in the appropriate places. After washing my hands and recording the measurement, I checked that the gentleman was alright and the site was not bleeding.

21.12.18 – 13.50 hours

This afternoon I was asked by staff to perform a blood glucose measurement on a young lady; having explained to her what I was going to do, she appeared quite relaxed about it. After gathering the equipment that I needed, I washed my hands and put on gloves. After I pricked her finger, she bled a little more than usual, I asked her to press on with the cotton wool I had given her and assured her it would stop shortly, as it did, by the time I had timed the reading, which was within normal range, recorded the measurement and informed the staff nurse.

I discarded all the used equipment in the sharps bin, washed my hands, and checked once more that the lady was feeling alright, she said her finger was a little sore.

21.1.19

I gathered together the equipment that I needed to perform a blood glucose test on a 75-year-old client. I washed my hands and put on some gloves. I then explained to him what I was going to do. I pricked his finger with an autolet pen, drew enough blood to cover the teststix and gave him some cotton wool to hold on the bleeding point.

After 1 min I wiped the end of the stick with cotton wool and waited a further minute, then recorded the result on the chart and told staff nurse what it was. I cleared away all the equipment and disposed of it in the appropriate places, and washed my hands.

I asked the gentleman if he was alright and checked that the bleeding had stopped.

Reflection

Today I performed a blood glucose test on a 75-year-old gentleman. Having known this gentleman for quite some time, as he has been staying with us for a while, I felt comfortable in performing this task. He, too, I think had confidence in me. I felt bad about having to stab his finger and maybe cause him pain, but this didn't seem to bother him too much. Having completed the test, recorded the outcome and passed on the information to staff nurse, I made sure that the gentleman was alright with the procedure and the bleeding had stopped and he was comfortable.

Fig. 7.5 Evidence log compiled by a student.

Date	Clinical Activites and Teaching/Learning Support
27.10.18	Difficulty with scrub technique. Trolley setting met performance criteria. Asepsis and uses of equipment discussed using question and answer with prompting from observer
	Discussed time for private study to review asepsis policy. Scrub poster and policy manual used to discuss equipment
2.11.18	Difficulty with scrub technique Trolley setting satisfactorily met performance criteria
	Highlighted scrub technique as major problem. Further session to be instigated
2.11.18	Practised scrub technique – applying gloves and gown
4.11.18	Practised scrub technique and applying gloves and gown. Improvement made
9.11.18	Improvement in scrub technique. Trolley setting satisfactory. Standard achieved. Further practice required. Asepsis and equipment usage discussed
13.11.18	Demonstrating competent performance. All learning outcomes achieved

Fig. 7.6 Evidence log compiled by the supervisor.

progress, consider whether the quality and quantity of clinical experiences the student has had are sufficient to enable development and therefore progress. Knowledge of the length of the placement, and the stage of education the student is at, will assist supervisors in deciding how much progression, within and across each of the levels (novice, advanced beginner, competent), can be expected.

MAKING ASSESSMENT DECISIONS

Formative Assessment—is the Student Progressing?

As discussed previously, the assessment activities of working alongside the student and observing practice, discussion with the student and checking the student's ongoing achievement record or portfolio and discussion with other supervisors are done both informally and formally to monitor progress. During the formal sessions, which should be planned and timetabled, the supervisor should formally review with the student the progress made and identify any difficulties at an earlier, rather than a later, stage of the placement. The number of formal progress review meetings you hold altogether during the student's placement would be dependent on the length of the placement and the progress the student is making, but typically, at least an initial and midpoint meeting are recommended. To enable a student to progress as a guide, you should consider holding a formal progress review session at least every two weeks. To decide whether the student is progressing, ask the following questions:

- Is the student achieving the required expected competencies or proficiencies?
- Is there a demonstration of a growing level of skill?
- Is performance consistent?
- Is there a demonstration of a growing understanding of the rationale underpinning practice?
- Is there a demonstration of development of the attitudes and values appropriate to professional practice?
- Is there a demonstration of a developing ability to engage in evidence-based and reflective practice?

Remember that the level of competence of new students can vary considerably because this is dependent on the opportunities they had during their education. During formative assessments, check that students are being provided with learning opportunities to enable the achievement of their learning outcomes. It is important for supervisors to remember that many factors can affect a student's progress and to explore reasons for the student's difficulties. Any judgement of a student's capabilities must consider the circumstances in which that student is performing.

Summative Assessment—Should the Student be Passed?

All assessments involve complex decision making where assessors must weigh the balance between different aspects of care. Providing a summative assessment, usually at the end of a student's placement, will require the assessor to consider evidence and to judge a student has met all the required criteria to provide an overall pass or fail grade.

A final meeting/discussion session should be arranged to take place during the last week of the student's placement. Additional time should be allocated to review and analyze fully the evidence of achievement, and time must be set aside for supervisors and assessors to liaise before meeting with the student. The meeting with the student should allow sufficient time to reflect, give feedback and complete the required records.

The following questions may assist in helping you judge and analyse evidence to establish whether there is sufficient assessment evidence to confer competence or successful achievement of proficiencies and skills. However you should be careful that responses to these questions alone do not influence your decision but instead back up and provide a sense check on the student's practice that you have already observed.

1. Has the Student Achieved the Expected Competencies?

Examine the student's assessment of practice document, which will contain the expected competencies and skills for the stage of the programme the student is at. All courses leading to registration with a professional body in the UK (whether as a nurse, midwife or allied health professional) will have been validated jointly by the professional regulator and the relevant university, and this will have included scrutiny of practice documents to ensure they are aligned with the requirements laid down by the professional body. In the UK, nursing and midwifery students must meet the progression criteria at progression points at the end of each part of the course, typically aligning with the end of year 1 and year 2, as well as at the end of the programme (NMC 2018c).

The NMC (2018a), and, likewise, the HCPC (2017a), require students, on qualification, to be able to practise safely and effectively without the need for supervision. If these education requirements are to be realised, it is generally accepted that only competent or not competent judgements can be made rather than a specific grade awarded. This has been the subject of debate over the past 30 years across many disciplines (Newton 2018), with moves from overall competency-based (pass/fail) assessments to more sophisticated standards-referenced assessments such as those used by the NMC and HCPC (HCPC, 2017a, NMC 2018b) and for a continuum or progression in learning to be recognised. The relative ease in grading theory compared with practice is accepted, and this has led to dual-outcome reporting (Newton 2018), with, for example, competence in practice and a degree classification based on

theory grades. Using the prespecified levels of supervision and practice (see Chapter 6), and conditions of practice discussed earlier in this chapter, criteria are put forward (Fig. 7.7) to help conceptualize the distinction between competent or not competent decisions as students progress. Levels 4, 5 and 6 (QAA 2014) correspond to students during years 1, 2 and 3 of a typical

LEVEL 4

Competence Achieved

Close supervision required

Participates and assists in care

Performs with few prompts

Can explain the rationale underpinning practice

Competence NOT Achieved

Direct supervision required

Has difficulty participating and assisting in care

Requires detailed and explicit instructions

Cannot explain the rationale underpinning practice

LEVEL 5

Competence Achieved

Minimal supervision required

Active participation in care

Beginning to prioritize care

Planning most activities and leading some

Performance is smooth and complete

Does not require prompting

Can explain rationale underpinning practice and
     discuss pertinent research

Competence NOT Achieved

Close supervision required

Participates and assists in care

Performance lacks completeness

Requires to be prompted

Cannot explain rationale underpinning practice

LEVEL 6

Competence Achieved

Indirect supervision required

Active participation in care

Planning all activities and leading most

Does not require prompting

Is organized and efficient

Is able to prioritize care

Critiques evidence-based practice and its implementation

Competence NOT Achieved

Close supervision required

Participates and assists in care only

Requires prompting

Unable to organize care

Does not consider evidence-based practice

Fig. 7.7 Criteria for assessing the achievement of clinical competence.

preregistration programme, respectively. However, actual decisions need to be made against detailed criteria within professional standards.

2. Is the Assessment Evidence Reliable and Valid?

Examine the student's practice document or portfolio. Has the student engaged in a sufficient number and range of care situations for you to be confident that validity has been achieved? And has the student demonstrated proficiency or skills on a number of occasions to suggest reliability and consistency? Does the student have the ability to actually care for patients? Remember that the narrower the base of evidence for the inference of competence, the less generalizable it will be to the performance of other tasks.

You need to consider whether there is sufficient performance evidence to confer competent practice. Performance evidence would have been gathered by the supervisor throughout the period of supervised practice and also generated from the testimonies provided by other members of the team. The NMC recommends that all assessments must be supported by a diverse and reliable evidence base (NMC 2019). Sources of evidence may include (NMC 2019):

- Direct observation of the student
- Communication with practice supervisors
- Student documentation, such as a PAD or ongoing record of achievement
- Communication with any other practice assessors
- Communication with anyone else who may be involved in the education of the student
- Communication with the academic assessor
- Student self-reflection
- Communication and an ongoing relationship with the student

Box 7.2 details the NMC and HCPC standards that relate to evidence-based assessment. Further information and guidance is also available from both regulators about how to apply and interpret their standards (HCPC 2017b, NMC 2019). The reader is referred to Chapter 5 for a discussion of validity.

3. Is there Sound Understanding of the Rationale?

Knowledge and understanding underpin competent practice. Students must be able to demonstrate that they understand the rationale for care activities. It is likely that the supervisor will have assessed the student's understanding through the use of questioning throughout the period of formative assessment. This may require supplementation through further questioning when assessment evidence is being reviewed and analysed. Additionally, at level 5, can the student discuss pertinent research underpinning evidence-based practice? Further, at level 6, can the student

---

> **BOX 7.2 Evidenced-Based Assessment: Nursing and Midwifery Council and Health and Care Professions Council Standards**
>
> Within the Nursing and Midwifery Council (NMC) and Health and Care Professions Council (HCPC) standards, the following criteria relate to evidence-based assessments:
>
> **NMC Standards**
> Approved education institutions, together with practice partners, must ensure that:
> - Practice assessors make and record objective, evidenced-based assessments on conduct, proficiency and achievement, drawing on student records, direct observations, student self-reflection and other resources (NMC 2018c: 7.3).
> - Practice assessors have an understanding of the student's learning and achievement in theory (NMC 2018c: 7.8).
> - Students are assessed across practice settings and learning environments as required by their programme (NMC 2018c: 5.10).
> - Practice assessment is facilitated and evidenced by observations and other appropriate methods (NMC 2018c: 5.12).
> - Students' self-reflections contribute to, and are evidenced in, assessments (NMC 2018c: 5.13).
>   - A range of people, including service users, contribute to student assessment (NMC 2018c: 5.14).
>
> **HCPC Standards**
> - Assessment throughout the programme must ensure that learners demonstrate they are able to meet the expectations of professional behaviour, including the standards of conduct, performance and ethics (HCPC, 2017a: 6.2).
> - Assessments must provide an objective, fair and reliable measure of learners' progression and achievement (HCPC, 2017a: 6.3).
> - The assessment methods used must be appropriate to and effective at measuring the learning outcomes (HCPC, 2017a: 6.5).

discuss and critique pertinent research underpinning evidence-based practice?

4. Is the Student Developing the Attitudes and Values Appropriate to Professional Practice?

Before being accepted as a student in either nursing or the health professions, potential candidates are now assessed through a values-based recruitment process (Health Education England 2016), which is described in more detail in Chapter 1. Throughout their studies, professional socialisation will continue, with attitudes and beliefs being refined and remodelled as the professional practitioner is developed.

The assessment of attitudes and values is not easy. Although several methods of assessment can be used to 'assess' the attitudes and values of another (see Chapter 4), it nevertheless leaves this crucial aspect of competent professional practice open to personal biases and subjectiveness. It is important that you are aware of the potential for unconscious bias to influence your assessment. There has been increasing attention with regard to unconscious bias affecting progression and employment opportunities in nursing and physiotherapy students from Black, Asian and minority ethnic backgrounds (BAME) (Hammond et al 2017). However, because of the challenges of assessing values, it also stands in danger of not being assessed at all (Miller 2010). Miller proposes that clustering the various affective issues under the headings of "presentation", "preparedness" and "interaction" may assist nursing students to understand what is required of them and may aid clinical educators and preceptors in assessing the student.

A tool termed the *professional behaviours inventory* to assess prespecified behaviours expected of a professional exhibiting the accepted conduct of practitioner is proposed in Chapter 3. These behaviours are assumed to be underpinned by the attitudes, values and beliefs of the person. The use of such a tool is likely to assist the assessor in being more objective.

MANAGING ASSESSMENT ISSUES

Students Experiencing Problems Learning During Clinical Practice: The Unsafe Student

Students who experience problems learning during clinical practice are a cause for concern because they are unsafe (Luhanga, Yonge & Myrick 2008). They use and defined the term *unsafe student* to refer to: "students whose level of clinical practice is questionable regarding safety, and who exhibit marked deficits in knowledge and psychomotor skills, motivation, or *interpersonal* skills … [unsafe clinical practice is] any act by the student that is harmful or potentially detrimental to the client, self, or other health personnel." (Luhanga, Yonge & Myrick, 2008:1).

They go on to state that a grave issue in these situations is that of giving the student the benefit of the doubt and failing to fail these students (e.g., see Dudek, Marks & Regehr 2005, Scholes & Albarran 2005, Luhanga, Yonge & Myrick 2008, Jervis & Tilki 2011, Duffy 2013, Hunt et al 2016b, Cassidy, Coffey & Murphy, 2017, Adkins and Aucoin 2022).

Any student who is either not progressing or failing to meet the required standard needs to be identified by assessment systems so that opportunities can be provided for that student to improve. It is suggested here that the use of the assessment activities to monitor progress discussed earlier in this chapter will help the supervisor to identify those students who require extra help and support. A number of authors (e.g., see Scholes & Albarran 2005, Luhanga, Yonge & Myrick 2008, Hunt et al 2016b, Cassidy, Coffey & Murphy 2017, Davenport et al 2018) provide some criteria for recognising these students early. They remind us that, although some of these behaviours are exhibited by many students at some time during clinical practice, the student who is either not progressing or failing exhibits these behaviours to such a degree and extent that learning is interrupted. These behaviours are listed here:

- Inconsistent in meeting the required level of competence for the expected stage of education; lacks practical skills, for example, care is not complete, patients are not left comfortable or the student may avoid direct patient contact and/or spend excessive time in distractions away from the client/patient;
- Lacks caution and is not careful;
- Inconsistent in clinical performance;
- Does not respond appropriately to constructive feedback and appears unable to make changes in response to feedback—therefore, clinical skills do not improve;
- Poor preparation and organizational skills for example, if doing a handover or on a ward round may be unable to respond to questioning;
- Limited interactional and poor communication skills with patients/clients and with team members; fails to ask questions
- Continual poor health perhaps exhibited by multiple short (1- to 2-day) sicknesses and showing signs or stating feelings of depression, anger, withdrawal, sadness, tiredness or high levels of anxiety;
- Uncommitted and unenthusiastic; may dismiss certain learning opportunities with the rationale of having done that before and not wanting repetition;
- Unethical behaviour, for example, failure to disclose and discuss clinical errors because this jeopardizes the communication needed for safe care—when challenged, is defensive with a range of excuses rather than embrace a culture of challenge and support;
- Poor punctuality and frequent changes requested to duty pattern (shifts) to avoid working with the allocated supervisor.

How can the supervisor manage the situation when a student is either not progressing or failing? In Chapter 2, there is a discussion of the professional responsibility and accountability of the supervisor in these situations. It is acknowledged here that people are generally reluctant to pass negative judgements on fellow workers. Supervisors also experience the handling of the assessment of weak students as great challenges, both professionally and personally (Luhanga, Yonge & Myrick 2008, Duffy 2013, Cassidy, Coffey & Murphy 2017). However, the implications of poor/unsafe students "slipping through the net" to become registered practitioners are grave because a minority of incompetent professionals can do untold damage. Appropriate management includes using intelligence, sensitivity, understanding and insight when dealing with these students. It is reiterated here that the use of the strategy of triangulation to collect assessment evidence (see Chapter 4) will increase the confidence of the practice supervisor or assessor when dealing with these students. Although the following plan of action is offered, the supervisor should be clear of the policy laid down by the higher education institution of the student for dealing with these situations so that the correct procedure is followed:

- Arrange to have a meeting with the student as soon as possible. Explain the reason for the meeting to the student.
- Consider and discuss the evidence that has led to concern. Give honest, unambiguous feedback (see section earlier in this chapter). Some students will react positively and be relieved when their shortcomings are openly discussed, allowing them to articulate their lack of understanding and plan strategies to extend their learning and increase their clinical skills.
- Document the concern in the assessment of practice document at an early stage, and certainly no later than the point at which formative midplacement assessment takes place. The nature of the problem should be carefully, clearly and explicitly documented. Include specific examples of incidents/clinical care situations to illustrate the nature of the problem. The written word gives a visual record of problems and actions taken.
- Make sure the student understands the nature of the issues(s) and has heard accurately what you are saying. The most difficult cases are those students who are clearly not succeeding but do not recognize this. Some students who are failing may lack insight of their weak areas of practice and therefore not perceive any necessity for extra support (Duffy 2013, Cassidy, Coffey & Murphy 2017). Supportive measures may then be ineffective if they are not recognized as such. Students should thus be provided with the opportunity to give their own perception of their performance. Help students identify what they already know and what they need to focus on to learn and overcome their weaknesses. Help students identify resources they can use to improve knowledge and skills.
- Jointly, with the student, draw up a targeted detailed action plan which provides a clear and unambiguous learning and assessment plan with clear, explicit goals (see Chapter 6) to enable success; set deadlines and make sure the student understands these.
- Make arrangements to work closely with the student.
- Arrangements should also be made for the student to work with other supervisors so that testimonies can be provided; this will increase the validity and reliability of the assessment. Furthermore, students have the right to be protected from unfair or biased assessment and should not be failed until they are judged by another assessor.
- Discuss the situation with the senior practitioner with overall responsibility for student learning. Following this, inform the student's personal teacher and/or the clinical link lecturer. Support from the higher education institution is essential in these situations.
- Establish clear and open communication between the student, practice supervisor, practice assessor, any organisational/trust education leads or practice facilitators and the university placement team and link lecturers.
- Make arrangements to conduct a progress review in 1 week. If, despite remedial action, there is little or no improvement, make arrangements for the clinical link lecturer to be present at a tripartite meeting to discuss the situation and develop another action plan. A weekly progress review is advisable for as long as the student's difficulties persist.
- Keep careful notes of all discussions; there may come a time when you have to use these as evidence that you may have pointed out the same things again and again and that the student has repeatedly failed to meet the goals you have set. Remember that the report may be scrutinized by the external examiners and the examination board of the higher education institution. It therefore needs to be clear, accurate and well evidenced. Where students have appealed against "fail" decisions, the benefit of the doubt will be in the student's favour if there is lack of clear evidence to support the fail decision.

If, despite the actions and opportunities provided for the student to improve, improvement does not occur and standards are not achieved, failure decisions can be made with confidence, fairly and on the basis of a fully documented evidence base.

Managing the Situation when a Student Has to be Failed

There comes a time when you may have to fail a student. This is a challenging responsibility, and the ability to face and deal with this situation with confidence is critical (Scholes & Albarran 2005). The arrival at this assessment decision would have been procedurally and emotionally difficult. It would also have been time consuming because you would have had to build up a case to fail the student (Dudek, Marks & Regehr 2005, Duffy 2013). It is important that failure does not come as a surprise to the student. Correct use of formative assessment processes, including feedback, would have indicated to the student those aspects of learning that were consistently not achieved. Before making this critical fail decision, you must have followed the plan of action outlined previously for helping the student who is not progressing. These situations are demanding and sensitive to handle. Notwithstanding that, supervisors have professional responsibilities and accountability to make sound and accurate assessment decisions, which include failing students who have not met the standards of education. The legal and ethical issues surrounding not failing a student who has not met the education standards and is unsafe to practise are discussed in Chapter 2. Suffice here to remind ourselves by asking the following questions dubbed the 'old test' by Scholes and Albarran (2005):

Would I want the student, when qualified, to look after me?

If not, why not? If it isn't good enough for you, then why should it be good enough for clients/patients?

Would you want this student, when qualified, to be in your team?

Could you rely on this practitioner to support you when the workload is heavy or in times of crisis, or would this practitioner be a liability?

Considerable skill and confidence are required to manage these situations effectively (Scholes & Albarran 2005, Luhanga, Yonge & Myrick 2008, Jervis & Tilki 2011). The supervisor and assessor require the courage and strength to fail a student and, importantly, the knowledge that their actions will be backed up and supported by the university. If assessment processes are fair, then decisions will be just, and assessors should have no fear that there will be reprisals for failing a student. However, remember that it is as wrong to fail to fail as it is to fail unjustly.

Consider the scenario shown in Activity 7.2. How would you deal with it?

The decision to fail a student is never an easy one to make, but when another supervisor or assessor disagrees with your decision, it becomes even more tricky. The starting point is perhaps to consider both your assessment evidence objectively. Are both of you using the same criteria for assessment so that assessment evidence is reliable? Therefore, evidence of achievement or nonachievement is based on the same criteria. The next question you may wish to consider is the validity of the assessment; for example, have both of you been assessing what you should be assessing? Has too much or too little been expected of the student? Other aspects of validity will also need to be considered (see Chapter 5).

Assuming that individual personal biases are not implicated and feasibility (see Chapter 5) within the assessment process has received due attention, and you still cannot agree with each other, as the supervisor, you may wish to take the following action(s):

- Arrange a meeting with the senior practitioner with overall responsibility for the student learning to discuss the situation.
- Arrange a meeting with your clinical link lecturer or the student's academic advisor to discuss the situation.
- Arrange a joint meeting with the senior practitioner and clinical link lecturer to discuss the situation.

The final point to remember is that, as the practice assessor, you are responsible for making the final assessment decision and are accountable for passing or failing the student at the end of the period of practice placement. The grade you award should reflect the student's standard of practice in the latter part of the placement. When making the summative assessment decision, refer to the documented evidence in the student's assessment of practice document to support your decision.

Failure to Fail

Having to fail a student causes many of us considerable anguish. At the other end of the continuum is the abuse of the power to fail, using it as a tool to exert control and punish "difficult" or unpopular students. This complex problem of failure to fail is not new and appears to be a continuing challenge for assessors of students on professional courses (Dudek, Marks & Regehr 2005, Scholes & Albarran 2005, Jervis & Tilki 2011, Hughes, Mitchell & Johnston 2016, Hunt et al 2016a). References are made to assessors giving students the benefit of the doubt in marginal situations instead of awarding a fail when it was clearly warranted. What is also of concern is that students may use coercive behaviours (see section later) to try to get around weak areas of practice (Hunt et al 2016b).

There are no straightforward answers as to why assessors find it difficult to assign a fail grade, but it would

---

Activity 7.2 **Practice Supervisor and Assessor Disagreement**

Mark is the practice supervisor to a student called Mary who has struggled considerably to achieve the required standard in three areas. He has been reviewing progress with her weekly. She is now approaching the end of the placement and has not achieved the required standard and, in Mark's opinion, should be failed. A fellow registered practitioner in the team, Nazeen, is Mary's practice assessor. She has also worked with Mary and argues strongly that Mary's practice is up to standard, and she intends to assess her as passed. What should Mark do?

appear that professional and strong affective and personal factors influence assessors' decision-making process when confronted with having to make a fail decision. This is a multifactoral issue, with some or all of the following having a bearing on assessors' failure to fail:

- Additional work for the assessor plus having to deal with the rancour of the student means some assessors may be loath to fail a student, especially if it is anticipated that the student may take out a grievance (Dudek, Marks & Regehr 2005, Luhanga, Yonge & Myrick, 2008, Jervis & Tilki 2011).
- Stress for the assessor around failing a student, with feelings including anxiety, guilt, distress, self-doubt, regret and relief. For some assessors, emotions were so strong that a pass grade was awarded over a fail because the failure to fail seemed the less stressful option, but it often engendered its own degree of guilt and shame in the assessor (Ilott & Murphy 1999).
- Assumptions that the focus is on the supervisor to provide good experience and support and therefore enable any student to pass. This locus of failure around the mentor (Hunt et al 2016b), rather than around the student's performance and behaviours, can influence the failure to fail decision.
- The caring role of health care professionals leading to a personal dilemma for many assessors that failing a student is incongruent with central role to care and nurture (Ilott & Murphy 1999; Luhanga, Yonge & Myrick 2008, Duffy 2013).
- The benefit of the doubt is more likely to be given where assessors lack confidence in assessing, have poor preparation for their role, have not worked alongside the student sufficiently or where they did not have sufficient documented assessment evidence (Luhanga, Yonge & Myrick 2008, Jervis & Tilki 2011, Duffy 2013)
- Students manipulate assessors or the system to avoid failure (Hunt et al 2016a, 2016b)
- Lack of support from colleagues, managers and lecturing staff made it more difficult to make fail decisions, with assessors even experiencing considerable pressure to pass students (Jervis & Tilki 2011, Timmins et al 2017).
- Reluctance to fail students in their third year because assessors do not want to be responsible for ending students' careers so late in a programme but also, paradoxically, difficulty failing first-year students because there is the held notion that problems will resolve later (Luhanga, Yonge & Myrick 2008).
- The subjective nature of assessing attitude and unprofessional behaviours and the need for assessment tools for the affective domain to mitigate this.

Student Reactions to Being Failed and How to Manage Them

Students at risk of failure on a placement may react in a number of ways. These behaviours need to be recognized for what they are—that is, the student's reactions to the news of failure and not a personal vendetta against the assessor. Extra time needs to be factored into these situations because the student needs time to process the information and should not feel rushed. They also need time to grieve the loss of what might have been long-held ambitions and consider the implications that the placement failure might have on progression or continuation in terms of their own expectations as well as family, friends and fellow students. Students need time, and assessors should listen attentively, show concern and provide the appropriate support if students respond with denial, anger and aggression or sadness at being failed.

Hunt et al (2016a) have suggested that there is growing evidence of a culture of expectation among nursing students, who view themselves as customers expecting success, which can lead to disrespectful, rude and manipulative behaviour when challenged by lecturers or mentors for not meeting the required standards for practice. They found that student nurses used coercive and manipulative behaviour to elicit a successful outcome in their practice assessment, and they noted four types of associated student behaviour (Hunt et al 2016b), which are shown in Fig. 7.8. These student behaviours led to varying degrees of fear and guilt in mentors. To increase resilience amongst practice supervisors and assessors in these situations, the following were suggested:

Ensure students understand that they may fail by changing their expectations, which are often along the lines that "as long as they have a good mentor on a good placement", they will automatically pass;

Help assessors to accept that it is the student's performance and/or behaviour which is failing, and not the assessor failing to adequately teach or support the student. This change in locus of the fail is needed to reduce assessor guilt;

Ensure assessors are able to recognize the coercive behaviours (see Fig. 7.8) because the effect of the behaviour is immediately reduced once recognized and counterstrategies can be considered;

Provide support and contacts, for example, informal team support and also formal protection and advice from education leads, human resource departments, occupational health departments.

In contrast, failure may be a positive experience for some students. Some may be quite relieved to have the decision to discontinue taken out of their because a career as a nurse, midwife or allied health professional may not be what they want after all, and they may not have the courage

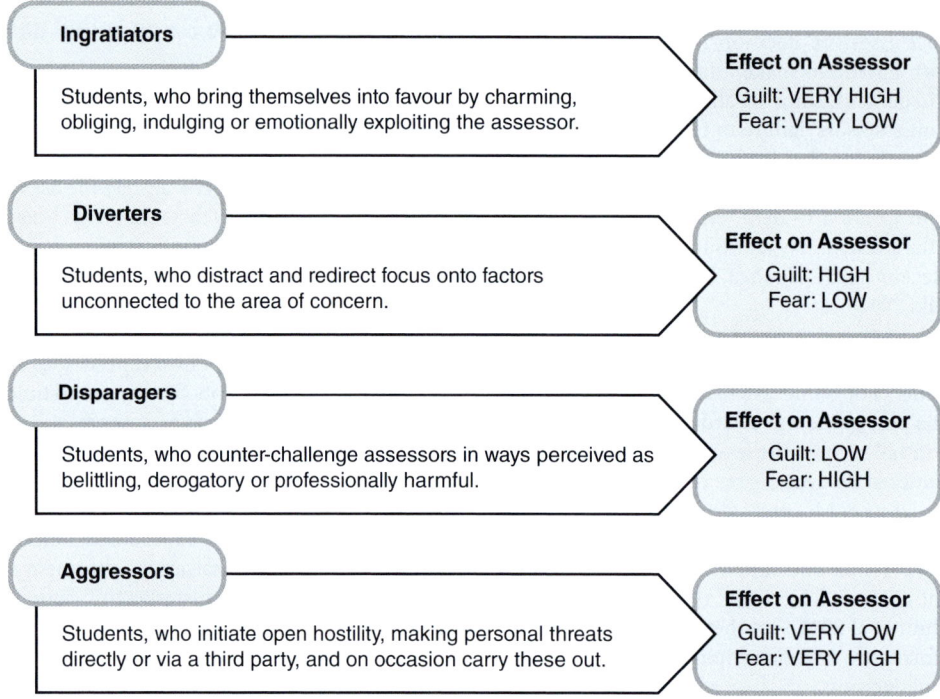

Fig. 7.8 Types of coercive students and their effect on mentors.

to make that decision. Equally, some students learn from the experience of failing a placement and go on to achieve success in other fields. Case Study 7.1 reflects the experience of a former medical student who learned from failure and feedback.

CASE STUDY 7.1 Learning From the Experience of Failure

A university medical lecturer was surprised when approached at a social function by a confident young woman who had recently been making her name in art design. She thanked him for helping her to make 'the most important decision of her life!' To his baffled enquiries, she told him that his "help" had been failing her in a first-year medical subject and taking the time to discuss her failure with her. She realized that she had, in fact, only done medicine because of her high university academic entrance mark and not through deep commitment. The result made her rethink her future and decide to follow her real area of interest and skill. Thus, this failure was a very effective part of her learning.

(From McAllister L et al. Facilitating Learning in Clinical Settings, Nelson Thornes Ltd:1997. With permission.

For some, failing a placement and failing to progress can be a devastating experience and can appear to be a scar carried for life. In his study of the kinds of failure people remembered, Cannon (2002) found that, with few exceptions, each experience of failure was still recalled with feelings of anger and sadness. He concluded that failures are 'anxiety-raising experiences [which] are simply difficult to delete from memory' (Cannon, 2002:76). This painful situation may be averted if lack of progress is determined early and appropriate support and help put in place.

An awareness of the factors that contribute to failure to fail may be a first step to understanding why we experience difficulties when dealing with a failing student and may thus end up passing a student when a fail is clearly warranted. It may also help us to identify the support we need when dealing with these difficult situations.

CONCLUSION

When working with students, it is important to be able to indicate to them the progress they are making. Progress during clinical practice needs to be tracked carefully and feedback given so that students may be able to learn and develop further. A discussion of the four assessment activities—working alongside the student and observing practice for development in the level of the student's competence, discussion with the student, examination of the student's portfolio and discussion with other supervisors—shows how they can be used to monitor the progress of students. Based upon what we know about the nature of expertise (Benner 1984, Glaser 1990, Benner, Tanner & Chesla 1996), a model that outlines the performance characteristics of novice, advanced beginner and competent practice is proposed here to monitor and assist with progression during clinical practice.

Monitoring progress is not about policing the student. It is very much about finding out the quality and quantity of learning that has taken place and any difficulties the student may be experiencing so that further assessment activities can be discussed and planned to further learning and development. It is inevitable that there will be instances when students do not succeed; for these students, early identification of difficulties and taking the appropriate remedial action may prevent failure and thus eliminate the trauma of failure for them.

If progress is carefully tracked through the four assessment activities discussed here and done throughout the student's placement, it becomes much easier to make assessment decisions that are also more likely to be based on a valid and reliable evidence base, which means that students have a fairer deal. It also makes the task of making assessment decisions easier for the assessor—easier although it is never easy to make fail decisions. Assigning a fail grade is something that is rarely done lightly or without misgivings. It is a formidable responsibility. Passing a student is an equally formidable responsibility.

KEY POINTS FOR REFLECTION

When monitoring progress, the role and responsibilities of the supervisor centre on answering these key questions:
- What has the student done and learned so far? How will I know?
- Is the student having any difficulties? How will I know?
- What can be done to facilitate further learning and development?

Answers to these questions may be obtained through the use of the assessment activities in Fig. 7.3.

The period of formative assessment allows the supervisor to monitor progress. Answers to the following questions will enable the assessor to decide whether there is progress:
- Is the student achieving expected competencies?
- Is there a demonstration of a growing level of skill and competence (see the criteria in Fig. 7.7)?
- Is performance consistent?
- Is there a demonstration of a growing understanding of the rationale underpinning practice?
- Is there a demonstration of development of the attitudes and values appropriate to professional practice?
- Is there a demonstration of a developing ability to engage in evidence-based and reflective practice?

The occasion of summative assessment centres on making a pass or fail decision. Answers to the following questions will enable the assessor to decide whether the student should be passed:
- Has the student achieved the expected competencies?
- Does the assessment evidence achieve validity and reliability of assessment?
- Is there a demonstration of a sound understanding of the rationale underpinning each competency?

- Is the student developing the attitudes and values appropriate to professional practice?

Students who are either not progressing or failing to meet the required standard need identification by assessment systems so that opportunities can be provided for them to improve. The following behaviours could be indicative of this:
- inconsistency in meeting the required level of competence for expected stage of education
- inconsistency in clinical performance and lacks clinical skills
- does not respond appropriately to constructive feedback
- inability to make changes in response to constructive feedback—therefore, clinical skills do not improve
- exhibits poor preparation and organizational skills
- has limited interactional and poor communication skills; does not ask questions; is unable to answer questions about care
- demonstrates unethical behaviour such as not disclosing/owning up to clinical errors made
- is uncommitted and unenthusiastic
- has poor punctuality
- may experience continual poor health or feel depressed, angry, uncommitted, withdrawn, sad, emotionally labile, tired or listless.

The following actions should be taken:
1. Document the concerns.
2. Discuss the situation with a senior practitioner and the higher education institution.
3. Discuss the concerns with the student.
4. Make sure the student understands the problems.
5. Jointly, draw up a targeted detailed action plan.

A fail decision should not come as a surprise to the student. Students may react with denial, anger, aggression and sadness or may try to bargain for a pass.

Responsibility and accountability for making assessment decisions lies with the assessor. It is a remarkable duty. Failing a student should not be done lightly or without misgivings. Equally, passing a student is crucial and must be done in a responsible way that fully recognises the professional status and role that passing can confer.

REFERENCES

Adkins DA, Aucoin JW. Failure to fail – Factors affecting faculty decisions to pass underperforming nursing students in the clinical setting: A quantitative study. *Nurse Educ Pract.* 2022;58:103259. Available at: https://doi.org/10.1016/j.nepr.2021.103259

Baillie L, Fish J, Barclay J, et al. Assessing nursing students in practice: a mixed method evaluation of a unified assessment document. 2016. *HEA Health and Social Care conference, Glasgow.* Available at: https://www.researchgate.net/publication/308077744_Enter_titleAssessing_nursing_students_in_practice_a_mixed_method_evaluation_of_a_unified_assessment_document (Accessed: 13 March 2020).

Benner P. From Novice to Expert: Excellence and Power in Clinical Nursing Practice. Menlo Park, CA: Addison-Wesley:1984.

Benner P, Tanner CA, Chesla CA. *Expertise in Nursing Practice.* New York: Springer:1996.

Bulman C, Schutz S. Reflective Practice in Nursing. 5th edn. Chichester: Wiley-Blackwell:2013.

Cannon D. Learning to fail: learning to recover, in Peelo, M. and Wareham, T. (eds) *Failing Students in Higher Education.* Buckingham: Open University Press:2002.

Cassidy S, Coffey M, Murphy F. "Seeking authorization": a grounded theory exploration of mentors' experiences of assessing nursing students on the borderline of achievement of competence in clinical practice, *J Advan Nursi,* 2017;73(9): 2167-2178.

Clynes MP, Raftery SEC. Feedback: an essential element of student learning in clinical practice, *Nurs Educ Pract,* 2008;8:405-411.

Davenport R, Hewat S, Ferguson A, et al. Struggle and failure on clinical placement: a critical narrative review, *Int J Lang Communic Disorder,* 2018;53(2):218-227.

Dudek NL, Marks MB, Regehr G. Failure to fail: the perspectives of clinical supervisors, *Acad Med,* 2005;80(Suppl):S84–S87.

Duffy K. Providing constructive feedback to students during mentoring, *Nurs Stan,* 2013;27(31):50-56.

Earl LM. *Assessment as Learning.* 2nd edn. Thousand Oaks CA: Corwin Press (Sage):2013.

Embo MPC, Driessen EW, Valcke M, et al. Assessment and feedback to facilitate self-directed learning in clinical practice of midwifery students, *Med Teach,* 2010;32(7):e263–e269.

Ferrell G, Gray L. *Feedback and feed forward: using technology to support students' progression over time.* 2013. Available at: https://www.jisc.ac.uk/guides/feedback-and-feed-forward (Accessed: 16 July 2019).

Fitzgerald M, Gibson F, Gunn K. Contemporary issues relating to assessment of pre-registration nursing students in practice, *Nurs Educ Prac,* 2010;10(3):158-163.

Giles TM, Gilbert S, McNeill L. Nursing students' perceptions regarding the amount and type of written feedback required to enhance their learning, *J Nurs Educ.* 2013;53(1):23-30.

Glaser R. Towards new models for assessment, *Int J Educ Research,* 1990;14(5):475-483.

Hammond J, Marshall-Lucette S, Davies N, et al. Spotlight on equality of employment opportunities: a qualitative study of job seeking experiences of graduating nurses and physiotherapists from black and minority ethnic backgrounds, *Int J Nurs Stud,* 2017;74:172-180.

Headlee C. *Ten ways to have a better conversation, TEDx presentation.* 2015. Available at: https://www.ted.com/talks/celeste_headlee_10_ways_to_have_a_better_conversation?language=en (Accessed: 13 March 2020).

Headlee C. *We Need to Talk: How to Have Conversations That Matter.* New York: Harper Collins:2017.

Health and Care Professions Council. Standards of Education and Training. London:2017a. Available at: https://www.hcpc-uk.org/globalassets/resources/standards/standards-of-education-and-training.pdf (Accessed: 13 March 2020).

Health and Care Professions Council. Standards of Education and Training Guidance. London:2017b. Available at: https://www.hcpc-uk.org/globalassets/resources/guidance/standards-of-education-and-training-guidance.pdf (Accessed: 13 March 2020).

Health Education England. Values Based Recruitment Framework. London:2016.

Hughes LJ, Mitchell M, Johnston ANB. "Failure to fail" in nursing – a catch phrase or a real issue? A systematic integrative literature review, *Nurs Educ Prac,* 2016;20:54-63.

Hunt LA, McGee P, Gutteridge R, et al. Failing securely: the processes and support which underpin English nurse mentors' assessment decisions regarding under-performing students, *Nurs Educ Today,* 2016a;39:79-86.

Hunt LA, McGee P, Gutteridge R, et al. Manipulating mentors' assessment decisions: do underperforming student nurses use coercive strategies to influence mentors' practical assessment decisions? *Nurs Educ Prac,* 2016b;20(Sept):154-162.

Ilott I, Murphy R. Success and Failure in Professional Education: Assessing the Evidence. London: Whurr:1999.

Jervis A, Tilki M. Why are nurse mentors failing to student nurses who do not meet clinical performance standards? *Br J Nurs,* 2011;20(9):582-587.

Lara RF, Mogensen KM, Markuns JF. Effective feedback in the education of health professionals, *Support Line*, 2016;38(2): 3-8. Available at: https://www.bu.edu/familymed/files/2016/08/1472-April-p1_dk_3_8.pdf (Accessed: 13 March 2020).

Luhanga F, Yonge OJ, Myrick F. Failure to assign failing grades, *Int J Nurs Ed Scholar*, 2008;5(1):8.

Miller C. Improving and enhancing performance in the affective domain of nursing students: Insights from the literature for clinical educators, *Contemp Nurs*, 2010;35(1):2-17.

Mruk CJ. Defining self-esteem: an often overlooked issue with crucial implications', in Kernis MH. (ed.) Self-Esteem: Issues and Answers - A Sourcebook of Current Perspectives. 2nd edn. New York: Psycology Press (Taylor and Francis):2013, Section 2.

Myall M, Levett-Jones T, Lathlean J. Mentorship in contemporary practice: the experiences of nursing students and practice mentors, *J Clin Nurs*, 2008;17(14):1834-1842.

Neary M. Responsive assessment: assessing student nurses' clinical competence, *Nurs Educ Today*, 2001;21(1): 3–17.

Newton PE. Grading Competence-Based Assessments: Notes from a Small Literature. Coventry.2018. Available at: https://assets.publishing.service.gov.uk/government/uploads/system/uploads/attachment_data/file/755765/Grading_competence-based_assessments.pdf (Accessed: 13 March 2020).

Nikos Mattheos, Nattestad A, Falk-Nilsso E, et al. The interactive examination: assessing students' self-assessment ability, *Med Educ*, 2004;38(4):378-389.

Nursing and Midwifery Council. Future Nurse: Standards of Proficiency for Registered Nurses. London:2018a.

Nursing and Midwifery Council. Realising Professionalism: Standards for Education and Training Part 1: Standards Framework for Nursing and Midwifery Education. London:2018b.

Nursing and Midwifery Council. Realising Professionalism: Standards for Education and Training Part 2: Standards for Student Supervision and Assessment. London:2018c.

Nursing and Midwifery Council. Supporting Information on Standards for Student Supervision and Assessment. 2019. Available at: https://www.nmc.org.uk/supporting-information-on-standards-for-student-supervision-and-assessment/ (Accessed: 15 July 2019).

QAA. UK Quality Code for Higher Education. Gloucester:2014. Available at: https://www.qaa.ac.uk/docs/qaa/quality-code/qualifications-frameworks.pdf (Accessed: 13 March 2020).

Rohatinsky N, Harding K, Carriere T. Nursing student peer mentorship: a review of the literature, *Mentor & Tutor: Partnership in Learn*, 2017;25(1):61-77.

Royal College of Nursing. Nursing our future: an RCN study into the challenges facing today's nursing students in Wales. London:2008. Available at: https://www.rcn.org.uk/-/media/royal-college-of-nursing/documents/publications/2009/november/pub-003309.pdf (Accessed: 13 March 2020)

Royal College of Nursing. RCN Guidance for Mentors of Nursing and Midwifery Students. 2017. London. Available at: https://www.rcn.org.uk/professional-development/publications/pub-006133 (Accessed: 13 March 2020).

Sanzero-Eller L, Leva EL, Feure A. Key components of an effective mentoring relationship: a qualitative study, *Nurs Educ Today*, 2014;34(5):815-820.

Scholes J, Albarran J. Failure to fail: facing the consequences of inaction, *BACCN Nurs Crit Care*, 2005;10(3):113-115.

Timmins F, Cassidy S, Nugent O, et al. Reluctance to fail nursing students in practice-implications for nurse managers, *J Nurs Manage*, 2017;25(7):489-90.

Valizadeh L, Zamanzadeh V, Badri Gargari R, et al. Self-esteem challenges of nursing students: an integrative review, *Res Develop Med Ed*, 2016;5(1):5-11.

Vandal N, Leung K, Sanzone L, et al. Exploring the student peer mentor's experience in a nursing peer mentorship program, *J Nurs Educ*, 2018;57(7):422-425.

Walsh D. The Nurse Mentor's Handbook: Supporting Students In Clinical Practice. 2nd edn. Maidenhead: McGraw-Hill:2014.

8

Clinical Learning Environment as a Setting for Learning and Professional Development

CHAPTER CONTENTS

INTRODUCTION

The clinical environment, stated simplistically, is where patient/client care and clinical activities take place. These activities may involve the interaction of a variety of health and social care professionals, each bringing their own skills and expertise to an unpredictable, volatile and dynamic environment. In modern day health care, the challenge is that the clinical environment is not solely confined to an in-hospital setting but may be in a variety of community, voluntary and independent sector locations, including the patient/client's own home.

The clinical environment is considered the real world of health care practice. Practice learning and immersion into the clinical environment are recognized as a significant component of the health care professional student's learning. The theoretical curriculum introduces students to the skills, knowledge, attitudes and behaviours required to be a health care professional, but it is the clinical environment that offers the student the opportunity to further develop, apply and integrate the learning (Newton et al 2010). Students have identified that they value the opportunities within the clinical environment that enable them to grow and become a professional nurse (Papp et al 2003). The current Standards for Preregistration Nursing Programmes from the Nursing and Midwifery Council (NMC) (2018a) make it clear that the students are to learn and be assessed in the clinical environment, with the extent of clinical learning amounting to at least one-half of the total training duration.

It is important to recognize and acknowledge that the clinical environment provides the authentic context in which students from health care professions can learn about care and clinical practice, and therefore it becomes the learning environment. The clinical learning environment is multifaceted and should not be viewed as "just a classroom" outside a school. Flott and Linden (2015) identify that the clinical learning environment contains four characteristics that can influence the student learning and outcomes: the physical space, psychosocial and interaction factors, organizational culture and teaching and learning components.

These attributes establish a relationship between the clinical learning environment and the learner, indicating a shared responsibility to ensure an effective clinical learning environment and positive student outcomes.

This chapter examines the components of the clinical learning environment and those factors that contribute to a positive learning environment. Strategies for creating this type of environment are suggested.

CLINICAL LEARNING ENVIRONMENT

The learning environment for any formal education setting is complex. It is suggested here that the clinical environment is a formal educational setting where the practice educators are the teachers and the students are required to learn. Ford et al (2016) identify that an environment that facilitates mutual respect and shared expectations will enable meaningful learning to occur. A quality learning environment could be considered as an environment that not only supports the students' learning experience but also supports the staff who are enabling the students' learning. The complexity is captured by Parlett and Hamilton (1977:14-15), who noted that a learning environment in the formal education setting is:

'The social-psychological and material environment in which students and teachers work together… [it] represents a network or nexus of cultural, social, institutional, and psychological variables. These interact in complicated ways to produce, in each [clinical area], a unique pattern of circumstances, pressures, customs, opinions and work styles which suffuse the teaching and learning that occur there. The configuration of the learning milieu in any particular [clinical area] depends on the interplay of numerous different factors ….there are more constraints ….there are [also] the individual [practitioner's] characteristics … and then there are student perspectives and preoccupations.'

In a clinical environment where enhanced employee work engagement is evident, enhanced effective performance, job satisfaction, caring behaviours from nurses and improved health care quality outcomes can be seen (Tomietto et al 2016). The findings of Tomietto et al's (2016) work emphasizes the positive impact of the organizational climate and having work-engaged staff on the learning experience of students. The clinical environment as a formal educational setting is thus much more than the physical environment where patients/client care and other clinical activities take place; it is inclusive of the material resources within it; the formal requirements; the culture, procedures, practices and standards of particular clinical areas; the expectations and interactions of all the people who are in it; as well as the personal characteristics of individuals who are part of the environment. The richness of the clinical environment provides a rich texture for learning during clinical practice. The setting provides the context and events within which the student operates and learns (Mariet 2016).

The environment for teaching and learning outside of the hospital opens another world for students. Although they do not have to work within the constraints of a hospital environment, students have to learn a different set of factors that influence practice. Professional carers are visitors in the client's own home—caring and teaching/learning activities are carried out in the client's domain. The client's lifestyle, values and health priorities could challenge the student's value systems. Students need to learn to respond sensitively in these situations as they learn about the complex forces that influence health care (Sjogren Forss et al (2019)).

You may wish to try Activity 8.1.

> ### Activity 8.1
>
> Think about the clinical area where you work. This can be a ward, your community "beat" an outpatient's clinic, day care, critical care environment, a care home and so on.
> 1. Make a list of all the people who you think influence the learning ethos on the environment. How do they exert that influence?
> 2. What other factors influence your clinical environment as a learning environment?

This chapter examines the components of the clinical learning environment and their associated factors that contribute to a positive learning environment.

It is necessary to take into account several factors and the interaction between these when considering the clinical environment as an educational environment. These components and factors can be grouped into the following categories:

1. The people
   a. The leader of the team
   b. The members of the team
   c. The students
   d. The practice educators
2. The learning opportunities experiences "provided by":
   a. Patient/client care
   b. Other clinical activities
3. Staff commitment to teaching and learning
   a. Support and supervision of learners
   b. Continuing professional development
4. Material resources

The People

Team Leader

Over the years, there have been significant changes in structure and roles and responsibilities within the ward environment. Until the mid-1980s, the role of the ward manager was to teach, supervise and assess student nurses and midwives, therefore playing an integral role in creating the clinical learning environment. Up until that time, the training of student nurses and midwives was the responsibility of the hospital; they were employees responsible to the ward manager who, in turn, was responsible for the students' education. In the mid-1980s, pre- and postregistration education moved into colleges, removing the responsibility from the ward manager (Bradshaw 2010).

With further changes and developments in roles and responsibilities, ward managers have taken on a wider responsibility for management, moving the ward manager further away from direct patient care and student contact. Nevertheless, the importance of the ward managers' indirect influence on the learning climate should not be underestimated. A positive learning environment is promoted by a leader who is aware of the learning needs and skills of their team and who positively encourages continuous learning for the benefit of all. With the support of a ward manager who is committed to the learning and development of students and staff, team members are more likely to be motivated in their role of practice supervisors and assessors to students, and to the development of the clinical environment into an educational environment (Tomietto et al 2016).

The Members of the Team

Each member of the team can contribute to an environment that fosters learning. Within The Code, the NMC (2018b) makes it clear that they expect all registrants to support the learning and development of students and colleagues, and they reinforce this by stating within the Standards for Student Supervision and Assessment (2018c) that all NMC-registered nurses and midwives are capable of supervising students, serving as role models for safe and effective practice. They also identify that any health care professional can take on a supervisory role for students in the clinical learning environment.

The staff–student relationship is acknowledged by Levett-Jones et al (2009) as a significant influence on the learning experience of students. Students identified that feeling "included" was important; they valued staff who were willing to share their knowledge, skills and insights while delivering patient care. Levett-Jones et al (2009) identified that students felt part of the team culture when staff who, irrespective of whether they were responsible for supervising the student or not, wanted to support the student's learning. Doyle et al (2017) identified that a clinical environment where staff have a positive attitude to the presence of students and who are welcoming and willing to help is one that is valued by students. This commitment toward students is also professed to foster positive well-being in the workplace and ultimately contribute to positive patient outcomes.

Interprofessional learning and collaboration: Remember also that members of the multiprofessional team make up the team, even though they may not be as visible as nurses and midwives in the clinical area. The multiprofessional team's philosophy of patient/client care and their attitudes toward learning and students will also greatly influence the learning environment. It is important that they contribute to the educational environment so that not only do all members of the team learn with and from each other, but also a spirit of teamwork may be created for the benefit of the patient/client.

The delivery of high-quality health care requires partnership by practitioners within and between professions (Lait et al 2011). According to Watkins (2016) Illingworth and Chelvanayagam (2007), interprofessional learning helps students to develop an appreciation of diversity. It can help ensure students are aware of the overlapping professional functions and the common knowledge between disciplines, better preparing them for encountering the complexities of real-life interprofessional work-based problems. Students should therefore gain, where possible, experience as part of a multiprofessional team so that they learn to function as an effective team member (Lait et al 2011). A relevant resource for interprofessional learning, which is time-efficient and practical, is an interprofessional team meeting (Nisbet et al 2015).

Now you may wish to try Activity 8.2.

Activity 8.2

How do you help your students fit into the team?
 What opportunities are available in your setting to help students fit into the team?
 What opportunities are available to enable students to work and learn with members of the multiprofessional team?

With recent changes to the NMC guidance on the assessment of students and with the implementation of the NMC Standards for Student Supervision and Assessment, students may now be supervised and given feedback relevant to their assessment by any health or social care professional (NMC 2018c); it is therefore essential that they learn to relate and work with the wider team.

The health care team is a complex one, but students need to learn to relate and work with the team members. Students are often nervous about being on placement and express how important feeling part of the team means to them (Ford et al 2016, Doyle at el 2017). Levett-Jones (2015) identified that theory-based preparation for working in teams can often heighten a student's anxiety before placement. Practice supervisors should ensure that students have opportunities to experience teamwork through working as a member of the team and observing different members of the team at work.

The following ideas, based upon and extended from the work of Lait et al (2011), Ford et al (2016) and Doyle et al (2017), are offered to help students fit into the team and to learn about multiprofessional teamworking:

1. Ensure that students have opportunities to fit into their own professional team—the "home team". Initially, this can be done informally by introducing the student to these team members. Students should be invited to attend staff meetings, journal clubs, training days, seminars, social events and so on. Arrangements can also be made to enable students to observe the team members; this need not involve any teaching. In preparation for the observational activity, students should be briefed on those specific aspects of the job role that are pertinent to the student's learning and development at the time. It is important that students demonstrate the ability to fit into the home team before they are expected to become a member of the multiprofessional team.

2. Meeting members of the multiprofessional team. Introducing students to members of the multiprofessional team informally—in the corridor, during coffee and meal breaks and in the staff room—can help others recognize new students. Later on, students can be gradually introduced to the work of these team members by making arrangements for students to observe them providing care for patients and being involved in situations that do not make any professional demands on the student, such as attending a team meeting and case discussion. These activities will increase the student's understanding of the roles of the multiprofessional team and also give students opportunities to interact with these professionals.

3. Meeting, working and learning with students from other professions. Health care students are used to interprofessional learning in their university. If your setting has students from the other professions, explore opportunities for these students to meet and perhaps work together in practice as well (e.g., discussing a patient/client they have looked after). These sessions will require to be facilitated to ensure that learning is collaborative (Holland 2002). Each student will be able to contribute to the discussion of care given, viewed from the perspectives of that particular professional group. Students will also be able to learn about the roles of some of the other professionals in this way. Respect for each other's professional roles is likely to be engendered. Students are thus engaging in interprofessional learning because they will be learning from and about each other to improve collaboration and the quality of care (Barr et al 2005, in Lait et al 2011). This strategy sows the seed

for good teamworking because students who have such positive experiences of the multiprofessional team are likely to carry this into their professional practice.

4. Working with members of the multiprofessional team. Plan graded steps to team involvement. As students' confidence increase, they can be placed in situations where they are required to work alongside a member of the multiprofessional team. In the first instance, be careful to involve the student with professionals who are patient and cooperative. The student should gradually become independent in interacting with all team members and develop the confidence to participate in care.

5. Learning actively from members of the multiprofessional team. Encourage students to talk to these team members to gather information or discuss management of specific patients/clients who have required multiprofessional input. The practice supervisor can assist the student to draw up the aims for the meeting and, subsequently, hold a debriefing session on the conduct and outcome of the meeting. Students will then be able to learn about the contribution that each professional makes to the care of that patient/client. This type of experience will make interprofessional collaborative care real for students. Lait et al (2011) cited the example of a physiotherapy student who participated in the care of a patient with traumatic brain injury. The student interacted with and interviewed the nine types of professionals involved in the care of this patient to understand their contributions.

6. Explore ways information is communicated within the multiprofessional team. As well as the use of formal letters, written reports and documentation in the patient/client's case notes, discuss other ways that communication takes place within the team, such as chats over coffee, telephone calls, during ward rounds and verbal reports.

Students

Students bring their own personalities, dispositions, hopes and aspirations, past experiences and backgrounds, and also worries and anxieties, to the clinical setting. For many beginning students, the impact of the clinical environment can be strong (Levette-Jones et al 2009). They have to deal with the unpleasant experiences such as sights, smells and cries of pain and challenging situations such as the abusive or disturbed patient/client. Many will not have done shift work or been on their feet for long hours. Students will have to learn to cope with the realities of social and economic differences, particularly when in the community setting, and come to grips with cultural diversity. Students may only spend short periods of time within a clinical environment, so making the most of the learning available is essential. If a student is not made to feel welcomed or, worse, if they are made to feel a burden (Ford et al 2016), their plans, hopes and aspirations can be thwarted and any worries and anxieties compounded by an uncongenial environment. In an environment where students are fearful of underperformance and negative evaluations, they are more likely to have difficulties in meeting the expectations of the placement supervisor (Levett-Jones et al 2015).

White and Ewan (1991) think that the differences between learning in the classroom and in the clinical setting are profound; in the classroom setting, students can "hide" behind the mantle of the group, which shields them from the close attention of the teacher. In the clinical setting, students are visible as they work closely with their practice supervisor/assessor and members of the team. Patients and clients may be observing their performance. They can feel threatened and vulnerable because their performance and behaviours are visible and open to the scrutiny of a range of people.

Recognize that students will bring with them their own diversity and life experiences and therefore have different learning styles. On entry into the environment, students create interactions that become learning experiences for themselves and others. Although being an active learner can be an advantage within the clinical setting, making use of the variety of learning opportunities available will be of value (Flott & Linden 2015). Not only will students have different learning styles, but they will also have different learning needs (Shivers et al 2017). Ford et al (2016) identified that students found it frustrating if the practice supervisor was not aware of the learning needs of the student, and likewise, the practice supervisor found it frustrating if the student lacked insight into their own needs and the learning opportunities available.

Wu et al (2015) identified that health care professionals, and nurses in particular, join their professions for altruistic reasons because they want to help others who are sick. Clinical practice provides the opportunity for students to experience caregiving and helps them to put into practice the theory they have learned—they will be learning how to care and to develop the competencies required of a professional. Following on from the Willis Report (Willis Commission 2012) and Francis Inquiry (Francis 2013), there has been an emphasis on teamwork, leadership, mentorship, supporting students and role modelling within the clinical environment, all being key attributes of the learning environment (Flott & Linden 2015). Wanting to feel a valued member of the team is a theme that is often identified as an anxiety for students, potentially impacting on their learning experience before commencing placement and while in placement (Levett-Jones et al 2009, Levett-Jones et al 2015, Ford et al 2016, Doyle et al 2017). They need to be viewed as valuable student members of the team with specific clinical learning needs rather than a burden.

A clinical environment that is an educational environment will be able to support students so that they achieve their personal and professional goals in the best possible ways. Professional socialization is seen as process through which students go to learn and develop the characteristics, attitudes and values of the profession; this is a requirement to be accepted into the profession (Norman 2015). It relates to the need for students to internalize and develop their occupational identity. The process of professional socialization is predominantly seen as one that takes place in the "real world" (Mariet 2016), led by those responsible for the students learning and all in the position of being a role model (Norman 2015, Mariet 2016).

The positive impact of professional socialization can be seen as a sense of belonging to the profession along with personal and professional growth and pride. Norman (2015) suggests that this fosters the values, beliefs and attitudes fundamental to planning and delivering excellent patient care. A clinical environment that is also an educational environment needs to espouse a philosophy of care, reflected in practice, which will enable students to develop into professionals who can truly meet the needs of society for care and caring. High standards of care need to be modelled; staff who are engaged and dedicated to their work are identified as significantly contributing to strong clinical learning environment and therefore effective in supporting student learning (Timietto et al 2016). However, as identified earlier, students need to actively engage in their learning (Flott & Linden 2015). It is not enough for the student to just be immersed in a positive learning environment; they need to be active in experiencing, discussing and evaluating professional behaviours and care to extract personal meaning. The NMC (2018c) also advocates that students need to be proactive and take responsibility, through empowerment, for their own learning in practice.

Practice Educator

In 1986, the United Kingdom Central Council for Nursing, Midwifery and Health Visiting (UKCC 1986) challenged the way students were expected to learn. Up to that point, students had been employees of the hospital, following what is often referred to as the "apprenticeship"-style training, counted and treated a member of ward staff, not a student.

Project 2000 (UKCC 1986) challenged the ways that students were expected to learn during clinical practice. As a consequence, students currently undertaking preregistration nursing and midwifery programmes enjoy supernumerary status. The NMC (2008) made it a mandatory requirement for all students on approved educational programmes to be supervised by a practitioner who is capable of supporting learning and assessment in practice, making judgements on fitness for practice to enter the register or to record a specialist practice qualification. These practitioners were accountable to the NMC for such judgements and referred to as mentors or practice teachers.

In Greek mythology, Mentor was the wise and faithful advisor to Odysseus. Today, the mentor is a friend, role model, an able advisor and the person who supports in many different ways. The NMC (2008) required the mentor to have skills of effective supervision, support and facilitating learning in addition to the ability to make a sound judgement of the students' competence in the role of the assessor for practice. Ratification of these prerequisite skills for a mentor was achieved by taking a NMC-approved course for the preparation of mentors.

With the implementation of the Standards for Education and Training Part 2: Standards for Student Supervision and Assessment (NMC 2018c), the mentor role has been replaced by other roles. There is no evidence as yet of the effectiveness of these roles, so many of the citations within this chapter refer to research undertaken with mentor roles that still has relevance. Students can now have their practice supervised by a "practice supervisor" and assessed by a "practice assessor". The role of the practice supervisor is predominantly to enable students to learn and safely achieve proficiency while acting as a role model for safe and effective practice. The practice assessor role is to carry out an evidence-based, robust and objective assessment of the students' performance and confirmation of proficiency.

Practice Supervisor: All NMC-registered nurses and midwives are now acknowledged as capable of supervising students, and the standards recognize that any other registered health and social care professional can also supervise the learning of students within their sphere of competence (NMC 2018c).

Although there is no mandated preparation for the role, the standards (NMC 2018c) do identify that the supervisor must:

1. receive ongoing support to prepare, reflect and develop for effective supervision and contribution to student learning and assessment, and
2. understand the proficiencies and programme outcomes they are supporting students to achieve.

This is to support them in their role to:

1. Act as a role model
2. Support learning and provide feedback
3. Contribute to the student's record of achievement and assessment
4. Raise and respond appropriately to concerns about student conduct and competence (NMC 2018c).

Practice Assessor: All students on an NMC-approved programme must be allocated a nominated practice assessor for a practice placement or series of placements in line with local and national policy. For nursing students, the assessor must be a registered nurse, but not necessarily from the same field of practice as long as they have appropriate equivalent experience for the student's field of practice. For midwifery students, however, the practice assessor must be a registered midwife, and for specialist community public health nurse (SCPHN) students, practice assessors must be a registered SCPHN with appropriate equivalent experience for the student's field of practice (NMC 2018c).

Unlike with the previous mentor role, there will be no NMC-approved course to be completed before undertaking the role of practice assessor, but the NMC have identified preparation requirements which include that they must undertake preparation or evidence before learning and experience that enables them to demonstrate achievement of the following minimum outcomes:

1. interpersonal communication skills, relevant to student learning and assessment
2. conducting objective, evidence-based assessments of students
3. providing constructive feedback to facilitate professional development in others, and
4. knowledge of the assessment process and their role within it (NMC 2018c).

Although the role of the practice assessor is primarily to conduct assessments to confirm student achievement of proficiencies and programme outcomes for practice learning, the role does have other aspects to it to enable them to undertake the assessment. These activities include:

1. Seeking feedback from practice supervisors, other practice assessors and relevant people
2. Making and recording evidence-based assessments on conduct, proficiency and achievement
3. Having sufficient opportunities to periodically observe the student across environments to make an informed decision for assessment and progression
4. Communicating and collaborating with the academic assessor (NMC, 2018c).

The practice assessor will have a key role to play in coordinating the feedback from supervisors to make an assessment on practice and to work with the student's academic assessor to make recommendations for progression (NMC 2018c).

Irrespective of whether a practice supervisor, assessor or relevant other (e.g., patient/client, member of multidisciplinary team), what students are looking for is someone who is willing to support their learning and who is approachable (Levett-Jones et al 2015, Ford et al 2016, Doyle et al 2017). Jarvis (1983) and Rogers (1983) believe that teaching is not essential to learning. Many learners acquire knowledge, skills and attitudes independent of any formal teaching. This is not to say that teaching is unimportant, but, given certain conditions, most adults engage in much more learning than is often realized and acknowledged. One way that students learn in the clinical setting is by observing staff as they work alongside each other. No formal teaching is done here. The work of Tomietto et al (2016) identifies that learning experience of students can be enhanced through having engaged work teams. Having an environment where staff are absorbed in their practice, students will remain focussed on their nursing care and relevant learning opportunities. By working and talking with the student, the practitioner is teaching as well as getting the work done.

Read the following modified extract (Examples 1 and 2) from Ogier (1989:25-26), and then tackle Activity 8.3. The scenarios took place on a busy general surgical ward. Mary is a second-year student nurse. Postoperative analgesia was being prepared.

1. Staff nurse: "Mary, can you come here and check this controlled drug with me? Mrs Gavey last had pethidine at 6.00 AM; it is now 10.00 AM, so she can have more.' The practice educator and Mary can be heard preparing syringes, counting the stock and administering the drug to Mrs Gavey. Following documentation, they clear up and go their separate ways.

2. Staff Nurse: "Mary, can you check this controlled drug with me? As you heard at the report, Mrs Gavey had a cholecystectomy yesterday afternoon. She last had pethidine 75 mg at 6.00 AM; it is now 10.00 AM, and the physiotherapist is due to see her at about 10.30 am. If we give her more pethidine now, it will be working by the time the physiotherapist comes to help Mrs Gavey with her deep-breathing exercises." While the practice educator is talking, the injection is being prepared, and the sound of syringes being unwrapped and drug cupboards being unlocked can be heard. They administer the drug and sign the documentation, and, while clearing up, the practice educator asks Mary, "How are you getting on?"

Activity 8.3

Imagine you are the staff nurse. List the information imparted in the interaction described in Example 1, and then do the same for Example 2. What types of interaction took place?

Preparing and giving the drug took the same length of time in each example, but in Example 2, the staff nurse was sharing her decision-making process—why the

pethidine was being given. Mary also gained an insight into the planning of more effective pain relief. She has learnt through experience, which was triggered by the staff nurse's explanation while they worked together. The staff nurse also showed interest in how Mary was progressing.

Ask yourself the following questions:
1. How can work be planned so that having students is a help rather than a hindrance?
2. How can students be involved in care so that they are learning while contributing to the work of the team?
3. How can the work be turned into dynamic learning experiences?

Learning Opportunities and Experiences

Patients and Clients and Opportunistic Teaching and Learning

In practice-based health care professions, the best place for learning about care delivery is in the direct context of patient/client care. Burnard and Chapman (1990:48) made this important statement, the basis of clinical learning should be the process of carrying out [care] with patients. The one thing that is always missing in the [academic setting] and always present in the clinical setting is the presence of patients. Encounters with patients, whatever the clinical setting, should always form the basis of learning, these learning opportunities are difficult to control, as the presence of which patients or clients in the clinical area cannot be prescribed. However, the nature of the conditions, illnesses or problems of patients and clients who require care in any given clinical setting are known. On this basis, the learning opportunities and clinical experiences that can be provided for students in each setting can be determined. Using these learning opportunities, learning contracts and assessment plans can be developed to meet the needs of the student. Although these plans provide the structure to assist the student achieve learning outcomes, the control and predictability of experiences are unlikely to be possible. Each patient or client is different, and each has varied needs that require different care and management. The condition of the patient/client could alter, sometimes dramatically. These differences and the unplanned and unpredictable events are learning opportunities that can be capitalized upon. The way that an unprecedented clinical event is responded to is a learning opportunity in itself.

The complexities of the healthcare environment means that learning opportunities may not always be planned or immediately recognised as a learning opportunity. Opportunistic learning or teaching does not have to be just about the practical aspect of doing and responding to experiences as they emerge in the realities of clinical practice. Newton et al

(2015) identify that 'learning by doing' is not the only way to learn, that conversation and discussion are key to supporting a student's learning and development. White and Ewan (1991) say that the 'ability so see opportunities and use them distinguishes [practice educators] as persons with ingenuity and flair' (White & Ewan 1991:138). For example, during the course of performing "routine" pressure area care with the student, there are opportunities for involving the student actively in the care of the patient/client by, for example, inviting the student's opinions on the condition of the skin and how the student would manage the situation, pointing out the warning signs of impending pressure sore development, which the student may not have seen, or discussing evidence-based management of pressure areas to prevent pressure sores, the policy of the clinical setting or hospital for the management of patients/clients at risk of developing pressure sores and so on. If a relative is present who wishes to be involved in the care of the patient/client, involving the relative with caregiving will show the student how this is done and the role of family members when a relative requires care. Subsequently, discussions with the student on this aspect of care will reinforce learning.

You may wish to try Activity 8.4 to help you consider the vast range of activities related to direct patient/client care, which are some of the learning opportunities present in your clinical setting.

Activity 8.4

Make a list of the patients/clients you have looked after during your last three spans of duty. Make a list of their conditions, illnesses and problems that they had presented you with. How did you deal with their range of needs? Think about one patient/client and identify the learning opportunities available around the different aspects of their care.

Remember that it is not only the direct encounters with patients and clients that are the learning opportunities for students. Other examples of learning opportunities provided by patient/client encounters could be the way you plan and manage your workload, the way you plan care, how you make decisions and how you handle different situations—particularly difficult ones. Chamberlain (1997) found that one strategy by which student midwives used to obtain information was to listen to their midwives' interactions with each other, clients and doctors. Total patient/client care gives students the opportunity to observe and participate in the provision and delivery of holistic care. Providing opportunities for students to look after the same patients/clients will enable them to learn more about this aspect of care delivery. There is then also the opportunity for students to follow the progress of those patients/clients and their response to care and treatment. Patient/client and staff satisfaction is generally higher with this method of care delivery, which can only contribute to a positive learning climate. Students can also learn, for example, the importance of good teamworking within a multiprofessional team, the range of caregiving activities a patient/client requires and how to coordinate these, and how to meet the total needs of a patient/client. These are also opportunities for students to realize that an acquisition of technical competence is not enough for professional practice as a health care professional. In the case of nurses, Virginia Henderson (1966) said, very profoundly, that 'nursing is of the head and of the hands and of the heart'. The skills of the practice supervisor/assessor in using the richness of the clinical learning environment will enable the development of a well-rounded health care practitioner as envisioned by that author.

Other Clinical Activities

Other than the learning opportunities provided by direct patient/client contact, there is generally a huge range of activities in any clinical setting that are learning opportunities for student participation. More often than not, engagement in these activities can generate evidence of competence. Students need to be directed to these activities and assisted to draw up the aims and learning outcomes to derive meaningful learning from participating in these activities.

You may wish to try Activity 8.5 to help you consider the vast range of other activities that can be learning opportunities for students working in your clinical setting.

Activity 8.5

Make a list of those activities and events that have taken place during the last 3 days you were on duty. Go on to make another list of those activities and events that you consider to be learning opportunities for students.

White and Ewan (1991) made the observation that students make the surprising but not infrequent comment that they have "nothing to do" during clinical placements. Pause to consider the undertones of this comment. Students frequently equate real learning with actively "doing". When the pace is slower and events less dramatic, students may wonder how such experiences contribute to their preparation for developing competence. Students may not be aware of activities that are not directly related to patient/client care or may not be aware that such activities are accepted as learning opportunities. Harrison-White and

King (2015) identified that activities that may take the student away from the allocated clinical placement area are often referred to as "spoke" learning opportunities, with the allocated clinical placement area referred to as the "hub". By supporting students to undertake spoke learning opportunities, Harrison-White and King (2015) identified that students achieved a richer learning experience. Such experience would prepare them to work confidently in a modern health care system, with a greater understanding of the patient journey and the roles and responsibilities of members of the multidisciplinary team.

To direct and support students to other sources of learning that would contribute to their overall professional development, a list of activities and events could be provided. Some suggestions of activities and events to which students can be directed in most clinical settings, and which should be considered to be part of the educational environment, are given here. There will be others that will be specific to your own clinical environment.

1. Learning and gaining insight about the work of the multiprofessional team. The activities for the student could be to:
   a) Observe several different professionals working—specialist nurses, allied health professionals, social care staff.
   b) Liaise and communicate with a number of different professionals.
   c) Go on ward rounds.
   d) Attend case conferences and seminars.
   e) Attend staff meetings
   f) Follow the patient on their journey through various departments/settings.
2. Learning communication skills within the profession specific team, the multiprofessional team and with other carers. Encourage students to practice and use communication tools such as Situation, Background, Assessment and Recommendation (SBAR) (NHS Institute for Innovation and Improvement 2010) when communicating with others to reduce the anxiety such communication may provoke. The activities for the student could be to:
   a) Liaise and communicate with a number of different team members; professionals in the multiprofessional team, including those who provide support services such as pharmacists and technicians and other carers such as relatives and friends of the patient/client and members of voluntary organizations.
   b) Use the telephone to communicate with a range of people. This activity may appear simple but can provoke anxiety for the student who has to speak in public to someone they do not know, and the student may fear not having the answers and thus feel foolish.
   c) Participate in ward handovers, ward rounds, case conferences, seminars and staff meetings. The requirement to speak during these events may also be anxiety provoking—students need to be encouraged and supported to develop the courage and skills of speaking and voicing their opinions during these events.
   d) Report back to staff on the outcomes of treatment and care given, both verbally and through written reports.
3. Acquiring administrative and management experience. Deficits in management and organization skills among newly qualified nurses and midwives in the UK are well documented and cause considerable anxiety and stress. These have been observed since the 1980s in several studies (Gerrish 1990, 2000, Whitehead & Holmes 2011). The nurses in Gerrish's studies found the management of self and a team of nurses problematic. They also found prioritizing care especially difficult. Whitehead and Holmes study identify that students felt unprepared for their new status and anxious about their new level of accountability. The following activities could assist students to develop organization and management skills:
   a) Organize the transfer of patients/clients to other units and agencies.
   b) Organize the discharge of patients/clients, including hospital transport if required.
   c) Order equipment.
   d) Manage own workload. Workload should be incremental and commensurate with the student's experience and stage of training. Senior students should be given the responsibility for the care of a group of patients/clients, including making the decisions for their care. The aim is to prepare the student so that transition to the professional role is accomplished at the point of registration.
   e) Coordinate the work of the team where appropriate. This activity could include delegating work to the team.
4. Learning about records and record keeping. The activities for the student could be to:
   a) Find out about the handling and storage of case notes.
   b) Retrieve case notes.
   c) File patient/client reports.
   d) Write in the patient's/client's care records.
   e) Extract from and input into computerized record systems.
   f) Observe or participate in audit activities.
   g) Find out about complaint management and the significance of documentation.

5. Learning to use equipment. The use of equipment should be demonstrated and followed by immediate supervised practice. Opportunities to handle and use the equipment during patient/client care should be provided as soon as possible following demonstration of their use. Repeated practice will help the student acquire dexterity, confidence and consistent performance.

6. Accessing teaching/learning sessions. Many clinical areas have these sessions, such as scheduled lectures, seminars, case conferences, demonstration of new equipment by company representatives and teaching ward rounds. Students should be directed to these sessions as appropriate and time made available for them to attend these sessions.

When considering the learning opportunities in your clinical setting, it may be useful to remember that 'while students have control over what they want to learn, they have limited control over access to opportunities for learning' (Chamberlain 1997:85). This means that opportunities for learning should be planned so that students can be directed to them and supported while they are learning. This strategy can only contribute to the educational environment in creating an ambience for learning.

Staff Commitment to Teaching and Learning

Support and Supervision of Learners

Doyle et al (2017) identified that clinical environments not only enable the student to gain clinical skills but they support them to become culturally acclimatized. The experience they have though is greatly influenced by the approach of staff and educators toward their development; student success in clinical placement was attributed to units that were welcoming and affirming. It is widely acknowledged that during clinical placements, students experience anxiety and stress for a wide range of reasons. Jimenez et al (2009) reported that nursing students perceived clinical stressors more intensely than academic and other sources of stress. Several studies in the UK (Deary et al 2003, Lindop 1999) found that third-year students experienced greater stress than in the earlier years of the programme. In a Canadian study, Beck & Srivastava (1991) found that, when compared with the general population, nursing students were at greater risk of having a physical or psychological illness. Sources of anxiety and stress reported in some of the literature include:
- Working with dying patients and death (Bagcivan et al 2015, Timmins & Kaliszer 2002)
- Interpersonal conflict with mentors and other practitioners (Ford et al 2016, Levett-Jones et al 2009, Timmins & Kaliszer 2002, Jackson & Mannix 2001)
- Insecurity about personal clinical competence and a perceived lack of practical skills (Admi et al 2018)

- Performing intimate care and caring for someone of the opposite sex (Seed 1995)
- Being assessed (Lefevre 2005) and fear of failure (Bagcivan et al 2015)
- Fear of making mistakes (Bagcivan et al 2015)
- Changes in ward allocation (Phillips et al 2000).

Many of these studies also found that stress and anxiety were heightened when staff members were unfriendly, unsupportive and did not make the students feel welcomed. It is important to remember that during clinical placements, students are usually removed from their peer support group. Levett-Jones et al (2009, 2015) and Doyle et al (2017) highlighted that a real concern for students was the feeling of belonging, being made to feel welcome and valued. Students in Ford et al's (2016) study identified that the sense of belonging or not affected the level of confidence they had to ask questions or seek out information and therefore impacted on their learning experience. One student quoted:

'I found that everyone was supportive and welcoming on the ward which makes a difference in how confident you feel in seeking advice and getting help' Ford et al (2016: 99)

Indeed, we should be perturbed if students had no concerns at all before beginning a placement or throughout a placement. However, there is a curvilinear relationship between anxiety and learning. Decreased learning occurs in the presence of high anxiety (Spielberger 1966 in Kleehammer et al 1990). In the context of clinical learning, Levett-Jones et al (2009) identified that students felt that the negative attitudes of staff diminished their confidence and their enthusiasm for learning. The concept of challenge and support was a positive one, although it was acknowledged that for some students who were insecure, challenge could be confrontational, causing students to doubt their ability and withdraw. Work on humanistic approaches to facilitating learning tells us that adults learn best in an environment that is psychologically comfortable where there is mutual trust and respect for their own worth and that of others (Knowles 1990, Rogers 1983). Powerful feelings such as anxiety, vulnerability, underconfidence, powerlessness, hope and dependence appeared not to interrupt students' learning if support, openness and encouragement were provided as these constructive measures allow mistakes in a trusting and safe learning environment (Lefevre 2005).

The following are some typical questions that students will ask before a clinical placement. These questions are based upon and extended from the work of Stengelhofen (1993) and Boud et al (1985).
- What will my role be?
- What will be expected of me?

- How much am I expected to know?
- How much am I expected to do?
- How much help and support will I get?
- What if I am asked to do something I cannot do?
- How will I know how I am doing?
- What are the demands of that setting?
- What will I learn?
- What will the people be like?
- Will they like me? Will I like them? Will I get on with my supervisor/assessor?

The answers that students seek to these questions could form the basis for the support and supervision that will contribute to the clinical placement being an educational experience for students.

You may wish to try Activity 8.6.

Activity 8.6

Ponder for a few minutes upon the questions above posed by students. What is the reputation of the learning ethos of your clinical area? How do you think a student new to your clinical area might feel?

Information Pack

Work that has been done into what helps students to learn during clinical placements tells us that making students feel welcome is a prerequisite to creating an atmosphere conducive to learning. Ideally, this 'welcome' should start before the commencement of the placement in the form of an information pack sent to the student. Stengelhofen (1993:73) makes an important point:

> 'Providing students with a clear picture of the clinical setting and the cases within that setting, as well as identifying the learning outcomes for them, appropriate to the stage of the course, will be a way of reassuring them that they will not be required to do anything or take responsibility beyond what can legitimately be expected.'

An information pack could include, for example:

- A welcome letter; this letter can also contain information to encourage the student to visit the placement before starting to meet the practice educator and find out what learning opportunities are available
- Maps of the locality and/or the hospital
- Facilities such as catering, parking, social and sporting
- Staff profile, including members of the multiprofessional team
- The allocated practice educator with contact details
- Clinical area profile, such as the philosophy, any nursing/midwifery model in use (for nursing and midwifery

students), the types of patients/clients seen and treatments offered
- A list of learning opportunities – teaching sessions, spoke opportunities, interprofessional learning
- A list of learning outcomes
- The roles and responsibilities of students in that clinical setting (this may need to be tailored to individual students depending on their prior experiences and stage of training)
- The shift hours
- Guidelines on dress.

When preplacement information packs are provided, important points can be assimilated by the student before commencement of the placement. This helps to reduce information overload during the early stages of the placement. Subsequently, the information is on record for reference.

Box 8.1 is an example of a welcome letter extracted from Stengelhofen (1993:68). There are other examples in her text. It is suggested that you draft one to suit your own clinical setting.

Receiving the Student

Some placement providers have practice placement facilitators/learning environment leads who make arrangements to meet all students on the first day of their placement. A programme of orientation for the day introduces the student to the placement provider and its various departments/services, their key functions and personnel.

BOX 8.1   Example of a Welcome Letter

Dear

We hope that you enjoy your placement with us.

The attached information pack is designed to help you understand how our service works, what we have to offer you while you are with us and what we expect from your university. Please read it before your first day. We will go over any queries you may have when we see you, but if you have any urgent questions you can telephone on_____. Please confirm that you are starting your placement with us on_____. We suggest that you arrive at_____. Before your arrival, it would help us in planning your time if you could send us some information about yourself. We would like to know a little about your background, your academic interests, previous clinical experience and your objectives for this placement. We look forward to meeting you. Involvement in study training is an enjoyable and stimulating, as well as a time-consuming, experience for us. We expect to learn from you as well as with you, and we hope that you will be happy with us. (From Stengelhofen 1993.)

The supervisor and/or practice assessor has a particular role in receiving the student and orientating the student to the work setting. When the placement is the first one for a student, supervisors and practice assessors are reminded to take particular care, as the student may be highly anxious. There is no doubt that first impressions will influence the student's enjoyment of the placement (Chesser-Smyth 2005) and may even shape the student's views of the profession (McKenna et al 2010). Make time for the crucial activity of orientation, which is seen to be the "gateway to a successful placement" (Beskine 2009). This might help students feel that they belong because nursing students say that a sense of "belongingness" is a prerequisite for clinical learning (Levett-Jones et al 2009). There should be a plan for the first day. This might include:

- Setting some time aside to welcome the student. It is sensible to start the student on a first shift at a later time than is the routine, preferably after the hustle and bustle of the shift has been dealt with.
- Orientation to health and safety matters.
- Orientation to the workplace, such as the general layout of the clinical area, working patterns—shift hours, meal breaks.
- Introduction to team members.
- Showing where information sources are kept, such as placement philosophy and policy and procedure manuals.
- Showing communication systems, such as telephones and answering protocols, patient/client buzzer system and emergency call system.
- Spending time to discuss the student's learning needs and previous experiences. Find out at which stage of training the student is. Students' self-esteem is increased if they feel they can share any previously acquired learning with practitioners (Stengelhofen 1993). It should be made clear to students what their roles and responsibilities are and when they should or should not help or participate. Most beginning students breathe a big sigh of relief when they are told that they are not expected to start to give care immediately and are reassured that they will be asked to do only what they are capable of doing.
- Taking prior learning into account, identify learning opportunities available and experiences that are required to enable the achievement of learning outcomes. Jointly develop an action plan for the duration of the placement. It may be necessary to allow students to settle into a placement first and delay this activity.

Providing Ongoing Support and Supervision

Gray and Smith (2000) identified that a good mentor was not only one that involved students in activities, spending time with the student and showing a real interest in the students' learning but one who also trusted the students' ability and withdrew supervision as appropriate. This can be equally applied to the new practice supervisor role. The students identified that the gradual distancing from the mentor came with the increase in their self-confidence but that the mentor still played a crucial role in supporting and facilitating their learning, confirming that ongoing support and supervision should aim to facilitate learning. The development of competence is linked to the effectiveness of support (Lauder et al 2008). Stengelhofen (1993) and White and Ewan (1991) suggest the following activities for the facilitation of learning by practice supervisors in the clinical setting:

1. Answer questions—make students feel free to ask questions and to seek help without loss of confidence or self-esteem.
2. Offer suggestions—be careful to foster students' self-confidence. Rogers (1983) suggested that when the student is moving from exploration into understanding, the facilitator responds directly to the content the student is struggling with (e.g., by giving direct answers). When the student starts to focus on actions to be taken during care, the facilitator moves into guiding further development of the student's skills and knowledge. Vygotsky's (1930, in Spouse 1998) theory of the "zone of proximal development" states that the potential of a learner to progress to the second stage of development could be capitalized upon by support and guidance from a more experienced other.
3. Allow students to make choices about care to be given—do not limit and constrain the student to your experience.
4. Facilitate development of desired behaviours—the practice supervisor is reminded that role modelling is one powerful tool for this purpose.
5. Encourage self monitoring and evaluation—help students to identify where they have reached in their learning and help them to develop the ability to assess their performance accurately and subsequently set realistic learning goals.
6. Provide opportunities and guidelines for students to observe care activities.
7. Learn from the students—listen to the students and facilitate two-way discussions. Rogers (1983) suggested that facilitators need to be able to respond to the feelings of students as learning experiences are explored together.
8. Give students time to reflect on what is happening and has happened—promote discussion about patient/client care.
9. Give students time to prepare—when assigning work to students, spend time briefing them and allocate time for them to prepare to give care.

10. Allow students to make mistakes in the confines of patient safety—show confidence in students and give positive reinforcement; reinforce the expectation of success. Allow 'hands-on' experience even when you think the task is complex. Manipulate the session to allow students to experience success.

11. Encourage students to think for themselves—structure and sequence questions so that students are led through their own paths of thinking to show how they came to a certain conclusion. Questions should therefore challenge students to trace their own thinking strategies and to explain how they drew inferences or came to certain conclusions.

The following questions may help you evaluate whether students are receiving adequate support and supervision:

1. How do I help students settle into the workplace?
2. What do I do to make their first days more enjoyable?
3. How do I make their placement an educational experience?
4. How do I help students feel confident about their role?
5. Do students in my area feel valued and respected?
6. When students are unhappy at work, do I know the contributory factors?

Continuing Professional Development

When the clinical environment provides a culture where learning and professional development take place, it becomes a positive learning environment where the atmosphere becomes one where there is a commitment to lifelong learning and continuing professional development (CPD) activities. Staff members are more likely to develop the commitment to seek to learn for themselves and to share their learning with one another. There is encouragement to undertake CPD activities through further formal education, accredited courses and informal in-house training. This kind of environment will assist nurses and midwives who are practice supervisors and practice assessors to preregistration nursing and midwifery students to fulfil the requirement of revalidation to develop their own knowledge, skills and competency beyond that of registration through CPD—either formal or experiential learning (NMC 20018b).

"Lifelong learning" is the term used to refer to the planned or unplanned learning that occurs throughout the life, usually the working life, of an individual (Hinchliff 1998). The undertaking of further education is indeed necessary, as professionals of health care cannot hope to practise safely and effectively in a context of continuous change without undertaking updating activities. The importance of CPD is clearly articulated by the NMC in The Code (2018b) and in alinement with NMC Revalidation Process (2019) for Registrants and for Health and Care

Professionals Council (HCPC) in its Standards of Continuing Professional Development (HCPC 2018). In The Scope of Professional Practice, the UKCC (1992) stated:

'Pre-registration education prepares nurses, midwives and health visitors for safe practice at the point of registration … [It] is therefore a foundation for professional practice … This foundation education alone, however, cannot effectively meet the changing and complex demands of the range of modern health care. Post-registration education equips practitioners with additional and more specialist skills necessary to meet the special needs of patients and clients.'

This statement is applicable not only to nurses and midwives but to all professionals of health care. It is also as applicable today as it was in 1992.

Pause to review how CPD can be encouraged in the clinical setting. Are there activities in your clinical area that you think would contribute to the CPD of staff? It is important to use learning opportunities in the workplace; not only is such learning directly relevant to practice, but also there can be many constraints on the availability and accessibility of formal courses in a resource-limited system. It is my belief that you and your colleagues, including members of the multiprofessional team and unqualified staff members, are the most important teaching and learning resource in your work area.

The following questions are intended to help you explore how the "human resource" for learning can be used to contribute to your clinical setting as one that motivates staff to engage in CPD:

- How can you contribute? How much do you contribute? Remember that your contributions such as developing a teaching/learning pack can be used as evidence of CPD.
- How can your colleagues and members of the multiprofessional team contribute? How much do they contribute? Do not forget unqualified staff members – someone may have a personal health experience which they can talk about.
- Are there planned teaching programmes? When this is an established routine, staff will be encouraged to contribute and attend.
- After staff members have been on study days and courses, is there a mechanism for the dissemination of information? This can serve several purposes; it helps the individual learn further through teaching or preparing a paper, and brings what is learned to the clinical area to improve professional practices.
- Are there staff support groups where staff members get together to debrief and reflect? Sharing ideas and experiences in a group is an effective way of developing

practice wisdom—wisdom being the distillation of knowledge and experience (Hull 1998).

- Are there activities such as case discussions and conferences and seminars? If you have cared for the patient/client featured in the case, you will be able to contribute to the discussion. Subsequently, if what you have learnt is written up, preferably with reference to literature as appropriate, it is again evidence of CPD.

Material Resources

Having examined how the human resource can make direct contributions to the learning environment of the clinical setting, go on to consider those nonhuman resources that can contribute to the learning environment.

You may wish to try Activity 8.7.

Activity 8.7

Have a good look around your clinical setting. Taking a look in the form of walking around may prove to be revealing. What material resources are there to contribute to the learning environment?

The following questions may guide you in your "walkabout".

- Do you have a resource room/area where text material such as books and journals are housed? If not, is it possible to make space for one? This resource area could also house contributions such as learning packages and posters developed by staff after they have been on study days, conferences and courses.
- If you have a resource room/area, is the area conducive to reading, browsing and study? For example, is text material shelved and filed in some kind of order, is it up to date, is the area generally tidy, is there some fairly comfortable seating and so on?
- Is there someone who is designated to maintain this area and keep resources up to date? Staff could take it in turns and be given time out to perform this function, such as going to the library to seek out relevant journal articles/relevant professional material and do the general housekeeping.
- Is there a file that contains information specifically for students and new staff members? This file could have information about the learning opportunities in your setting, core experiences that students should participate in, names and designations of specialist members of the team and so on.
- Are there places such as notice boards where information, such as flyers about courses, teaching/ learning events and so on, can be displayed? If not, is it possible

to find a suitable wall space for a notice/pinboard to be installed? These are generally not too costly.

- Are policy and procedure manuals up to date? Are they in an accessible location? If on the intranet, do students have access?
- Is there a philosophy of care/values statement for your area? If there is, where is it displayed? Are staff members aware of its intentions?
- Is there a collection of material such as health promotion leaflets and so on from both charitable and government organizations relevant to your clinical area? These are frequently free and provide useful information for both patients/clients and staff.
- If there are audiovisual aids such as DVDs and CDs, are they still up to date? Is the equipment for using these aids in good working order?
- Are there other teaching/learning aids such as models and mannequins? Are they in good order?
- Are information technology facilities available to access electronic sources of information from the internet, databases or e-learning packages?

QUALITY ASSURANCE

Quality assurance can be viewed simply as comprising all those activities in an organization that help to identify and promote good practice and prevent poor practice (ENB 1993). From an education perspective, the NMC (2018d) describes it as the approach they take to ensure their standards are achieved and maintained by all approved educational institutions. The NMC stipulates that approved education institutions, in partnership with practice partners, are responsible for the quality assurance of all aspects of the programme. Since the 1990s, it has been accepted that quality can be achieved and maintained through the use of audit, which has become the most prominent and important mechanism for improving the quality of health and education sector services (Nicklin & Kenworthy 1995).

In its Standards Framework for Nursing and Midwifery Education, the NMC (2018a) identified the importance of effective governance systems to ensure quality of education provision. It specifically goes on to identify that to confirm that all learning environments are suitable, safe and effective, regular reviews must be undertaken of the learning environment. Although this does not specifically identify the need for educational audit, as was the case previously, this could still be considered an appropriate approach to be taken. The English National Board for Nursing, Midwifery and Health Visiting (ENB) and Department of Health (2001) suggest that the outcomes of audit and monitoring should lead to the dissemination of good practice and joint action planning between placement providers and approved education institutions to address any areas of concern or those needing enhancement. When attempts are made to judge the quality of the students' experiences, White and Ewan (1991:160) say that 'only the students are capable of judging the value of the experience because they are the ones having the experience'.

Student feedback is sought by approved education institutions through their own internal quality monitoring processes and also via external sources, such as the National Student Survey that asks students to give feedback on academic and practice experience, and Health Education England's National Education and Training Survey that looks at placements experience. Actively soliciting feedback should contribute to the ongoing evaluation of the learning environment. As can be seen from the exploration of the clinical setting as an environment for learning, there are many factors that influence and interact with each other to impact on this learning environment. These factors and the concomitant processes arising consequent to the interaction of these factors should not be left to chance—they need to be worked at to ensure that there are positive influences. Approved education institutions, in partnership with their service colleagues, need to work together to ensure that high-quality practice placements, in a supportive environment, help students achieve the learning outcomes of their educational programme and ensure that they are able to provide the safe care needed by patients and clients (NMC 2018a).

An essential element of the legislation establishing the NMC and the HCPC as health professions regulators is the role of the quality assurance of the education of aspiring professionals. As guardians of the professional registers and with their duty to protect the public, it is essential that regulators are able to judge whether a health care student is fit to join the register once they have completed their pre-registration education and training. Within the wider context of quality assurance, the regulators' activities should be considered in conjunction with the other quality assurance exercises that education providers engage in.

At the institutional level, the Quality Assurance Agency (QAA) award higher education institutions with degree-awarding powers. This can be awarded indefinitely or for a period of up to 6 years, and the QAA may also undertake intermittent quality monitoring visits (QAA 2018a). The four main areas of quality assurance activity of the NMC and HCPC are:

- new programme approval
- ongoing monitoring of approved programmes
- approving major changes to programmes
- programme reapproval.

Approval is the process of validation and accreditation that leads to decisions about whether a programme is approved so

that it can be launched or is reapproved/reaccredited so that it may continue. Through the systematic process of approval, decisions are made about the ability of the proposed programme to meet, over a period of time, the requirements of regulatory bodies, education providers, health and social care providers, service users and education commissioners. Ongoing quality monitoring and enhancement is the process by which education providers and external stakeholders satisfy themselves that the quality of educational programmes is being maintained and improved upon. It includes all activity that occurs on an ongoing basis in both the academic and practice-based settings; for example, practice placement audit and regular monitoring (normally annually or every 2 years) by the regulatory bodies. The quality assurance approach of the NMC has previously been one focusing on risks to be controlled in the delivery of programmes (NMC 2013). These risks were:

- inadequate resources
- inadequate safeguards for monitoring student conduct
- inadequate governance of practice learning
- failure to provide learning opportunities of a suitable quality
- unreliable conformation of achievement
- failure to address required learning outcomes
- failure of internal quality assurance systems to provides assurance against NMC standards.

With the implementation of the current Standards Framework for Nursing and Midwifery Education (2018e), the focus on risk management will continue against the new standards criteria:

- Learning culture
- Educational governance and quality
- Student empowerment
- Educators and assessors
- Curricula and assessment

The Quality Assurance Agency

In the UK, the QAA will use the Quality Code for Higher Education (2018b) as a basis for guiding the educational practices of higher education institutions. In particular, the UK Quality Code for Higher Education Advice and Guidance Work-Based Learning (QAA 2018c) outlines the precepts that programmes have to meet to provide quality placement experiences for students to meet programme learning outcomes. The following principles to support and monitor placement learning are specified in the code:

1. Work-based learning courses and opportunities are designed and developed in partnership with employers, students and other stakeholders (where appropriate) and contain learning outcomes that are relevant to work objectives.

2. Work-based learning consists of structured opportunities for learning and is achieved through authentic activity and is supervised in the workplace.
3. Work-based learning opportunities are underpinned by formal agreements between education organizations, employers and students.
4. Education organizations and employers consider any specific issues in relation to the workplace environment and deal with them appropriately, including informal agreements where appropriate.
5. Work-based learning is delivered through a meaningful partnership between students, employers and the education organization.
6. Work-based learning opportunities enable students to apply and integrate areas of subject and professional knowledge, skills and behaviours to enable them to meet course learning outcomes.
7. Parties understand and respect the respective roles, responsibilities and expectations of the education organization, employer and student, and appropriate training and support is provided where required.
8. Education organizations and employers acknowledge individuals have unique needs within the education organization and in the workplace, and collaborate to ensure opportunities are inclusive, safe and supported.
9. Work-based learning opportunities are designed, monitored, evaluated and reviewed in partnership with employers.

CRITERIA FOR EDUCATIONAL AUDIT

You may wish to try Activity 8.8.

Activity 8.8

Obtain a copy of the tool for the educational audit of your clinical area. What are the aspects of the clinical environment that are audited? How well do they reflect the clinical environment that is an educational environment?

In 1993, the ENB proposed the use of the following eight aspects, with their associated criteria, for auditing practice placements. Although published in 1993, these aspects are still relevant today as the guiding principles for the audit.
1. Ethos of the placement:
   • general climate
   • channels of communication
   • approachability of staff
   • relationships between the higher education institution and the placement
   • commitment to teaching and learning.

2. Organization of care:
   • philosophy and approach to care
   • the organisation of workload so as to promote continuity (e.g., team nursing)
   • involvement of students in multiprofessional teamwork.
3. Supervision and assessment:
   • effectiveness of supervision and assessment activities by first-level practitioners
   • contribution by academic staff
   • fulfilment of clinical contact hours
   • compliance with regulations in supervision and assessment of students.
4. Teaching programme and assessment:
   • planned programmes
   • opportunities for students to achieve competencies through continuous assessment
   • learning outcomes set at appropriate academic and professional levels n patient/client groups support achievement of learning outcomes.
5. Research basis of care planning and delivery:
   • evidence of the application of research in teaching and implementation of care.
6. Academic and professional qualifications of staff.
7. Staff development programmes.
8. Physical environment. The following three aspects should be added:
9. Teaching/learning resources and strategies:
   • a designated study area
   • a range of teaching/learning resources are provided
   • there is availability of information technology with access to electronic sources of information
   • teaching/learning strategies practised to help students relate theory to practice and reflect on care given.
10. Management of the learning environment. There is a designated learning environment manager who:
    • has overall responsibility for all teaching/learning activities and the learning environment
    • liaises with the clinical link lecturer and/or academic assessor
    • supports supervisors and assessors.
11. The clinical link lecturer/academic assessor. There is a designated clinical link lecturer and/or academic assessor from the approved education institution who liaises with placement staff to ensure effective implementation of the curriculum by:
    • providing support and guidance for staff and students
    • acting as a resource for educational activities such as compiling a profile of learning opportunities.

The Process of Educational Audit

Generally, before a clinical area being used as a placement area for preregistration students, an educational audit of that area is required to ensure that it is able to support student learning. Subsequently, the area is audited annually. Typically, this is done by the learning environment manager and a representative from the approved educational institution, for example, the clinical link lecturer or academic assessor. However, it should also be conducted whenever the circumstances of the clinical setting changes, such as a reduction of bed numbers and the type of patients/clients cared for.

You may wish to try Activity 8.9.

> ### Activity 8.9
>
> How do you, your colleagues and students contribute to the educational audit of your clinical area? How is your clinical link lecturer/academic assessor involved?

CONCLUSION

What helps students learn and develop into the professionals we desire them to be? Clinical settings provide unique learning experiences and opportunities for students; these must be planned, structured, managed and coordinated (ENB & Department of Health 2001) so that students undergo professional socialization positively and develop the competencies for professional practice that cannot be readily acquired elsewhere. The clinical experience for students should be much more than just learning what to do and how to do it—it should be about the education of students who will one day be our professional peers, colleagues and co-learners. Clinical placements for students should contribute to their education so that they become self-directed learners who will also engage in lifelong learning.

Thoughtful and informed development of a clinical environment so that it is also an educational environment will enhance the learning of students and the professional development of staff. The challenge for practitioners is to create this type of environment. It is important to have a good understanding of the characteristics of an educational clinical environment and those factors that contribute to or detract from it. The educational audit of clinical placements helps to monitor and maintain the quality of placement areas. This mechanism may also be helpful in the acquisition of resources to support the continuing development of a learning environment.

Underpinning the success of any effort to develop a positive learning climate is a commitment by all staff to contribute not only to their own learning but also to that of others; the key to engendering this positive learning climate is the people who work in the setting. Students will tell us what does and what does not help them learn during clinical placements, and their feedback should be used to inform changes that are made.

A quote from Helen Orton's book titled *Ward Learning Climate* will be used to conclude the chapter. Although the book was published in 1981, it could be suggested that what she wrote in this excerpt is equally true, if not more so, for today's health care climate (Orton 1981:67).

'… patient well-being and student well-being have been shown to be inextricably bound together. In terms of potential improvement for either group it is probably not important whether the motive for change stems from a desire to enrich ward experience for patients or for students. What is now certain is that the encouragement and development of 'good' learning climates would bring improvements for all those involved in ward life and that the benefits could be measured not only in economic terms but also by the increase in human happiness and well-being.'

KEY POINTS FOR REFLECTION

When considering the clinical environment as an educational environment, several groups of factors and the interaction between them need to be taken into account. These factors can be grouped as:

1. The people: The leader of the team: the creation of a democratic and nonhierarchical structure promotes teamwork and good communication because facilitating learning cannot be divorced from competent management and humane leadership. The members of the team: each team member contributes to the creation of the learning environment. The clinical setting provides opportunities for students to learn and work as part of a multiprofessional team so that each learns to function as an effective team member. The students: students bring their own personalities, dispositions, hopes and aspirations, past experiences and backgrounds, and also worries and anxieties to the clinical setting. They should be viewed as valuable student members of the team with specific clinical learning needs while being socialized into the profession. The practice educator: to facilitate learning effectively, the practice educator needs good

teaching and interpersonal skills as well as being clinically competent and knowledgeable.

2. Learning opportunities and experiences "provided by": patient/client care: in any clinical setting, encounters with patients/clients should always form the basis of clinical learning. Other clinical activities: a list of activities and events with their potential for learning can be useful in directing and guiding students to sources of learning other than participating in direct patient/client care.

3. Staff commitment to teaching and learning: support and supervision of learners: this starts with sending learners an information pack that includes a welcome letter. Be ready to welcome and receive the learner on the first day. Subsequently, provide adequate ongoing support and supervision to enable students to maximize their learning. The following questions may be helpful in guiding the activities of the supervisor:
   - How can work be planned so that having students is a help rather than a hindrance?
   - How can students be involved in care so that they are learning while contributing to the work of the team?
   - How can the work be turned into dynamic learning experiences?
   - How do I make their placement an educational experience?
   - How do I help students feel confident about their role?
   - Do students in my area feel valued and respected? CPD: to meet the changing and complex demands of the range of modern health care effectively, practitioners must develop their own knowledge, skills and competence beyond that of registration. CPD can be either formal or informal (e.g., through experiential learning).

4. Material resources: text information needs to be kept up to date, and teaching aids need to be in good repair. Quality assurance processes ensure that the quality of educational programmes is being maintained and improved. It includes all activity that occurs on an ongoing basis in both the academic and practice-based settings.

Generally, before a clinical area being used as a placement area for preregistration students, an educational audit of that area is required to ensure that it is able to support student learning. Subsequently, the area is audited formally at least annually so that institutions can demonstrate that they can provide quality placement experiences for students.

REFERENCES

Admi H, Moshe-Eilon Y, Sharon D. Mann M. Nursing students' stress and satisfaction in clinical practice along different stages: a cross-sectional study. *Nurs Educ Today,* 2018;68:86-92.

Bagcivan G, Cinar FI, Tosun N, Kormaz R. Determination of nursing students' expectations for faculty members and the perceived stressors during their education. *Contemp Nurs,* 2015;50:1:58-71

Barr H, Koppel I, Reeves S, Hammick M, Freeth D. in Lait, J., Suter, E., Arthur, N., Deutschlander., S. (2011) Interprofessional mentoring: enhancing students' clinical learning. *Nurs Educ Prac.* 2005;11(3):211-215.

Beck DL, Srivastava R. Perceived level and sources of stress in baccalaureate nursing students. *J Nurs Educ.* 1991;30(3); 127–133.

Beskine D. Mentoring students: Establishing effective working relationships. *Nurs Stand,* 2009;23:30, 35–40.

Boud D, Keogh R, Walker D. Promoting reflection in learning. In: Boud, D., Keogh, R., Walker, D. (Eds.), Reflection: Turning Experience into Learning. Kogan Page, London:1985, 18–40.

Bradshaw A. Is the ward sister role still relevant to the quality of patient care? A critical examination of the ward sister role past and present. *J Clin Nurs,* 2010;19:3555-3563.

Burnard P, Chapman CM. Nurse Education: The Way Forward. Scutari Press, London:1990.

Chamberlain M. Challenges of clinical learning for student midwives. *Midwifery,* 1997;13: 85–91.

Chesser-Smyth PA. The lived experiences of general student nurses on their first clinical placement: a phenomenological study. *Nurs Educ Prac,* 2005;5, 320–327.

Deary IJ, Watson R. Hogston R. A longitudinal cohort study of burnout and attrition in nursing students. *J Advanc Nurs,* 2003;43:1:71-81.

Doyle K, Sainsbury K, Cleary S, et al. Happy to help/happy to be here: identifying components of successful clinical placements for undergraduate nursing students. *Nurs Educ Today,* 2017;49:27-32.

English National Board. Guidelines for Educational Audit. English National Board for Nursing, Midwifery and Health Visiting, London:1993.

English National Board, Department of Health. Placements in Focus. The English National Board for Nursing, Midwifery and Health Visiting and The Department of Health, London: 2001.

Flott EA, Linden L. The clinical learning environment in nursing education: a concept analysis. *J Advanc Nurs,* 2015;72:3:501-513.

Ford K, Courtney-Pratt H, Marlow A, Cooper J, Williams D, Mason R. Quality clinical placements: the perspective of undergraduate nursing students and their supervising nurses. *Nurs Educ Today,* 2016;37:97-102.

Francis R. Report of the Mid Staffordshire NHS Foundation Trust Public Enquiry: Executive Summary. 2012. https://www.gov.uk/government/publications/report-of-the-mid-staffordshire-nhs-foundation-trust-public-inquiry Accessed on 28/01/2019.

Gerrish K. Fumbling along. *Nurs Times,* 1990;86:35-37.

Gerrish K. Still fumbling along? A comparative study of the newly qualified nurse's perception of the transition from student to qualified nurse. *J Advanc Nurs,* 2000;32:2:473-480.

Gray MA, Smith LN. The qualities of an effective mentor from the student nurse's perspective: findings from a longitudinal qualitative study. *J Advanc Nurs,* 2000;32:6:1542-1549.

Harrison-White K, King E. Hub and spoke model for nursing student placements in the UK. *Nurs Child Young Peop,* 2015;27:2:24-29.

Health and Care Professions Council. Standards of Continuing Professional Development. HCPC, London:2018, Online. Available: https://www.hcpc-uk.org/standards/standards-of-continuing-professional-development/ Accessed on 28/01/2019.

Henderson V. The Nature of Nursing. Macmillan, New York:1966.

Hinchliff S. Lifelong learning in context. In: Quinn, F.M. (Ed.), Continuing Professional Development in Nursing. Stanley Thornes, Cheltenham:1998, pp. 34–58.

Holland K. Inter-professional education and practice: the role of the teacher/facilitator (editorial). *Nurs Educ Prac,* 2002;2: 221-222.

Hull C. Open learning and professional development. In: Quinn F. (Ed.), Continuing Professional Development in Nursing. Stanley Thornes, Cheltenham:1998, pp. 182–204.

Illingworth P, Chelvanayagam S. Benefits of interprofessional education in health care. *Br J Nurs,* 2007;16(2):121-124.

Jackson D, Mannix J. Clinical nurses as teachers: insights from students of nursing in their first semester of study. *J Clin Nurs,* 2001;10:270-277.

Jarvis P. *Adult and Continuing Education: Theory and Practice.* Croom Helm, Beckenham:1983.

Jimenez C, Navia-Osorio PM, Diaz CV. Stress and health in novice and experienced nursing students. *J Advan Nurs,* 2009;66(2):442-455.

Lait J, Suter E, Arthur N, Deutschlander S. Interprofessional mentoring: enhancing students' clinical learning. *Nurse Educ Prac.* 2011;11(3)211–215.

Lauder W, Watson R, Topping K, et al. An evaluation of fitness for practice curricula: self-efficacy, support and self-reported competence in preregistration student nurses and midwives. *J Clin Nurs,*20 08;17:1858-1867.

Lefevre M. Facilitating practice learning and assessment: the influence of relationship. *Social Work Educ,* 2005:24(5):565-583.

Levett-Jones T, Lathlean J, Higgins I, McMillan M. Staff – student relationships and their impact on nursing students' belongingness and learning. *J Advan Nurs,* 2009;65(2):316-324.

Levett-Jones T, Pitt V, Courtney-Pratt H, Harbrow G, Rossiter R. What are the primary concerns of nursing students as they prepare for and contemplate their first clinical placement experience? *Nurs Educ Prac,* 2015;15:304-306.

Lindop E. (1999) A comparative study of stress between pre- and post- Project 2000 students. *J Advanc Nurs,* 1999;29(4):967-973.

Mariet J. (2016) Professional socialisation models in nursing. *Int J Nurs Educ,* 2016;8(3):143-148.

McKenna L, McCall L, Wray N. Clinical placements and nursing students' career planning: a qualitative exploration. *Int J Nurs Prac,* 2010;16:176-182.

National Health Service Institute for Innovation and Improvement. Safer Care, SBAR Implementation and Training Guide. National Health Service Institute for Innovation and Improvement, Coventry:2010.

Newton JM. Jilly BC, Ockerby CM, Cross WM. A clinical learning environment scale: a factor analysis. *J Advanc Learn,* 2010;66, 1371-1481, Cited in Bjork IT, Berntsen K, Brynildsen G, Hestetun M. Nursing students' perceptions of their clinical learning environment in placements outside traditional hospital settings. *J Clin Nurs,* 2014;23:2958-2967.

Newton J M, Henderson A, Jolly B, Greaves J. A contemporary examination of workplace learning culture: An ethnomethodology study. *Nurse education today,* 2015;35(1):91-96

Nicklin PJ, Kenworthy N. Teaching and Assessing in Clinical Practice. 2nd Edition. Baillière Tindall, London:1995.

Nisbet G, Dunn S, Lincoln M. Interprofessional team meetings: opportunities for informal interprofessional learning. *J Interprof Care,* 2015;29:5:426-432.

Norman K. How mentors can influence the values, behaviours and attitudes of nursing staff through positive professional socialisation. *Nurs Manag.* 2015;22:8;33–38.

Nursing and Midwifery Council: Standards to Support Learning and Assessment in Practice. 2nd Edition. Nursing and Midwifery Council, London:2008.

Nursing and Midwifery Council. Quality Assurance Framework for Nursing and Midwifery Education. Nursing and Midwifery Council, London:2013.

Nursing and Midwifery Council. Standards for Education and Training. Part 3: Standards for Pre-registration Nursing Programmes. Nursing and Midwifery Council, London:2018a.

Nursing and Midwifery Council. The Code. Professional Standards of Practice and Behaviour for Nurses, Midwives and Nursing Associates. Nursing and Midwifery Council, London:2018b.

Nursing and Midwifery Council. Standards for Education and Training. Part 2: Standards for Student Supervision and Assessment. Nursing and Midwifery Council, London:2018c.

Nursing and Midwifery Council. Quality Assurance Framework for Nursing, Midwifery and Nursing Associate Education. Nursing and Midwifery Council, London:2018d.

Nursing and Midwifery Council. Standards for Education and Training. Part 1: Standards Framework for Nursing and Midwifery Education. Nursing and Midwifery Council, London:2018e.

Nursing and Midwifery Council. How to Revalidate with the NMC. Requirements for Renewing Your Registration. Nursing and Midwifery Council, London:2019.

Ogier M. Working and Learning. Scutari Press, London:1989.

Orton HD. Ward Learning Climate. Royal College of Nursing, London:1981.

Parlett MR, Hamilton DF. Evaluation as illumination. In: Parlett MR, Dearden GJ. (Eds) Introduction to Illuminative Evaluation: Studies in Higher Education. Pacific Soundings Press, Cardiff-by-the-Sea, California:1977, pp. 9–29.

Papp I, Markkanen M, Von Bonsdorff M. Clinical environment as a learning environment: student nurses' perceptions concerning clinical learning experience. *Nurs Educ Today,* 2003;23:4:262-268.

Phillips T, Schostak J, Tyler J. Practice and Assessment in Nursing and Midwifery. Doing it for Real. The English National Board for Nursing, Midwifery and Health Visiting, London:2000.

Quality Assurance Agency. The Right to Award Degrees. Guidance. 3rd Edition. Quality Assurance Agency, UK:2018a.

Quality Assurance Agency. The Revised Quality Code for Higher Education. Quality Assurance Agency, UK:2018b.

Quality Assurance Agency. *UK Quality Code for Higher Education. Advice and Guidance, Work-Based Learning.* Quality Assurance Agency, UK:2018c.

Rogers, C., (1983) *Freedom to learn for the 80's.* Charles E. Merrill, Columbus, Ohio.

Seed A. Crossing the boundary – experiences of neophyte nurses. *J Advanc Nusr,* 1995;21:1136-1143.

Shivers E, Hasson F, Slater P. Pre-registration nursing student's quality of practice learning: Clinical learning environment inventory (actual) questionnaire. *Nurs Educ Today,* 2017;55: 58–64.

Sjogren Forss K, Persson K, Borglin, G. Nursing students' experiences of caring for ethnically and culturally diverse patients. A scoping review. *Nurse Education in Practice,* 2019;37: 97-104

Spielberger CD. (Ed.), (1966) Anxiety and Behaviour. Academic Press, New York. In Kleehammer K, Hart AL, Keck JF. Nursing students' perceptions of anxiety producing situations in the clinical setting. *J Nurs Educ,* 1990;29:40:183-187.

Spouse J. Scaffolding student learning in clinical practice. *Nurs Educ Today,* 1998;18: 259–266.

Stengelhofen J. Teaching Students in Clinical Settings. Chapman & Hall, London:1993.

Timmins F, Kaliszer M. Aspects of nurse education programmes that frequently cause stress in nursing students – fact-finding sample survey. *Nurs Educ Today,* 2002;22:203-211.

Tomietto M, Comparcini D, Simonetti V et al. Work-engaged nurses for a better clinical learning environment: a ward-level analysis. *J Nurs Manag,* 2016;24: 475-482

United Kingdom Central Council for Nursing, Midwifery and Health Visiting. Project 2000: A New Preparation for Practice. United Kingdom Central Council for Nursing, Midwifery and Health Visiting, London:1986.

United Kingdom Central Council for Nursing, Midwifery and Health Visiting. The Scope of Professional Practice. United Kingdom Central Council for Nursing, Midwifery and Health Visiting, London:1992.

White R, Ewan C. *Clinical Teaching in Nursing.* Chapman & Hall, London:1991.

Whitehead B, Holmes D. Are newly qualified nurses prepared for practice? *Nurs Times,* 2011;107(19):20-23.

Willis Commission. Quality with Compassion: The Future of Nurse Education. Royal College of Nursing, UK:2012.

Wu LT, Low MMJ, Tan KK, Lopez V, Liaw SY. Why not nursing? A systematic review of factors influencing career choice among healthcare students. *Int Nurs Rev,* 2015;62:547-562.

9

Learning Through Clinical Practice: Unearthing Meaning from Experience

CHAPTER CONTENTS

INTRODUCTION

Practice-based learning is an important part of any health care professional's preregistration experience, with at least 50% of the preregistration nursing and 60% of the midwifery curriculum taking place in practice placements. Within these settings, students learn through the provision of opportunities to engage in patient care, learning from colleagues, and reflecting on these experiences. This chapter aims to discuss how students can learn from practice experience supported by practice assessors and supervisors and outlining models and approach which can be applied.

The introduction of the Nursing and Midwifery Council (NMC; 2018a) Standards for Student Supervision and Assessment is part of a wider revision of the role of the Nurse or Midwife as a practice-based educator, assessor and supervisor in the modern UK health care workforce. Changes to nursing proficiencies required for registration (NMC 2018b) set the scene for learning from practice. Previous concepts of "Mentorship" have framed practice-based learning as a one-to-one relationship, with both supervision and assessment being performed by the nominated mentor. However, conflicts in delivering both supportive and assessment roles were well documented (Bray & Nettleton 2008), and led to laissez-faire attitudes toward mentor development, alongside mentorship occurring in silos with little reference to the wider team (MacLaren 2018).

The recent NMC (2018a) standards formalize a team approach to supporting students with recognition that all team members have a contribution to and are accountable for student learning and the safety of the general public. Workplace learning is reframed as a participatory, collaboratively constructed and socio-culturally situated activity (Lave & Wenger 1991, Hager 2004, Fenwick 2008). Learner-centred facilitation of learning rather than teacher-led transmission of knowledge and skills form the focus of learning in practice, mirroring strategies, such as problem-based learning, and clinical simulation, common within the taught curriculum (Andrews & Reece Jones 1996, Haigh 2007).

Benner (1984) provided a phenomenological exploration of the development of nursing expertise and the knowledge embedded within practice. She conducted initial interviews with 21 expert and novice (newly qualified) nurse pairs, using shared experiences of a clinical situation as the basis of the interviews. Further interviews and observation with nurses at all career stages bolstered the data. Application of the Dreyfus skills acquisition model (Dreyfus & Dreyfus 1979: cited by Benner 1984) with its five stages of skill acquisition (Novice, advanced beginner, competent, proficient and expert) allowed Benner to identify clear differences in the ways that experts and newly qualified staff practice. Novices appeared rule-bound and task driven, whereas experts appeared not to rely on the same analytical principles as their junior colleagues to guide their course of action. This was reported in terms of changes in learners' perceptions of task demands from a series of equally relevant components as novices, to a more holistic overview where only some aspects are relevant. Furthermore, it is attributed to practitioners' moves from detached observer to involved performer, reflecting an apprenticeship or Communities of Practice (CoP) model, such as that outlined by Lave and Wenger (1991).

CoP theory advances learning in the workplace as a gradual enculturation into working practices of a group (Lave & Wenger 1991). Wenger (1998) identifies that mutuality, joint endeavour and a shared repertoire are key assisting factors in socialization into a community of practice. Thus, nurses working in an acute ward environment might be considered as working within a community of practice, with nurses sharing a sense of public service, professional belonging, working practices and goals in patient care (Levett-Jones & Lathlean 2008, Jensen & Lahn 2005). As identified in Benner's (1984) study, newcomers to practice experience a period of socialization which draws them more centrally into the nursing work of the practice area. This occurs not only with students, but also when a registered nurse enters a new area of practice.

The focus of learning in this context is individual skill acquisition (psychomotor and decision-making/judgmental skill) through mastery, and experience of a wide range of patient-centred episodes. Benner foregrounds the use of reflection for making sense of practice experiences, identifying patterns and testing formal and informal theories

(Benner 1984, Innes 2004). This offers nurses a powerful tool for personal learning and professional development which has almost become a competency in its own right. Reflective practices are organizationally attractive as they do not require further resources to manage, but crucially it does not demand that knowledge and experience are formally shared with colleagues. Reflection is instead considered a personal professional capacity and responsibility (NMC 2018c, Newman 2011). With reflective outcomes regarded in terms of personal capacity rather than 'learning' and enshrouded in a body of codified and propositional knowledge, more complex aspects of workplace learning can become difficult to elucidate (Billett 2008, Eraut 2004, Brown 1991). For example, the Dreyfus model does not necessarily provide a mechanism for explaining how learning towards specific outcomes happens in practice or the relationships that foster learning. The influence of others is recognized in that learning is constructed over many patient episodes or experiences, but the role of the team or assessor in practice-based learning or developing expertise is not fully explored in this model. This chapter therefore attempts to fill this void by exploring the roles of student, assessors, supervisors and the university in facilitating learning through practice-based experience.

Studies of student nurse learning in practice provide some insight. These tend to focus on the notions of participation and belongingness as prerequisites for learning. Jensen and Lahn (2005) frame this as the development of a "binding" professional identity as a nurse. Further, full team membership, a common perspective on reality, conforming to norms of practice and collaborating to uphold working practices have been suggested as both key predictors of a social identity (Haslam & Platow 2001), and prerequisites for a community of practice (Wenger 1998). Meanwhile Levett-Jones and Lathlean (2008) foreground the interpersonal relationships required in socializing into practice, where students' orientation, intellectual capacity and willingness to learn appear the most influential indicators of learning.

Likewise, Thrysoe et al (2010) recognized that student proactivity played an important role in final year students' assimilation into the ward as a community of practice. Similar findings were discussed by Newton et al (2009) in their longitudinal interview study of eight Australian student nurses, whereas O'Driscoll et al (2010) from a UK perspective indicated that assertive students are better placed to negotiate learning opportunities, than less assertive colleagues. Although these studies have focused on students developing a sense of belonging and sameness, nurses are not a homogenous group. Different expectations of students emerged from Newton et al's (2009) study of several generations of nurses.

Newton et al (2009) identified that valuing of practitioners' own modes of initial training and education and differing work expectations and experiences led to negative stereotyping of nursing students. This mediated against invitational aspects of clinical practice experiences, leaving student nurses feeling that they are used as "glorified" health care assistants rather than team members. Student conformity and dissembling in the face of incorrect nursing practices of assessors and qualified registered nurses, is noted by Levett-Jones and Lathlean (2009) and mediates against belongingness: maintaining student reputation is paramount for progression into registered practice. Each of these studies identifies the process of socialization by which newcomers are introduced to and become more significant individuals within practice settings.

It can be argued that student nurses in these studies represent professional learning communities where the shared endeavour is to gain entry to the nursing profession. However, the CoP framework is criticized as offering a view of workplace learning as merely socialization and situational determinism (Bierema 2001, Hodkinson & Hodkinson 2004). Several factors are influential here. Firstly, the forced heterogeneity of team members within a ward means that team membership necessarily includes colleagues from other professions and occupations. It is shaped by contractual working obligations rather than a community developing out of explicitly shared practice values. The aim of apprenticeship in Lave and Wenger's (1991) conception of situated learning is full engagement with practice, however lack of invitation to participate and the generational differences identified by Newton et al (2009) would mediate against learning and community engagement.

Secondly, the motivation to participate within a CoP is broadly unchallenged by Lave and Wenger (Lave and Wenger 1991, Wenger 1998), with an understanding that peripheral participation can lead to more central engagement with the work of the community. Just as sitting in a classroom does not guarantee learning, peripheral engagement in the practicum requires cognitive stewardship through the invitational practices of others (Newton et al 2009, Spouse 2001). Similarly, Kupferberg (2004 [cited by Andrew et al 2008]) argues that the CoP model does not explain why some individuals are fast-tracked into a more central position, whilst others never fully participate. Finally, Andrew et al (2008) identify that although influential in other professions, CoP have not been widely acknowledged within British acute nursing settings. Instead work premising CoPs has focused on experienced nurses involved in small-scale strategic project working (Lathlean & Le May 2002, Attenborough, Knight & Brook 2018) or wider-scale practice development (Tolson et al 2005).

The CoP concept appears most successfully applied where group learning is based on an area of uncontested agreement. This may account for the relative unpopularity of this theory in the nursing literature. A fundamental critique of both Benner (1984) and CoP models of workplace learning is that they suggest a relatively unproblematic enculturation of group norms and ideals based on a power differential between "old-timers" and newcomers. They do not account for how existing members of a group are influenced to engage in learning and supervision of others. In addition, the professions studied by Lave and Wenger (1991) do not fit with contemporary understandings of professionalism. The increasingly technologic, managerial and regulatory world of contemporary nursing practice is not reflected in either research. The role of relationships and the individual dispositions that orient individuals to act in certain ways is not explored in these approaches.

Therefore learning from experience in the practice setting needs to rely on more than just models of socialization and role modelling from established colleagues. It equally relies upon the delivery of a set of prescribed theory, rules, routines and behaviours in a prepackaged and predetermined curriculum influenced by the professions and health care practice regulators. The argument for preparing practitioners in this manner is that it reduces the risks of professionals failing to provide a reliable service and limits the unwarranted variation in practice and outcomes identified as compromising care in the National Health Service (NHS) England document *Leading Change: Adding Value* (2016).

The "technical–rational" view of professionalism which foregrounds theory, rules and regulations has received much criticism from writers, such as Schön (1987, 1983) who stated that such simple offerings do not prepare practitioners to meet the real situations of practice, as this model makes assumptions that practice is a relatively simple interaction in which the practitioner gives, and patients and clients receive. Hence a more recent move towards collaborative partnership between education, and clinical practice providers is documented in the development of apprenticeship modes of preregistration preparation, which use work-based learning opportunities and foreground reflection on and in practice (Attenborough, Abbott, Brook, Knight, 2019).

An important "hallmark" of the health care professional is generally acknowledged to be the need to be aware of, and to deal with, complex human issues as part of practice (Fish & Twinn 1997). These essential human interactions between professionals and patients/clients make the detailed knowledge and skills needed in each interaction unpredictable. Professional practice involves complex decision-making and elements of professional judgement and practical wisdom guided by moral principles, as well as ethical codes of conduct (e.g., NMC 2019c). These however, cannot be set down in absolute routines (Fish & Twinn, 1997), for although they provide many opportunities and challenges for nursing students, these environments are continually changing (Hodges, 2011).

Organizations currently face challenges in maintaining efficiency and delivery of high-quality care. Several factors contribute to this such as advances in science, technology and new and more challenging emerging diseases and long-term conditions which may affect patient longevity and quality of life (Solman & Wilson, 2016). Changing patient and workforce demographics as society ages creates staffing challenges, such as workforce contraction because of issues, such as the introduction of course fees for nursing programmes, changes to European recruitment and general shortage of nursing staff. Virkstis et al (2019; 580), from a US perspective, refer to an "experience-complexity gap" where the retirement of older nurses, combined with a general shortage of nursing staff leads to the loss of experience or organizational memory within the practice area, which can affect care provision, patient experience and the learning of student and early career nurses. However, despite these issues practice areas remain the best place to learn and develop care, skills and practice, albeit supported by opportunities for simulated practice. Illustrating this, in a study exploring the efficacy of the ward as a practice placement area, Lewin (2007) identified that over a 25-year period, wards remained stable learning environments, with staff rising to meet the demands of 21st century health care and facilitate its development amongst newer members of the workforce.

Health care professionals need to be able to exercise professional judgement and select, or even create knowledge necessary to the unique situation. Practitioners need to be prepared so that they are able to engage in these processes not only through their initial preregistration preparation but also through continuing postregistration education. The technical–rational model of professional preparation, and its consequent influences on how the practitioner practises, does not equip the practitioner fully to deal with those aspects of professional work that cause the greatest human concern and yet defy the use and application of rules and routines. Furthermore, prescribed professional knowledge and proficiencies are changing (NMC 2018b); requiring the practitioner to be motivated to refine and update knowledge and practices so that professional expertise and thus "practice wisdom" (Hull 1998) is continually developing. The introduction of the Student Supervision, Support and Assessment Standards (NMC 2018a) has reconsidered dyadic Mentorship relationships

in favour of more distributed roles in student support and assessment. This reflects the emergence in recent years of concepts, such as team or group mentorship in the literature surrounding support in (nonhealth) workplace settings (Chandler & Kram 2005, Higgins & Kram 2001, Kram 1983, Dobrow & Higgins 2005, Salami 2007, van Beek et al 2011), but have made little impact on the support and assessment of nursing students in practice settings until recently (MacLaren 2018).

What is therefore also needed is a model for preparing for professional practice that does not rely slavishly on the use and application of rules, schedules and prescriptions, but allows for student centred learning through experience and reflection. This model should be holistic in nature, catering for the initial preparation, as well as the continuing professional development of health care practitioners. It should have clinical experiences as a key focus. The Model for Learning from Experience proposed by Stuart (2000) is explored here as a framework to consider experience-based learning and how students can be assisted to interact with the clinical environment to learn through practice and unearth meaning from experiences. Stuart's model has four phases, with each phase of the model focusing on several factors and strategies that influence how the learner engages with the experience and can be supported to do so by supervisors and assessors. The phases, factors and skills/strategies are identified in Table 9.1.

EXPERIENCE-BASED LEARNING

Research focused on experience-based learning (Boud et al 1993, Boud & Walker 1990, Kolb 1984, Dewey 1963/1938) advises that learning from clinical experience is not as simple as "learning by doing". What students do, see, hear and smell during clinical placements can often remain at a superficial level unless they are stimulated to analyse critically their observations and to question the meaning of their experiences and their implications for future learning. Students need to actively engage with their learning and be stimulated to apply theory to practice.

Complexity is a particularly relevant consideration for health care student learning and the application of evidence to practice (Chandler, Rycroft-Malone et al 2016). Complexity theory addresses the development of increasing complexity in systems, similar to the increasingly complex range of knowledge, skills and attitudes that must be assumed by the student throughout their professional preparation and beyond. The student has to contend and learn to deal with the complex, unstable and uncertain worlds of practice, synthesize theoretical content from various fields, become familiar with the patients/clients and their needs and problems, learn to analyse those needs

TABLE 9.1. A Model for Preparing for Professional Practice

1. The preparatory phase: focusing on:
   - the student as a learner
   - developing noticing skills
   - developing intervening skills
2. The experiencing phase: during this phase the student "reflects-in-action". Several teaching/learning strategies will assist and influence how the learner engages with, and reflects during, the experience:
   - sharing, explaining and "pointing out" (including role modelling)
   - questioning and challenging
   - allowing to experiment
   - giving feedback on performance
3. The processing phase: the experience is systematically reflected on during this phase. There are three key stages in reflecting on experience:
   - description of the experience
   - processing through critical analysis
   - synthesizing and evaluating
   - Outcomes and action
   - linking learning to action

and problems and, during the course of needs analysis and problem solving, attempt to apply theories learnt and experiences gained previously. Subsequently, the student has to learn to evaluate the effectiveness of care given and make the appropriate changes that may be required.

Learning through clinical experiences is, then, far more diverse and pervasive than is usually conceived. Effective facilitation of learning in the clinical setting and the supervision and assessment of clinical practice are challenging. The most complex skills, such as the ability to translate theory into practice are likely to take longest to develop (Moriaty et al 2010). If students are to learn to "think", the thought patterns required by the practitioner need to be determined as successful clinical practice requires the highest level of intellectual functioning – namely that of application, synthesis and evaluation (Stengelhofen 1993).

Boud et al (1985:7) ask the following questions about experience-based learning:

- What is it that turns experience into learning?
- What specifically enables learners to gain the maximum benefit from the situations they find themselves in?
- How can they apply their experiences to new contexts?
- Why can some learners appear to benefit more than others?

In practice-based professions, such as (but not limited to) nursing and midwifery, it is particularly pertinent that

attempts are made to answer these questions so that students can be best assisted to extract maximum learning and achieve personal and professional development as a result of their experiences during clinical placements. Therefore to explore Stuart's (2000) Model for Learning from Experience in detail, each phase is considered in turn, focusing on those issues that are important in ensuring that the process of learning through experience is an effective one. First, some of the characteristics of the nature of experience for learning are explored.

THE NATURE OF EXPERIENCE FOR LEARNING: CONTEXTS AND RELATIONSHIPS

The fundamental assumption of experiential learning is that two types of processes are happening to facilitate learning. Firstly, an external interaction between the learner and their social, cultural and material environment coupled with an internal psychologic process or drive to acquire and elaborate on the results of prior learning (Illeris, 2007). It is perhaps appropriate to start by considering what the word "experience" could mean in the context of learning and the role of experience in learning. Within the clinical context, is it what a student has observed, encountered or undergone or is it what a student has done? Or is it all of these? Dewey considered that experience is not simply an event that happens, but rather than this event has meaning, pointing out that "events are present and operative anyway; what concerns us is their meaning" (Boydston 2008).

Drawing upon this perspective, there is now broad consensus (Illeris 2010, Eraut 2011, Newton, Henderson et al 2015) that to be labelled as experiential learning, there needs to be a sense of continuity and interaction within the learning environment. Experience is framed as a meaningful encounter. It is not just an observation, a passive undergoing of something, but an active engagement with the social and material forces within the environment, practice, and professional relationships (Fenwick 2014). Illeris considers experiential learning to contain elements of learner control, involvement of the learner's self (engagement) and correspondence of the learning environment to "real" conditions (fidelity). The ability of learning to be applied and involved in a very broad range of educational connections (Illeris 2010) reflects the issue of meaning within learning. Issues such as freedom from distraction, and elements of liberation or emancipation of the learner that Illeris also considers important, can be mapped to the concepts of engagement, navigating through communication and "entrustability" (the extent to which a student can practice with minimal supervision), which emerge from Newton, Henderson et al's (2015) fieldwork observations of 95 students and registered nurses in practice. However, this freedom to practice must always be considered in the context of an imperative to maintain public safety (NMC 2018c).

Experience is not singular or limited by time and place, as much experience is "multifaceted, multilayered and so inextricably connected with other experiences that it is impossible to locate temporally or spatially" (Boud et al 1993;7). Indeed, in 1938, Dewey pointed out that educational experiences have continuity and integrate with one another so that "every experience should do something to prepare a person for later experiences of a deeper and more expansive quality. That is the very meaning of growth, continuity, reconstruction of experience" (Dewey 1963/1938:47). Work on the cognitive learning theory (see, for example, Ausubel 1968) also tells us that learning always relates in some way to what has gone on before. Boud and Walker (1990) refer to the "personal foundation of experience" of a learner, which is the accumulation of previous experiences. Contributory sources to this personal foundation of experience may be the social and cultural environment of the learner, prior clinical placements and experiences. The social, cultural and professional norms and mores assimilated contribute to the formation of the perceptual lenses through which the learner views, and acts, in the world of work. The response of the learner to new experiences is determined significantly by these past experiences, as presuppositions and assumptions have been developed – the past creates expectations, which influence the present. The present context can serve to reinforce or counterbalance this.

What students bring to the clinical area: their expectations, knowledge, attitudes and emotions, will necessarily influence the construction and interpretation of what they experience. The way one learner reacts in a situation will not be the same as another. Boud et al (1993) believe that, in general, if an event is not related in some way to what the student brings to it, whether or not they are conscious of what this is, then it is not likely to be a productive opportunity. Even when starting a first clinical placement in a hospital, students will bring memories, feelings and knowledge of hospitals, whether or not they have been in one. It will be a rarity to have a clean slate on which to begin – unless new experience and ideas link to previous experience to form "new wholes" (Ausubel 1968), they will exist as abstractions, isolated and without meaning (Boud et al 1993).

Planning clinical learning experiences is therefore important: building on continuity rather than being separate and discrete events. Furthermore, students should be assisted to make links and connections between experiences to provide new meanings and enable them to "see" new whole pictures. This encourages a deep approach to learning (Marton & Säljö 1984) in which students seek an understanding of the meaning of what they are learning, relate it to previous material and interact actively with the material at hand.

Most people would agree with Boud et al (1985:7) when they state that "experience alone is not the key to learning". Dewey (1963/1938:15) was critical of how experiences were offered to students. He asked this question.

"How many acquired special skills by means of automatic drill so that their power of judgment and capacity to act intelligently in new situations was limited?"

Students were considered callous to ideas, thus losing the impetus to learn. Does this still happen in the education of health care professionals today? Boud et al (1993) believe that experience cannot be considered in isolation from learning – experience is the central consideration of all learning. Although experience is the foundation of, and the stimulus for, learning, it does not necessarily lead to learning unless there is active engagement with it. Aitchison and Graham (1989, in Critocos 1993:161) state that:

"Experience has to be arrested, examined, analysed, considered and negated to shift it to knowledge".

Working with experience in the manner suggested by Aitchison and Graham is the key to learning from experience. For learning to take place, the experience need not be recent. We may return to the same experience again and again and draw different meanings from each "visit". Boud et al (1993:9) believe that "learning occurs over time and meaning may take years to become apparent … learning from it can grow, the meaning can be transformed, and the effects of it can be altered". The meaning of experience is not a given: it is subject to interpretation. Only the person who experiences can ultimately give meaning to the experience. It is the learner's interaction with the learning milieu that creates the particular learning experience (Boud & Walker 1990). No matter what external prompts there might be—supervisors and assessors, interesting opportunities, resources—learning can occur only if the learner chooses to engage in, and with, the experience.

The emphasis in experiential learning is thus on the process of learning. It proceeds from the assumption that ideas are not fixed and immutable elements of thought, but rather are continuously derived from, and tested out, through experience (Kolb 1984). Kolb's well-known model of this learning process is termed an "experiential learning model" to emphasize the important part that experience plays in the learning process. Learning is conceived of as a four-stage cycle, as shown in Fig. 9.1. The here-and-now personal experience is real and concrete, and forms the focal point for learning "giving life, texture and subjective personal meaning to abstract concepts" (Kolb 1984:21). The core of the model is the translation of experiences into

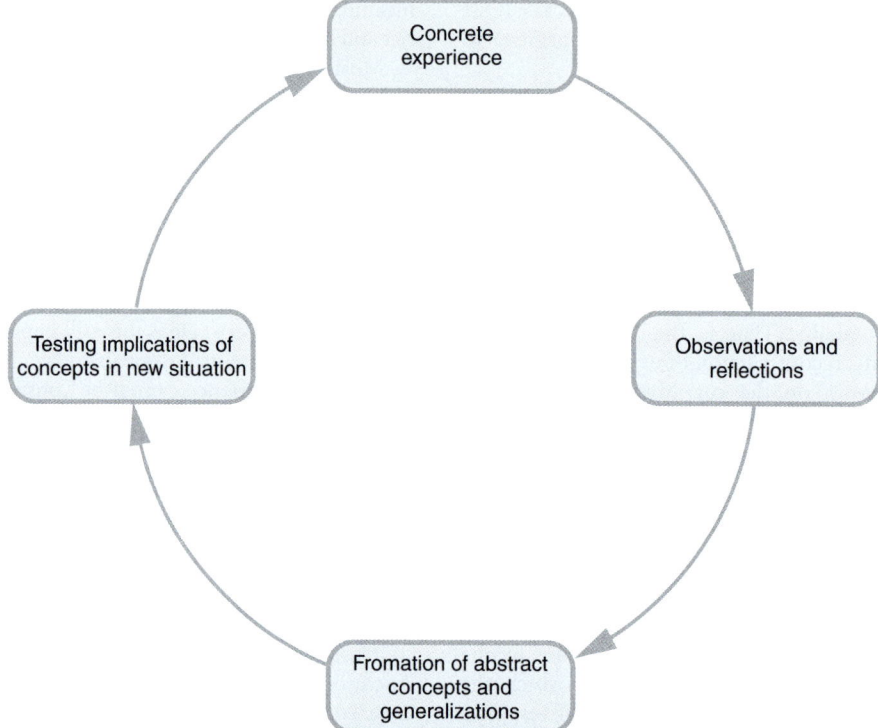

Fig. 9.1 The Lewinian–Kolb experiential learning model. (From Kolb, D.A. (1984). *Experiential Learning: Experience as the Source of Learning and Development*. ©1984. Adapted with permission of Pearson Education, Inc., Upper Saddle River, NJ.)

concepts through reflective activities. These concepts are subsequently used to guide and inform new experiences.

STUART'S MODEL FOR LEARNING FROM EXPERIENCE

Each phase of the "*Model for Learning from Experience*" (Stuart 2000) will now be considered in detail.

THE PREPARATORY PHASE

Advanced preparation helps address some of the challenges that students will encounter. The quality of the preparation before the experience also potentially determines the learning extracted during the experience and from later reflection and exploration. The preparatory phase at the start of a clinical placement would normally consist of a number of elements:

- An outline of the aims of the placement and a broad structure of what is to take place. These should be agreed jointly between the practice educator and the student after the first meeting/interview has taken place, as discussed in Chapter 6.

- An introduction to staff, resources and learning opportunities that are available to help the student during the placement. Suggestions on how these may be used to help the student learn are discussed in Chapter 8. Those resources and learning opportunities that are specifically required to enable students to achieve their learning intent should be identified.

- Students should have the opportunity to seek clarification.

Subsequent preparation for experience focuses on the student as a learner, integrating the student into the work of the practice area, beyond socialization, and on helping the student develop noticing and intervening skills, as these are two of the prerequisite skills required for learning through clinical experience.

FOCUSING ON THE STUDENT AS A LEARNER: BEYOND SOCIALIZATION

As discussed in an earlier section, what the learner brings to the clinical setting has an important influence on what is experienced and how it is experienced: these factors, including the individuality of the student, should be considered during the preparatory phase. The other important element to consider is "learning intent" (Boud & Walker 1990:64). Intent can be regarded as a personal determination; there is a clear reason for being there, which prompts learners to take steps to achieve their goals. The learning outcomes of a formal educational programme may influence the learning intent, but workplace learning needs to also meet the needs of the organization, for example, in developing the workforce of the future (Manley, Titchen et al 2009). Boud et al (1985) believe that intent to learn for a particular purpose can assist in overcoming many obstacles and inhibitions. Intent can be determined only by direct reference to the learner. For example, during a particular placement the student's intent may be to develop communication skills with very ill patients and their relatives. This intent will influence how the student is likely to experience these types of care situations; it acts to focus and intensify, or play down, perceptions in relationship to these experiences. "The intent can act as a filter, or magnifier" (Boud & Walker 1990:64); these authors give the example of the photographer who, when using a zoom lens, will see certain things more clearly but in the process of doing so eliminates other things from the frame.

Students may arrive at a clinical placement with little conscious learning intent or even commitment to being there. Unless the supervisor and assessor can assist the student to form an intent during the preparatory phase, opportunities for learning will not be well utilized owing to a lack of focus; this is likely to result in superficial learning. Skilled facilitators, such as assessors and supervisors, play an important role in helping students to clarify their intent and guide and direct students to the appropriate formal and informal learning opportunities in the clinical setting (Manley, Titchen et al 2009). Assessors should be careful that they do not impose their own intents on the student. A discrepancy in intent between the assessor and student may lead to unproductive experiences and considerable frustration for both parties (Boud & Walker 1990).

Typically, during the preparatory phase there will be a high level of anxiety. Based on the well-documented evidence of student anxiety and stress in clinical settings (see Chapter 8), time should be spent in assisting students to identify and voice their concerns so that ways may be found to reduce their stress and anxiety and increase their confidence. Knowledge that they will not be alone and will not be expected to do more than they are able to will provide reassurance and make students feel less vulnerable. Support, trust and confidence in students can help to overcome past negative influences and allow them to start to act and think differently. Similarly, conditions of threat or lack of confidence in the student are usually antithetical to any new motivation the student may have and serve to reinforce any negative images the student may already hold (Evison 2006). This is shown in nursing and midwifery research, where belongingness, engagement and entrusting of students are core features of positive learning environments (Levett & Lathlean 2009, Thrysoe et al 2010, O'Lúanaigh 2015).

During the preparatory phase, when students start to focus on their learning intent, they start to explore what is required of them, how they can contribute, what their role might be, what the demands of the setting are, what they can learn and how they can use their own resources, such as knowledge, skills and what they have learnt from prior clinical experiences. This model of increasing participation and eventually increasingly autonomous working is being advocated by the Pan London Practice Learning Group:

Year/Part 1 Guided participation

Year/Part 2: Active participation

Year/Part 3: Practicing independently (with minimal supervision)

(Pan London Practice Learning Group, 2019)

FOCUSING ON NOTICING AND INTERVENING SKILLS TO HELP STUDENTS LEARN THROUGH CLINICAL EXPERIENCE

Asking the following questions may prompt both assessor or supervisor and student to focus on how best to prepare for learning through particular experiences:

- Why has this particular experience (e.g., the care of a certain patient, a visit to another department) been arranged?
- What can be learnt through this experience?
- How can learning from previous experiences be linked to this experience?
- How can students be assisted to plan thoughtfully so that they "(act) deliberately, (observe) the consequences of actions systematically and (reflect) critically on the situational constraints and practical potential of the strategic action being considered" (Carr & Kemmis 1986:40)?
- How can students be assisted to engage in the clinical experience so that it means "living through actual situations in such a way that it informs (them) of the perceptions and understandings of (other similar) subsequent situations" (Benner & Wrubel 1982:28)?

Answers to these questions are of course not straightforward, as each clinical situation is different. However, if "coaching" (Schön 1987:20) of the students starts during the preparatory phase, they can be assisted to extract maximal learning through their experiences.

Boud and Walker (1990) believe that there are two aspects of experience–based learning that are necessary to enhance the working of the processes for learning through experience. The first aspect is noticing, by which the student becomes aware of the event or particular things within it. The second aspect is intervening, in which the student takes an initiative and is active in the event. We see noticing and intervening as two prerequisite skills for learning through experience.

DEVELOPING NOTICING SKILLS

Boud and Walker (1990:68) define noticing as "an act of becoming aware of what is happening in and around oneself". It is active and seeking and involves a continuing effort to be aware of what is taking place in oneself and in the learning experience. As well as paying attention to the happenings around the care-giving situation—the experience—it is equally important that students pay attention to what is happening in themselves. They need to be aware in three areas:

• How they are acting
• What they are thinking
• How they are feeling

Being aware of how they are acting and what they are thinking can alert students to what might be influencing them in the event. Being aware of how they are feeling will make students more aware of their emotional responses to the event for these to be attended to. Attending to feelings involves being sensitive to the situation: seeking to detect the nuances and the affective climate, as well as what is overt. Neglect of emotions can lead to a build-up of "stress and a numbing of awareness which can inhibit the ability to act and distort learning" (Boud & Walker 1990:69, Peters 2018). Stuart (2000) gave the example of midwives being in constant contact with women in pain during labour without acknowledging their own feelings and thoughts. This may eventually lead them to become less sensitive to the needs of women during this time, resulting in "compassion fatigue". Peters (2018) refers to this as a preventable phenomenon, although all health care professionals appear to be at risk. It is characterized as a "decline in energy and endurance, an emotional decline in empathetic ability and emotional exhaustion, and a spiritual decline as one feels hopeless and helpless to recover that results from chronic exposure to others' suffering" (Peters 2018: 470).

Noticing provides students with the basis for becoming more fully involved in a care-giving situation and enables them to "reflect-in-action" (Schön 1983) as they become more aware of the processes of how decisions are made to inform actions taken. It is essential to the initiation of the reflective processes during the third phase of the "model of experience" so that sufficient information is retained for retrospective analysis and interpretation of practice after the event. Noticing seems to be a skill that has to be present to cause the experience to be the basis for learning (Stuart 2001). Stuart

(2001) found that students in her study who did not know "how" and "what" to notice were unable to enter into experiences and subsequent reflective interactions with their experiences. As two frustrated student midwives said:

"I think it is very routine … what they did, I learnt in the first week … It's just like in the morning she [the community midwife] goes round and does the visits, and in the afternoon she does the clinics, and the clinics are all the same, and then going to houses is pretty much the same …" (p. 178).

"I think on community all your days are very much the same … so, no, basically I have nothing to talk about … " (p. 180).

As can be seen from the earlier excerpts, virtually every care event has the same meaning for these students. These students did not know how to notice. The starting point for the learning process to unearth meaning through experience is noticing; paying close systematic attention to detail, noticing exactly what occurred, including any thoughts, feelings, actions and reactions. Developing the skills of noticing will help students use their "observer" status to benefit; how this status can be used for learning is poorly understood and has robbed students of valuable learning opportunities (May et al 1997; Ashley & Stamp, 2014). This has contributed to the unpopularity of the observer status (Neary 2000). Paying attention to those aspects suggested in Box 9.1 will assist in the development of noticing skills.

BOX 9.1   Aspects to be Considered for the Development of Noticing Skills

Noticing while engaging in an experience:

• The context of the episode, such as the history of the patient/client; time of day; location; and team members involved
• Other factors in the environment, such as sights, smells and sounds
• What were the patient/client's needs/problems?
• What care was given?
• How were the patient/client, family and significant others involved?
• Personal thoughts during, and after the episode
• Personal feelings during, and after the episode
• Personal concerns at the time
• What was noticed about yourself and others, such as the verbal and body language; what you said; what others said; how you behaved; how the patient/client behaved/said; how the practitioner(s) behaved; the approach used by the practitioner(s)?

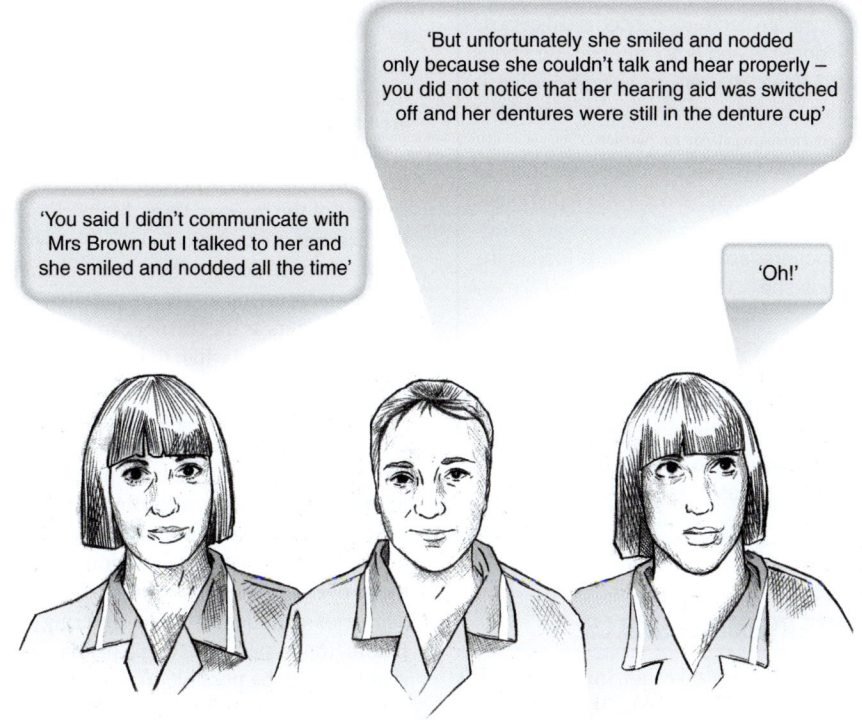

Fig. 9.2 Students have to learn how and what to notice.

Learners can be directed to use these aspects in a general way, which will lead them to notice things that might have gone unnoticed otherwise. Alternatively, the supervisor or assessor can indicate specific aspects to be noticed to help the learner achieve particular learning intents. For example, if a student wishes to learn how to assess the needs of clients at home following major orthopaedic surgery, the student could be directed to notice specific aspects about individual clients visited. The following example is based upon and extended from the work of Stengelhofen (1993).

THE SETTING

We are visiting Mrs Brown for the first time. She is known to be housebound; her general practitioner has referred her to district nursing team for a holistic (wellbeing) assessment. She is 82 years old, lives with multiple long-term conditions and lives alone on an inner-city local authority flat.

Students have to learn how and what to notice (Fig. 9.2).

Aspects for noticing are:

1. Start observing when we reach the house, are there stairs, ramps or lifts, and what floor does she live on (how would she cope if the lift was out of order)? Also the general repair and deprivation of the area could be considered:
   - How long does she take to answer the door?
   - Note the use of any walking aids – is she using them correctly?
   - What is her gait like and mobility?
2. Are there any trip hazards?
3. Does she have any occupational adaptations in situ?
4. How is she dressed?
5. What is the state of her personal hygiene
   How does her flat appear to you? (cleanliness, pets, damp/mould, can you see smoke alarms, is the flat smoky or in good repair)
6. During discussion with her:
   - How does she state she is coping?
   - Is she anxious/confident/confused?

7. What does she think are her major concerns/difficulties?
8. What are her concerns and is there anything she is struggling with? What matters to her, and what is important to her? Is there anything she would like to change about her situation or health?
9. What do you think are her major concerns and difficulties? What do you think can be done to help improve the situation?
10. Observe her functional activities. Is there food in the fridge, and how is she managing shopping and meal preparation?
11. Can she manage activities of living, such as washing, dressing, cleaning the house, independently?
12. What are your thoughts and feelings about someone like Mrs Brown living on her own?

Students should be encouraged to keep written records of what they have noticed, as these serve as valuable "memory joggers" for later critical reflection.

DEVELOPING INTERVENING SKILLS

Intervening is when the learner takes an initiative and is active in the event (Boud & Walker 1990). This can be any verbal or physical action taken by the learner within the learning situation. Learning through experience is an active process that involves the learner not only in noticing but also in taking initiatives to extend and test their knowledge. Looking on is no substitute for active involvement, as the learner who intervenes is adopting an active approach to the experience and is therefore likely to make more of the potential for learning from the event.

The learner's personal foundation of experience will influence interventions taken; it can either be limiting or act as a trigger for further actions. Boud and Walker (1990) believe that the greatest barriers to intervention are past failure and feelings of inadequacy or embarrassment, which inhibit clear thinking. Evison (2006) further categorizes these as performance anxiety blocks (relating to perceived shame at own performance), put down blocks (aggressive, sarcastic or highly critical comments from self or others), thinking blocks (unable to search out an answer the student knows), and powerlessness blocks (lack of self-belief in ability). These are further characterized by O'Lúanaigh (2015) as poor quality role modelling, learning supervision and support, influenced by increased workloads, role conflict and role uncertainty. These dysfunctional emotional responses and negative self-images can paralyse learners so that they are unable to perform or they act so maladroitly, or defensively that learning opportunities are lost. On the other

hand, past success and feelings of confidence and willingness to "give it a go" can carry the learner through initial periods of discomfort. During the preparatory phase, the best way to help learners to intervene is to attend to those feelings that are blocking their ability to act (Evison 2006).

Learners need to learn the skills to be players. They need to know how and when to intervene and the nature and content of the interventions. Many clinical situations require the exercise of technical skills. Knowing how to perform these, such as doing a bed bath, changing an intravenous infusion, removing a urinary catheter, can act as great confidence boosters as the learner can intervene directly. Learning how and what and when to intervene is learning how to cope with the experience, as one major concern of students is coping in clinical practice (White & Ewan 1997). Typical care events could be analysed and suitable responses rehearsed. The use of simulated practice, role plays, case studies or audio or video recordings of typical events, followed by rehearsal of intervention strategies, will enable learners to practise appropriate intervention sequences. This will help them overcome anxieties and uncertainties and develop a degree of confidence before entering unknown situations. Before the experience (e.g., before going to the patient/client) it may be possible to predict what common chain of events may arise and a range of strategies can be developed and discussed with the learner. The learner could be asked searching questions, such as "Knowing what you know about Mr Johns, what problems do you foresee? … What care do you think he needs? … What actions would you take?". The supervisor and assessor may suggest particular interventions that the learner could implement or ways in which the learner's own ideas could be put into practice.

Because of the uncontrollable and unpredictable milieu surrounding clinical situations, not all the possibilities available in practice can be anticipated. Boud and Walker (1991) believe that it is neither possible nor desirable to cover every eventuality—part of learning from experience is dealing with the unexpected when it arises. There should, however, be sufficient preparation to ensure that learners can act effectively and that they are able to remain conscious of what they want to learn.

THE EXPERIENCING PHASE

The experiencing phase draws upon Schön's (1987) three models of coaching for learning. Whilst there have been recent concerns about the multiple interpretations of Schön's work muddying its understanding by health care professionals (Comer 2019), it remains influential in helping to understand learning in practice settings. During the experiencing phase, the key role of the supervisor and assessor is to facilitate reflection and interventions of the learner within the situation. The learner needs to be assisted to make judgements about when and where to take the initiative and what should be the nature and content of the intervention. Boud and Walker (1990) believe that the most significant influence on the actions of the learner during the situation is the reflective process that run through it as this active working with the data of the situation by the learner influences actions taken. Reflection within the situation can also lead to a recognition of the feelings and thoughts that accompany intervention, which can significantly influence the quantity and quality of learning extracted from experiences. This, in turn, will influence the learner's ability to transfer learning from this event to other events. As Dewey (1963/1938: 51) pointed out:

> "We always live at the time we live and not at some other time, and only by extracting at each present time the full meaning of each present experience are we prepared for doing the same thing in the future"

This means that attentive care must be devoted to the conditions which give each present experience a worthwhile meaning. It appears that the "taking on board of what is going on" while "performing" needs to be accompanied by the "thinking" and the "feeling". Kolb (1984:34) suggests that learning develops from the interplay of environment and learner, necessitating careful consideration of the milieu in which the event is taking place at the time of the experience. The richness of the clinical environment is a facilitating factor for learning, but there are many demands that compete for the learner's attention, such as the patient/client condition (and even distress), and their need for care and attention, and other disturbing events in the immediate vicinity. At the same time, the supervisor and assessor may be expecting the learner to listen to an explanation or suggestion for intervention. Boud and Walker (1990) also point out that learners' engagement with an experience, and their level of reflection during it are influenced by their personal foundations of experience, learning intent, noticing and intervening skills and the learning milieu. During the preparatory phase, the learner's personal foundation of experience and learning intent would have been explored so that the learner is as "ready to learn" (Knowles et al 1998) as possible. Although the learner has been prepared to notice and intervene, these learning processes need to be actively facilitated.

How can meaningful learning during the "experiencing phase" be facilitated so that learners' "power of judgement and capacity to act intelligently in new situations" (Dewey 1963/1938:15) are developed further? The following guiding principles of Schön's three models of coaching for learning may be helpful.

THE GUIDING PRINCIPLES OF SCHÖN'S THREE MODELS OF COACHING FOR LEARNING DURING THE EXPERIENCING PHASE

Schön's three models of coaching have three distinct yet overlapping styles: joint experimentation, follow me and hall of mirrors. The coaching role adopted by supervisors and assessors may call on the use of the style of only one or all three models, depending on the level of experience of the student and the complexity of the event. These models are now described.

JOINT EXPERIMENTATION

Joint experimentation can succeed only when learners already know what they want to do to intervene. The learner must be willing to step into the intervention and "have a go" with the unfamiliar. The skill of the supervisor or assessor here lies in helping the learner formulate the interventions to be achieved and leading the learner to search for and decide on a suitable way of achieving the intervention. As different interventions are explored together, the supervisor and assessor work at "creating and sustaining a process of collaborative inquiry" (Schön 1987:296). The supervisor and assessor must resist the temptation to tell the learner how to intervene or intervene on behalf of the learner, but they may generate a variety of interventions and leave the learner free to choose and produce new possibilities for action. Joint experimentation is inappropriate when learners are unable to intervene or when the supervisor and assessor wants them to grasp a new way of seeing and doing things.

FOLLOW ME

When the supervisor and assessor want to offer a new way of seeing and doing things, the follow me approach is most useful. The supervisor and assessor provide detailed descriptions of interventions while they are being performed, being careful to give rationales for the interventions. Schön emphatically stated that the "relations between a whole performance and its parts, between the whole and aspects of the whole, are crucial" (Schön 1987:296) and should therefore be emphasized. During this "analysis in action", the supervisor and assessor draws on a repertoire of "media, languages and methods of description" (Schön 1987:297) because the ultimate aim is to present images that will "click" with the learner. While observing the supervisor and assessor, the learner will be attempting to remember the actions and explanations, and subsequently trying to derive meaningful learning through personal interventions. As the learner attempts to imitate the supervisor and assessor, there is great potential for ambiguity and confusion. Guidance and feedback from the supervisor and assessor are important, as the learner will be "testing by further words and actions how the meanings she (sic) has constructed are like or unlike his (sic) (supervisor and assessor)" (Schön 1987:297).

HALL OF MIRRORS

In this model of coaching, there is willing cooperation between the supervisor and assessor and learner as they try to grasp their own and each other's understandings of the clinical situation. As learners seek to exemplify their proposed interventions in practice, they are assisted to see their interventions from several perspectives. To achieve this, the supervisor and assessor and learner continually shift perspective; this may be carrying out the intervention proposed by the learner or having a dialogue about it or mutually redesigning the intervention. The supervisor and assessor's skill lies in having the courage to allow the student to experiment and take "risks". Schön believed that "to the extent that he (sic) can do so authentically, he models for his student a new way of seeing error and 'failure' as opportunities for learning" (Schön 1987:297).

Using Schön's (1987) three models of coaching to provide the underlying principles for learning during the experiencing phase, several strategies are suggested for use during this phase. These are shown in the framework in Fig. 9.3. The strategies in the framework may be seen as "coaching strategies". As indicated in Fig. 9.3, the central activity, which underpins these coaching strategies, is "talk during practice". This is an essential activity between supervisor and assessor and learner for meaningful learning to take place during the "experiencing phase". Each of the coaching strategies will now be discussed.

SHARING, EXPLAINING AND POINTING OUT

When supervisor and assessors work alongside learners, opportunities are provided to engage learners in "situated negotiation of their practice" (Phillips et al 2000:111). Informal on-the-job conversations take place that allow the sharing of ideas and understanding about care, which are then put into practice. These mutual exchanges not only value each other's ideas and understandings but also enable the learner's understandings of practice to be clarified. Phillips et al (2000) give the example of a supervisor and assessor and their student working together as they made a heavily sedated terminally ill patient as comfortable as possible. As they work, the supervisor and assessor and student discuss how best to position the patient. The student could see areas of tissue damage which the supervisor and assessor could not from her position.

The position that was planned to be used was modified using the information from the student's evaluation. The supervisor and assessor in this instance shared how they solved the problem and made the decision by "thinking aloud" thus:

> "Oh well, if you can see that and that's actually happening now, we really can't put her over on her side – well, not completely. If I take her through a bit more this way – I'll not come round to see. It means disturbing her more. So what if we just gently lift her through to me? What if I work your side next time we move her? That way I can get a look at it myself without disturbing her too much" (Phillips et al 2000:111).

It can be seen in this event how the opinion of the student is valued, which can only increase her confidence. As

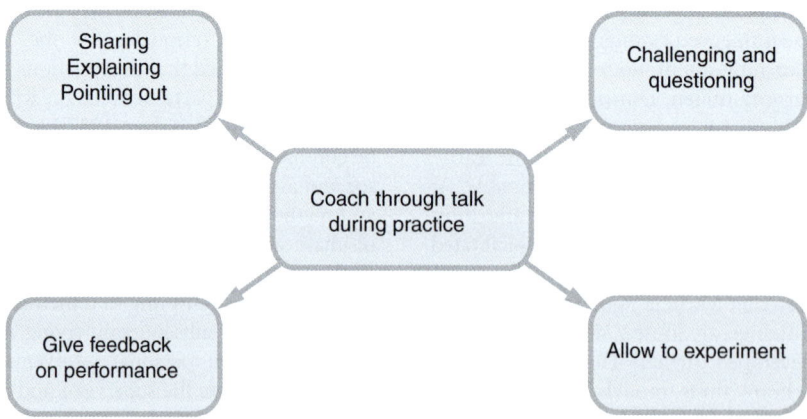

Fig. 9.3 The coaching strategies during the experiencing phase.

the supervisor and assessor talked through the rationale for the choice of new or better position for the patient, they were also sharing and pointing out other aspects of care that this patient required, such as not being unduly disturbed and the necessity to be gentle. For this student the event would probably have meant much more than merely changing the position of the patient. Through this experience the student may have learnt to "read" some of the needs that such patients require, thus deriving meaningful learning from what may appear to be the routine task of repositioning a patient.

Most students, even senior ones, need to be alerted to "signals" from patients and clients. They need to develop skills in interpreting the presenting signs and symptoms of patients and clients so that the physical condition and illness stages can be noted. They also need to become skilled in noting the emotional responses, such as fear, distress, withdrawal and other overt indications. White and Ewan (1997) point out that inexperienced practitioners, such as students are concerned that their performance should be accurate. They focus on following guidelines and rules. Consequently, they have difficulty in managing the competing demands of the situation. The subtler cues of response and reactions within a clinical event are often missed. Opportunities for learning through these experiences are thus lost to them.

As supervisors and assessors work alongside students, opportunities are provided for pointing out the messages and signals that patients and clients are overtly or covertly giving; exposing the learner and teaching them how to handle the sensitive moments which can represent some of the more difficult challenges of practice, such as breaking bad news. Based on such information, explanations can then be given on how care is tailored to meet the needs of the patient/client at the time. Learning through a clinical event is incomplete if a student focuses only on the "content" of the particular activity – to unearth the real meaning of the experience the student also needs to be aware of its "extension into the framework of the patient's situation and surroundings" (White & Ewan 1997) so that there is awareness of the context of the whole situation for the patient and the carer.

Sharing, explaining and pointing out can be in the form of overt physical guidance of actions, such as placing your hand on the student's at times to transfer the amount of pressure to be used in massage, or placing your hand on the student's to transfer the movements and manoeuvres which need to be made to deliver a baby, or listening with the "student" to body sounds through monitors, or seeing with the "student" fine discriminations of change in the patient's colour, or smelling with the "student" to note the odour characteristic of some body fluid or discharges.

White and Ewan describe these ways as "giving away skills – your skills" and guidance is provided by leading "behind" the student (White & Ewan 1997: 135).

Drawing from the work of Vykotsky (1930, in Spouse 1998) on the zone of proximal development, Spouse explored how students' learning during clinical practice can be improved. One of the conclusions she came to was that students who are cognitively ready to move to the next stage could be assisted to reach this potential through support and guidance from a more experienced other. Development is best facilitated if the supervisor and assessor's speech guide the student to a level beyond that currently in use or practised. Having an accurate assessment of a learner's level of capability is crucial in assisting a learner to develop a higher level of competence.

QUESTIONING AND "CHALLENGING"

The supervisor and assessor are advised not to give all the answers, which deprive students of the opportunity of carrying out some of the problem-solving and decision-making activities (Stengelhofen 1993). These cognitive processes foster deep learning, and thus help the student extract more meaningful learning through experiences (McAllister 1997). White and Ewan (1997) state that asking students stimulating and challenging questions helps them to uncover the hidden meaning of their clinical experiences and points them to the "hidden curriculum" of clinical learning, which may be missed by some students altogether as they are primarily concerned with the task to be completed. Students say they need the supervisor and assessor to think of things that might never occur to them (Windsor 1987). Skilful questioning and the challenging of thinking help "awaken" students to the otherwise unrecognized insights and discoveries. Also we "need to be challenged so that we do not fool ourselves with our own distorted assumptions or fail to consider new information which is outside our present range of experience" (Boud et al 1993:15).

Some suggestions on how to use questioning and "challenging" are made subsequently. These are based upon and extended from the work of Tilley et al (2007), Stengelhofen (1993) and White and Ewan (1997):

- Ask the student to explain and justify why a certain course of action has been chosen.
- Ask the student why you are proceeding in a certain way (e.g., "Why do you think I am doing this?")
- Ask the student what actions should be taken in certain situations (e.g., "What assessment should you be thinking of making?", "What actions do you need to take and why?", "How would you make Mr Johns more comfortable?", "What do you intend to do about Mr Johns' request to see his daughter?")

- Place the student in your shoes (e.g., "I have to make a decision as to whether to treat now or leave. What are some of the considerations that might be going through my head?") (Stengelhofen 1993:97).
- Invite the student to come forward with a diagnosis of what the problem may be and how that problem is best managed (e.g., "Have a look at Mr Johns then tell me what you think the major problem is and what we can do about it, then you can tell me how we can fix it") (White & Ewan 1997:141).
- Invite the student's opinions about a situation (e.g., "I would like you to take a look at the patient you looked after yesterday. I think there are some changes … see what you think" (White & Ewan 1997:141), or "What are the real issues here?", or "Do you think Mr Johns' request is reasonable? … Why do you say it is unreasonable?")
- The following questions will help the student synthesize data and identify a problem (e.g., "What is the problem?", "What complications could occur?", "What clinical data would lead you to believe that this complication will occur?", "What clinical data would indicate that the patient needs immediate intervention and why?", "What data are we going to give the doctor or social worker or another professional in the multi-professional team)?")

Questioning and challenging can be threatening for some students; any threat felt needs to be responded to. Supervisors and assessors have to be careful not to undermine students' self-confidence. This may be avoided by manipulating situations and questions to allow students to experience success. Be generous with positive reinforcement.

As the student's learning is actively facilitated by questioning and challenging, the supervisor and assessor needs to be able to facilitate further learning according to the responses of the student as they explore a learning experience (White & Ewan 1991). As the student moves from tentative exploration into understanding, the supervisor and assessor should respond to the content the student is struggling with. When the student's focus is on action, the supervisor and assessor move into guiding further development of the student's knowledge and actions.

ALLOW TO EXPERIMENT

According to Townsend (1990:67), the supervisor and assessor as facilitator will:

"… provide a secure environment in which everyone can experiment, take risks, increase their acceptance for uncertainty and develop mutual trust and commitment. Facilitators are creative, flexible, motivated and involved in mutual goal setting and achievement."

When being allowed to experiment, the student assumes control of clinical care. As in the joint experimentation coaching strategy put forward by Schön (1987), the supervisor and assessor support by helping the student formulate the care to be given by prompting the student in searching for, and deciding upon, the most suitable option of care; the final decision rests with the student.

There is prior agreement that the supervisor and assessor will intervene only if necessary (e.g., when the situation becomes too complex or there could be detrimental consequences for the patient). There is also agreement for the form of support to be given during care delivery; support may be in the form of verbal affirmation of correct performance or nonverbal by the use of body language or just being the "silent supporting presence" – "just standing by" – offering neither approval nor disapproval (White & Ewan 1991). Boud et al (1993:15) made the point that, as learners, we need "appropriate support, trust and challenge from others. This can enable us to continue our tasks when they seem too much for us or when we get blocked…".

If the supervisor and assessor is present during care giving, the temptation to take over and assume control must be resisted. Mutual trust must exist, with both the supervisor and assessor and student accepting any uncertainties.

Trust in the student's ability is necessary to enable the student to progress and develop clinical competence. Boud et al (1993:15) found that some of the most powerful factors influencing learning from experience are those relating to confidence and self-esteem, saying that "unless learners believe themselves capable, they will be continually handicapped in what they do". Many students have said that it is a "nice feeling" to know that they are trusted. The supervisor and assessor has to "step back" so that the student can have opportunities to experiment and assume control with confidence. This level of responsibility requires the student to be able to make clinical decisions with the guidance of the supervisor and assessor. When thus engaged in the thinking and the decision-making processes associated with clinical practice, namely "clinical reasoning" (Higgs 1997, Hunter & Arthur 2016), the student must necessarily use knowledge and higher order cognitive skills to make clinical decisions. From the perspective of the clinical educator Hunter and Arthur identify clinical reasoning as a developmental process rather than a single skill to be achieved. This can be supported by meaningful questioning and explicit criterion referenced assessment (using agreed national standards and policy). Further, they recognize this as an area where further research is required to ascertain enablers and barriers to developing clinical reasoning skills. Skilful facilitation of clinical reasoning will help students "see and read" the depth and breadth of clinical events so that much more meaning can be derived through clinical experiences.

Being allowed to experiment should also include being entrusted with responsibility (e.g., responsibility for planning and managing care for a single or a group of patients/clients). The delegation of responsibility for this aspect of care is necessary to assist senior students to develop the skills of prioritizing, decision-making and time management (Gerrish 2000, Fraser et al 1997). In their study of the effectiveness of preregistration midwifery programmes, Fraser et al found that many of the new midwives experienced a fall in confidence at registration. They concluded that this could perhaps have been reduced if more had been expected of them before registration.

GIVE FEEDBACK ON PERFORMANCE

Giving feedback to students during the performance of clinical activities presents invaluable opportunities to enhance learning and meaning derived from care activities. Whereas it is important to time feedback so that errors of care delivery are avoided, it is also important to allow the student enough scope to use individual skill and flair during performance. This requires the supervisor and assessor to have a degree of trust in the student while being a sensitive observer.

Giving immediate feedback on particularly commendable performances or pointing to where desired improvement could occur will help students extract more learning from clinical events. Remarking on the appropriateness of specific initiatives, or praising a demonstration of exceptional caring, or indicating to the student a grasp of principles underlying an action or a behaviour, not only reinforces the student's experience of success (White & Ewan 1991) but may also motivate the student to reflect on the actions taken and care given. As the student thinks through these, awareness of the feelings and thoughts associated with a particular action may develop; further learning and meaning may be extracted from the experiences if the student works on these feelings and thoughts to enhance future actions.

If the judgement of the client or patient is also solicited, this source of feedback may act as a direct indicator as to whether care given was appropriate and performed to enhance comfort – this additional information further helps the student to evaluate care skills and rethink clinical decisions and actions if necessary. Some more learning may take place, which can only allow the student to derive more meaning from a particular clinical experience.

THE PROCESSING PHASE

Looking back at the preparatory and experiencing phases, it can be seen that learners have to cope with a considerable amount of new information. Situations force them into active involvement whether they like it or not. They face, and have to deal with, many personal demands. Reflection

before and during the experience helps the learner deal with the vast array of inputs and feelings and thoughts generated. Boud et al (1985:26) point out that if "we are exposed to one new event after another without a break we are unlikely to be able to make the most of any of the events separately". In the *Four Quartets*, T. S. Eliot spoke of those who "had the experience but missed the meaning". Following the experience, it is equally vital, if not more so, to process the experience further through reflection, as reflecting after the event is "one of the most helpful means of drawing learning from experience" (Boud & Walker 1990:72). What is also significant is that reflection is not an end in itself – the outcome is that knowledge is created through the transformation of experience (Kolb 1984) so that we are "ready for new experience" (Boud et al 1985:34).

The processing phase is a complex one in which both feelings and cognition are closely interrelated and interactive (Boud et al 1985). Learning is influenced by the socioemotional context in which it occurs. The role of others in the present, such as support, trust and confidence in the learner, can help overcome negative feelings and allow the learner to act and think differently from the past (Stuart 2001, Boud et al 1993). The climate of the processing phase can act to reinforce or counterbalance both negative and positive experiences; it therefore needs to be planned and managed so that learners may be assisted to extract some more meaning and learning from their experiences. Students are likely to raise many questions and problems that have arisen from their experiences. In general, it is not possible to "process" every experience. It may be possible to identify a focus for reflection that addresses several clinical events (e.g., the care of patients who required pressure area care or discussing the cessation of smoking with clients). An alternative is to select discrete experiences identified by the student as significant clinical experiences.

When conducting the session, it is important to remember that this is not another typical group discussion or individual encounter, nor is it a simple reporting back of clinical events, nor an invitation to students to "rehash" what they did and to receive comment on how well or badly they performed and what to do about it. Particular care has to be taken to prevent a session from turning into a "moan session" where no learning takes place and feelings of frustration are heightened (Stuart 2001). Students' presentations of their observations, actions and behaviours, feelings and thoughts in their own words need to be acknowledged and actively worked through with the supervisor and assessor as facilitator. An interactive nonthreatening style of questioning and facilitation will assist the student in drawing out the meaning of what has been experienced. As both supervisor and assessor and student pose questions and attempt to solve problems that have arisen directly from the experience, previously unchallenged assumptions about theory and practice are likely to be explored (Bedford et al 1993, White & Ewan 1991). Learning through reflection needs to be actively facilitated for many learners (Stuart 2001). The reason may be that certain cognitive skills, which are developed to different stages in different people, are required to engage in reflection to learn through this process. Atkins & Murphy (1993) identified these skills as having the abilities to describe, critically analyse, synthesize and evaluate:

- Description involves the ability to recollect and replay the experience in its totality. A close attention to detail, noticing exactly what occurred and one's reactions, without making judgements, is required (Boud et al 1985). These authors suggest that this description should be written or verbalized to others.
- Critical analysis involves examining the components of a situation, identifying existing knowledge, challenging assumptions and imagining and exploring alternatives (Brookfield 2012, Bloom et al 1956).
- Synthesis is the integration of new knowledge with previous knowledge, to form a "new whole" (Bloom et al 1956). The new knowledge can then be used in creative ways to solve problems and to predict likely consequences of actions.
- Evaluation, according to Bloom et al, is the making of judgements about the value of something, for a given purpose. It involves the use of criteria. Mezirow (1981) argues that both synthesis and evaluation are crucial to the development of a new perspective.

These four cognitive skills will now be related to learning through the reflective process during the processing phase. The use of three stages incorporating these cognitive skills is proposed here:

- Description of the experience
- Processing through critical analysis
- Synthesizing and evaluating

Reflection on experience is treated in this format to aid exposition. It is not intended to imply that the stages must take place consecutively. Each stage may be visited and revisited. Reflective exercises within activity boxes are suggested to help the student extract more learning from care giving experiences – these are offered as a guide and not meant to be a prescription.

DESCRIPTION OF THE EXPERIENCE

Boud et al (1985) believe that one of the most useful activities for initiating reflection is to recollect what has taken place in as much detail as possible by:

- Replaying and describing the event as it happened chronologically; this replay of the event in the mind's eye may be done verbally or committed to paper

- Paying close attention to the details of the event
- Noticing exactly what occurred
- Noticing one's reactions to it in all its elements; of particular importance is an observation of the feelings evoked during the experience.

As far as possible, the description should be clear of any judgements because these tend to cloud our recollections and may blind us to some of the features that may need reassessing. As we "witness" the event again, it becomes available for us to reconsider and examine afresh; we may begin to realize how we were feeling and how these feelings may have prompted our responses, which in turn influenced our actions. Those aspects to be considered for the development of noticing skills outlined in Box 9.1 could be used here to assist with the recall of the details of the event. In recalling past events the nature of memory poses problems, as we inevitably forget. To capture the details and nuances of the event, recall should be done as soon as possible.

As students recall and describe their "lived experiences", it is important for supervisor and assessors to listen attentively and respond appropriately, without offering any interpretation or analyses of their own. Supervisor and assessors need to be highly aware of the ways in which language is used by the students to describe or interpret their experience. As the event is replayed and recalled, students will become aware of the feelings that were present during the experience. These feelings need to be acknowledged, as emotions and feelings can either be a significant source of learning or they can become barriers at times. An examination of feelings may reveal that emotional reactions had overridden rationality to such an extent that there was an unawareness of how behaviours and perceptions were blurred. For example, during an emergency situation, feelings of panic may have overtaken rational thoughts and actions so that the chain of events that ensued compromised the wellbeing of the patient. On occasions, resultant negative feelings become barriers and may inhibit the student from entering into further similar experiences. These negative feelings act as learning blocks and, unless they are recognized and addressed, further learning will not proceed. For example, if a student is overcome with anxiety and fear after encountering an aggressive client or a dying patient, this student is likely to shy away from these situations. There are also occasions when students are hurt and distressed after difficult and painful experiences. Phenix (1964:197) urged educators to take responsibility for "improving the quality of human meaning at the deepest personal level". As one student in Stuart's (2001:180) study painfully recounted during the processing phase:

"She's got it (terminal cancer) and she's going to die soon. She's only 44. I think because I'd never come into a situation like this before it hit me hard. I don't know ... I think the imagination goes. I just feel guilty myself ... just felt like I should not have been there, just don't know what to do. I don't want to go into a situation like that again. I went with (the community nurse) for three days and each time she had her on the list, I just dreaded going. It was just so horrible".

It is clear that such feelings must be acknowledged, explored and attended to so that undesirable, and even debilitating, influences are removed or the student may remain disabled. Boud et al (1993:15) emphasize that emotions and feelings strongly influence learning, saying that "denial of feelings is denial of learning". An increased awareness of emotions will help students to develop the sensitivity required to detect the nuances and the affective tone of the situation so that they can respond sensitively to the needs of the patient/client. In so doing, students will learn to give care as well as caring for the patient/client for "... care without caring is empty and meaningless ..." (Nordman et al 1998:161). Further, the point when students acquire this form of professional artistry is the point when they have begun to unearth meaning from clinical experiences. Positive feelings should be retained and enhanced so that confidence and self-worth are fostered; these can provide the impetus for students to pursue, or persist with, experiences they may previously have thought to be too difficult or even insurmountable. Unless we believe in ourselves and our capabilities, we can constrain ourselves to such an extent that we ultimately deny ourselves the learning opportunities for further learning and development.

PROCESSING THROUGH CRITICAL ANALYSIS

During this stage, the experience is thought about and mulled over further to examine and seek relationships among the components of the situation and subsequently to see it as a whole picture within the wider context of the care setting and health care. New knowledge and ideas are identified and related to that which is already known, with the aim of integrating the two sources of knowledge to form a "new whole". This "new whole knowledge" can then be used in creative ways to solve problems and predict likely consequences of future actions. Aspects to be considered to assist processing through critical analysis are suggested in Box 9.2. It is necessary to refer to the information provided from the description of the experience.

As students respond to the issues raised by asking the questions in Box 9.2, their responses and explanations could be prompted at times with further questions to probe more deeply and to expand on "glib" responses. In addition, they could be asked to reconsider the validity and

> **BOX 9.2 Aspects to be Considered for Processing Through Critical Analysis**
>
> Consider the following aspects about the experience:
> - The rationale of the care given
> - The effects on the patient/client/family of the care given
> - What aspect(s) of the episode had the most impact on you and why?
> - What, if anything, you found demanding?
> - What you did that was appropriate/inappropriate and the reasons for making the judgement
> - What others did that was appropriate/inappropriate and the reasons for making that judgement
> - Decisions/choices made by yourself and others and whether these were the "right" ones; what are the reasons for making that judgement?
> - In a similar situation, what were your thoughts, feelings and behaviours?
> - Is there a pattern?

reliability of their knowledge base and clinical data they have used as the basis for the decisions they have made and the care given. It is important to connect the ideas and feelings that arose during the experience and those that arise during the processing phase with existing knowledge and attitudes. Cognitive theorists, such as Ausubel (1968) regard this linking of new information with those relevant elements in our existing cognitive structure as one of the central features of the learning process.

This cognitive process has to be facilitated if we want to encourage learners to develop a deep approach to learning (Marton & Säljö 1984), an approach characterized by active interaction with the material at hand as the student searches for further meaning from the experience. This results in an integration of formal learning with personal experience and making links between components of knowledge. For example, the student referred to earlier in Stuart's study (2001) may be assisted to explore her knowledge about the care and support of young clients with terminal cancer and the support services available. The student may then evaluate how such care can influence the quality of life of these clients and start to realize that, although it is indeed sad that young people do die of cancer, a quality of life can still be achieved. She has to make connections between the needs of the client, the services available to support the client and her role in meeting the needs of this client and family. This student realized that the client had not had time to come to terms with her illness (Stuart 2001:182):

"These defence mechanisms (referring to the stages of the grieving process) we have – she found out at

Christmas that she had cancer and she was given a month to live and it's just come so quickly that I don't think she'd been able to go through these defence mechanisms; she hadn't been able to know that she's got it; she hadn't been able to come to terms that she got it. I think all her feelings are muddled up."

Knowledge and understanding of the stages of the grieving process will assist the student in helping the client work through the grief of having terminal cancer. The student needs to make connections between the formal theory of the grieving process and how this client may be best assisted. The student also needs to make links between what her needs are to enable her to carry out the care required and how they can meet those needs. For example, they may have to learn to come to terms with feelings of guilt and pity for these clients, which are present in their existing cognitive and affective structures. The student may realize that they can be a more effective carer if they have an attitude of empathy rather than pity.

The student's feelings of guilt and pity may be reflective of their assumption that clients with terminal cancer cannot have a quality of life; if this is the case that assumption can be challenged. This challenging may start to take place as the student realizes that, with care and support, these clients can be enabled to experience a quality of life. As the student learns of the strategies they can use to help these clients, and how these strategies may need to be adapted to meet the needs of individual clients, they are beginning to imagine and explore the alternatives for client-centred care.

SYNTHESIZING AND EVALUATING

As students draw conclusions and develop insights into the material they are processing—material from both formal theory and their personal experiences—they develop a set of ideas and perspectives about the management of the clinical situations they were involved with. They have, in effect, developed their own theory of practice through personal experiences. Students can demonstrate the knowledge, understanding and values that have informed their actions. A new set of ideas, concepts and/or "mindscape" (Bedford et al 1993) may emerge, "enabling them to appreciate the inherent contradictions within professional caring without incapacitating them to the extent that they are unable to act because of their awareness of those dilemmas" (Bedford et al 1993:141). This will lead to altered ways of giving care. Aspects to be considered to assist further processing through synthesis and evaluation are suggested in Box 9.3.

Boud et al (1985) suggest using the process of validation to test for consistency between the new appreciations and existing knowledge and beliefs, and between these and

BOX 9.3   **Aspects to be Considered for Processing Through Synthesizing and Evaluating**
Students should ask themselves the following questions: • What made me think, feel and act that way? • Could I have acted differently? • Did I have any choice? • Did I do anything that was different? • Why was the care given successful/unsuccessful? • Was the care given an accurate reflection of personal and professional philosophies? • Were there any conflicts between personal beliefs and values and the care that was given? • What conclusions can I draw? What ideas, concepts and generalizations can I form? • How do I know that my conclusions are valid?

parallel data drawn from others, such as those of the supervisor and assessor and the literature. The literature may be searched for written material that will shed further light on the various facets of the experience, such as data to support the care given. If there are any contradictions, the situation may need to be reappraised. These authors further suggest that, even if our new perception is not consistent with that held by others, it does not imply that we should reject it. Our idea may be breaking new ground or we may wish to hold a certain position regardless of conventional wisdom.

OUTCOMES AND ACTION

The aim of reflecting-on-experience during the processing phase is to make us ready for new experience. However, the benefits gained from reflection could be merely an exercise in abstract thinking if any resultant learning is not linked to action. Students will ask questions such as: "What do the ideas and concepts mean to me? … How can I make use of what I have learned?" This is an ideal time for assisting students to specify what actions they plan to take so that they can consider the changes in practice and behaviours they want to incorporate into future clinical experiences. The changes may be quite small or they may be large.

In some instances, before changes can be made to practice, students may be required to accept the new understanding and approaches into their own value systems. Changing their view of self is involved, as well as the values associated with self as practitioner. As students gain a better understanding of self and their professional practices, their confidence is likely to increase. They are then empowered to try out their new ideas in practice. As they do so, their practices are likely to be reshaped and they then enter into new experiences.

TABLE 9.2   A Framework to Review Learning Through Processing of Experience

Stages of Processing	Requires Further Development	Well Developed		
Description of situation including personal and others' thoughts and feelings	Relevance of description not demonstrated Lacks coherence, organization and clarity	Situation described, but lacks focus and omits sufficient detail	Recognizes and recollects key features of situations, including context, feeling and thoughts	High level of perception evident Subtle nuances in the situation noticed
Critical analysis of situation in relationship to personal and others' involvement	Minimal awareness	Begins to explore thoughts, feelings and behaviour of self and others triggered by the situation	Constructive exploration of thoughts, feelings and behaviour	Demonstrates insight into situation Shows an objective appreciation of how and why self and others felt, thought and behaved as they did in the situation, and how they affected the situation Sees the heart of the matter
Synthesizing and evaluating	Relevant underpinning values not identified No evidence of forming ideas nor drawing any conclusions	Identifies some values relevant to the situation Limited range of ideas formed Assumptions underlying practice are not explored Conclusions lack depth	Identifies the values, ideas and concepts relevant to the situation Explores some assumptions underlying practice and draws some meaningful conclusions	Critically analyses values, ideas and concepts and their relationship to practice Sees the wider professional implications Constructively challenges own and others' assumptions
Evidence of learning/ outcomes of reflection	No evidence of implications for own practice/ learning	Identifies some implications for own practice/learning Some explicit evidence of learning	Evidence of learning explicit Identifies implications for practice, and begins to specify how own practice can develop	Integrates "new" knowledge with previous knowledge to reach new/ different perspectives Specifies where and how own practice will develop Relates innovative practice development to the wider professional context

FRAMEWORK TO REVIEW LEARNING THROUGH PROCESSING OF EXPERIENCE

Proposed here is a framework (Table 9.2) to review learning that has arisen as a result of processing experiences. The treatment of learning in this format is to assist the learner and supervisor and assessor in deciding the quality of learning achieved and what further learning needs to take place. It is not intended to imply that learning through the processing

of experiences can be compartmentalized; nor can such learning be quantified (e.g., through the use of grading).

EXPERIENTIAL LEARNING AND CONTINUING PROFESSIONAL DEVELOPMENT

Professional knowledge and practices change constantly and require the practitioner to be motivated to refine and update knowledge and practices so that professional expertise, and thus practice wisdom (Hull 1998), is continually developing. Furthermore, it is essential to ensure that practitioners can maintain autonomous practice where they are capable of making their own decisions about their actions and the moral bases of those actions (Fish & Twinn 1997). The ability to exercise professional judgement is essential; professional judgement is seen as a complex skill requiring abilities to notice and analyse the patient's/client's problem, deciding what has to be done and evaluating the effectiveness of actions taken. Such ways of managing professional work cannot be laid down as absolute rules of practice and are termed "professional artistry" by Schön (1987), which is seen to be well beyond technical efficiency and the use of routine craft skills. The professional artistry view relies on frameworks and rules of thumb rather than rules. The practitioner is not less accountable, but is in fact more accountable, as moral accountability for all conduct is exercised (Fish & Twinn 1997).

A holistic model for the continuing professional development of health care practitioners, as is the case for preregistration education, will also have clinical experiences as one of its key points. Using the "model for learning from experience" explored so far in this chapter to structure the learning process will help the practitioner use clinical experiences as the key focus for continuing professional development. Although practice is of primary importance, its underlying theory is not set to one side. There is a close interrelationship between theory and practice; no professional action is devoid of theory, for theory involves beliefs, values, ideas and assumptions. Everything we do is thus influenced by theory. What may be absent is awareness of such theories. Many believe that unearthing the meaning of experiences comes after, or at best during, the action. This means that developing expertise (Benner 1984) in professional practice must begin with action. Often the most useful theorizing for action takes place during the activity and the most useful theory develops after the activity, if the activity has been carefully reconsidered during the processing phase (Schön 1987, 1983). The experience is the vehicle for enabling practitioners to consider what is involved in learning during and after professional activities, and how this learning can be used to develop professional practice.

The principles of learning from each phase of the model, in particular the experiencing and processing phases, will help the practitioner to derive more meaning and learning as professional activities are planned, entered into and reflected upon during and after completion of care. Practitioners enter into a continuum of learning, as this model shows; professional activity cannot be separated into the component parts of theory and practice. Using the principles of learning from the model for learning from experience, the following questions may aid the development of expertise through continuing professional development activities:

- What is the nature of learning through professional activities? For example, is it a practical problem-solving activity involving people? Is it refining and defining practical wisdom? Is it developing theory? Is it questioning and challenging established practices?
- What sorts of professional/clinical activities should be used for refining and developing professional practice? Should they be every aspect of your working life? Should they be some aspect of practice that catches your attention? Should they be incidents that are outright critical events, such as emergency situations? Should they be aspects of practice that have simply gone unexamined and unchallenged and are now accepted practices?
- What can you say about yourself as a learner seeking to develop your professional practices? Are you able to get on with it by yourself? Do you find it helpful to bounce ideas off your colleagues? Do your colleagues bounce their ideas off you?
- When was the last time you examined how you practised in a constructive way with others?

Bedford et al (1993) believe that as you enter into dialogues with others about your practice, not only do you make your understanding accessible to each other, but also you help to develop both the theory and the practice out of each other. If these dialogic debates are of sufficient depth and breadth, you will be able to explore and understand further the moral dimensions and the ambiguity, complexity and uncertainty of the practice settings.

Within their mandates for continuing professional development, the NMC and the Health Care Professions Council (HCPC 2012) require their practitioners to keep a record of continuing professional development activities by demonstrating competence and updating at revalidation. For Nurses and Midwives, this consists of reflections on practice alongside evidence of practice and sign-off from a fellow registrant (NMC 2019). The profile is to be created by documenting learning activities which are relevant to their practice and the ways in which they have informed and influenced practice. It is suggested here that the learning activities in Table 9.2 and those in the section on the processing phase can be used to assist practitioners to maintain this record.

CONCLUSION

Dewey (1963/1938) stated that all genuine education comes about through experience. Certainly, in practice-based professions, such as the health care professions, clinical experience should be the basis for learning. To extract learning from experience, we need to create meaning from our experiences as we interact with, and react to, them. We cannot allow any experience to be taken for granted; once we do so, actions become routine and habitual, we stop noticing and enter into a rut.

This chapter has attempted to portray some of the complexities of learning through clinical practice that can promote or hinder meaningful learning from experience. Learning from experience is not a simple rational process – not only do we need to know what and how to do, but also, we need to know what and how to think. Impacting on, and influencing, these psychomotor and cognitive processes are our feelings, values and beliefs. We therefore also need to exercise our affective self, which very frequently dominates our experience and may become either a positive or negative influence for learning. Forces around us also have their influences on how we engage with and extract meaning from an experience, such as the facilitative presence of others and our surroundings. Schön (1987) stated

that learning conditions that are not easily met are an awareness of each other's experience, the ability to describe it and a willingness to make it discussable.

Usher (1993) reminds us that experience always says less than it wishes to say: there are many readings of it, it is never exhausted, and total clarity may never be reached. Nevertheless, I hope that the discussion in this chapter has provided a range of perspectives to assist the learner and supervisor and assessor during clinical practice to unearth meaning from clinical experiences.

If professionals are to develop skills in learning through their experience so as to develop the professional artistry to deal with the complex human issues of practice (entering into complex decision making and elements of professional judgement and practical wisdom guided by moral principles) they need to be taught, and encouraged to do so, during their preregistration training.

KEY POINTS FOR REFLECTION

A model of preparation for professional practice that does not rely slavishly on the use and application of rules, schedules and prescriptions is more likely to equip practitioners to be able to deal with the complexities of clinical practice.

Stuart's Model for Learning From Experience considers experience-based learning and has clinical experiences as one of its key foci. This emphasizes experiential learning, which proceeds from the assumption that ideas are not fixed, and immutable elements of thought but rather are continuously derived from, and tested out, through experience.

The underpinning principle of the model is that, although experience is the foundation of and the stimulus for learning, it does not necessarily lead to learning unless there is active engagement with it. This model has four phases:

1. The preparatory phase. The following questions may assist preparation:
   - Why has this particular experience been arranged?
   - What can be learnt through this experience?
   - How can learning from previous experiences be linked to this experience?
   - How can students be assisted to plan thoughtfully?
   - How can students be assisted to engage in the clinical experience?

   The preparatory phase focuses on:

   The student as a learner: consider "learning intent", prior learning and the accumulation of previous experiences. The response of the learner to new experiences is determined significantly by these past experiences and

their learning intent, as presuppositions and assumptions have been developed – the past creates expectations, which influence the present. The present context can serve to reinforce or counterbalance this.

Developing noticing skills: noticing provides students with the basis for becoming more fully involved in a caregiving situation and enables them to "reflect-in-action" (Schön 1983) as they become more aware of the processes of how decisions are made to inform actions taken. As well as paying attention to what is happening around the experience, it is equally important to pay attention to what is happening in themselves. Students need to be aware in three areas: how they are acting; what they are thinking; how they are feeling.

Developing intervening skills: intervening is when the learner takes an initiative and is active in the event. This can be any verbal or physical action taken by the learner within the learning situation. Learners need to know how and when to intervene and the nature and content of the interventions.

2. The experiencing phase. During this phase the "taking on board of what is going on" while "performing" has to be accompanied by the "thinking" and the "feeling". One key aim is to facilitate development of learners' "power of judgement and capacity to act intelligently in new situations" (Dewey 1963/1938:15). Learners are assisted to "reflect-in-action". Several teaching/learning strategies influence how the learner engages with, and reflects during, the experience:

   Sharing, explaining and "pointing out": students who are cognitively ready to move to the next stage of development can be assisted to reach this potential through support and guidance from a more experienced other. Development is best facilitated if the supervisor and assessor's speech guides the student to a level beyond that currently in use or practised. Having an accurate assessment of a learner's level of capability is crucial in assisting a learner to develop a higher level of competence. Consider engaging learners in "situated negotiation of their practice": informal on-the-job conversations take place, which allow the sharing of ideas and understanding about care. Sharing, explaining and pointing out can also be in the form of overt physical guidance of actions.

Questioning and challenging: skilful questioning and the challenging of thinking help students to uncover the hidden meaning of their clinical experiences. Ask students to explain and justify why a certain course of action has been chosen; explain why you are proceeding in a certain way; come up with decisions and actions that should be taken in certain situations; place the student in your shoes; invite the student to come forward with a diagnosis of what the problem may be and how that problem is best managed; invite the student's opinions about a situation.

Allowing to experiment: the student assumes control of clinical care. Support by helping the student formulate the care to be given by prompting the student in searching for, and deciding upon, the most suitable option of care; the final decision rests with the student. Trust in the student's ability is necessary to enable the student to progress and develop clinical competence. Learn to "let go".

Giving feedback on performance: immediate feedback on particularly commendable performances or pointing to where desired improvement could occur will help students extract more learning from clinical events. Balance timely feedback to avoid errors of care delivery against giving the student enough scope to use individual skill and flair during performance.

3. The processing phase. The experience is systematically reflected on and actively facilitated during this phase, as reflecting after the event is one of the most helpful means of drawing learning from experience. There are three key stages in reflecting on experience:

4. Description of the experience: recollect and replay the experience in its totality, paying close attention to detail, noticing exactly what occurred and one's reactions, without making judgements.

5. Processing through critical analysis: the experience is thought about and mulled over further; assist to make links and connections among the components of the situation, and between other similar situations, and subsequently to see it as a whole picture; new knowledge and ideas are identified and related to that which is already known.

6. Synthesizing and evaluating: new experience and ideas/concepts formed are linked to previous experience to form "new wholes"; through the process of validation, test for consistency between the new appreciations and existing knowledge and beliefs and between these and parallel data drawn from others and the literature.

7. Outcomes and action: learning is linked to action; assist students to specify actions they plan to take so that they can consider the changes in practice and behaviours they want to incorporate into future clinical experiences.

REFERENCES

Aitchison, J., Graham, P., Criticos, C. (1989). Potato crisp pedagogy: experiential learning in formal and non-formal education. In: C. Criticos. *Experiential Learning in Formal and Non-Formal Education*. Media Resource Centre, University of Natal, Durban, p. 1–13.

Alexander, M.F. (1982a). Integrating theory and practice in nursing – part I. *Nursing Times, Occasional Papers*, 78 (17), 65–68.

Alexander, M.F. (1982b). Integrating theory and practice in nursing – part II. Nursing Times, *Occasional Papers*, 78 (18) (1982) 69–71.

Andrew, N., Tolson, D., Ferguson, D. (2008). Building on Wenger: communities of practice. *Nurse Education Today,* 28, 246-252.

Andrews, M., Reece Jones, P. (1996). Problem-based learning in an undergraduate nursing Programme. *Journal of Advanced Nursing*, 23 (2), 357-365.

Ashley, J., Stamp, K. (2014). Learning to think like a nurse: the development of clinical judgment in nursing students. *Journal of Nursing Education*, 53 (9), 519-525

Atkins, S., Murphy, K. (1993). Reflection: a review of the literature, *Journal of Advanced Nursing*, 18,1188–1192.

Attenborough, J., Abbott, S., Brook, J., Knight, R-A. (2019). Everywhere and nowhere: work-based learning in healthcare education, *Nurse Education in Practice*, 36, 132–138.

Attenborough, J., Knight, R-A., Brook, J. (2018). Developing and sustaining a community of practice through Twitter for work-based learning. *BMJ Evidence-Based Nursing*, 21 (4); 89–90.

Ausubel, D.P. (1968). *Educational Psychology: a Cognitive View*, New York, Holt, Reinhart & Winston.

Bedford, H., Phillips, T., Robinson, J. (1993). *Assessment of Competencies in Nursing and Midwifery Education and Training*, London, The English National Board for Nursing, Midwifery and Health Visiting.

Benner, P. (1984). *From Novice to Expert: Excellence and Power in Clinical Nursing Practice*. Menlo Park, Addison-Wesley.

Benner, P. Wrubel, J. (1982). Skilled clinical knowledge: the value of perceptual awareness, part 2. *Journal of Nursing Administration*, 12 (6), 28–33.

Bierema, L.L. (2001). Women, work and learning. *New Directions for Adult and Continuing Education*, 92, 53-62.

Billett, S. (2008). Learning through work: exploring instances of relational interdependencies. *International Journal of Education Research*, 47, 232–240.

Billett, S. (2015). Learning through health care work: premises, contributions and practices, *Medical Education*, 50, 124–131.

Bloom, B.S., Engelhart, M.D., Furst, E.J. (1956). *Taxonomy of Educational Objectives, Handbook 1: Cognitive Domain*. London, Longman.

Boud, D., Walker, D. (1990). Making the most of experience. *Studies in Continuing Education*, 12 (2), 61–80.

Boud, D., Walker, D. (1991). *Experience and Learning: Reflection at Work*. Geelong, Deakin University, Australia.

Boud, D., Walker, D. (1993). Barriers to reflection on experience. In: Boud, D., Cohen, R., Walker (Eds). *Using Experience for Learning*. Buckingham, The Society for Research into Higher Education and Open University Press, p. 73–86.

Boud, D., Cohen, R. Walker, D. (1993) Understanding learning from experience. In: Boud, D. Cohen, R. Walker D. (eds.), *Using Experience for Learning*. Buckingham, The Society for Research into Higher Education and Open University Press, p. 3–20.

Boud D., Keogh, R., Walker, D. (1985) What is reflection in learning? Reflection: turning experience into learning. In: Boud, D., Keogh, R., Walker, D. (Eds.) *Reflection: Turning Experience into Learning*. Kogan Page, London, p. 7–39.

Boydston, J.A. (Ed.) (2008). *John Dewey: The Later Works, 1925-1953, Volume I: 1925 'experience and nature'*, Carbondale, Southern Illinois University Press.

Bray, L., Nettleton, P. (2007). Assessor or mentor? Role confusion in professional education. *Nurse Education Today*, 27, 848–855.

Brookfield, S.D (2012). Teaching for Critical Thinking: Tools and techniques to help students question their assumptions. San Francisco, Jossey-Bass.

Brown, J.S., Duguid, P., (1991). Organizational learning and communities-of-practice: toward a unified view of working, learning, and innovation, *Organization Science*, 2 (1), 40–57.

Carr, W., Kemmis, S. (1986). *Becoming Critical: Education, Knowledge and Action Research*. The Falmer Press, London.

Chandler, D.E., Kram, K.E. (2005). Applying an adult development perspective to developmental networks. *Career Development International*, 10 (6/7), 548–566.

Chandler, J., Rycroft-Malone, J., Hawkes, C., Noyes, J. (2016). Application of simplified Complexity Theory concepts for healthcare social systems to explain the implementation of evidence into practice, *Journal of Advanced Nursing*, 72 (2), 461–480.

Comer, M. (2019). Rethinking reflection in action: what did Schön really mean? *Nurse Education Today*, 36, 4–6.

Criticos, C., Boud, D., Cohen, R., Walker, D. (1993). Experiential learning and social transformation for a post-apartheid learning future. In: Boud, D., Cohen, D., Walker, D. (1993) *Using Experience for Learning*. Buckingham, The Society for Research into Higher Education and Open University Press, p. 157–168.

Dewey, J. (1963/1938). *Experience and Education*. New York, Macmillan.

Dobrow, S.H., Higgins, M.R. (2005). Developmental networks and professional identity: a longitudinal study, *Career Development International*, 1 (6/7), 567–583.

Eliot, T.S. (2001). *The Four Quartets* (main edition). London, Faber and Faber.

Eraut, M. (2004). Informal Learning in the workplace. *Studies in Continuing Education*, 26 (2), 247–273.

Eraut, M. (2011). Informal learning in the workplace: evidence on the real value of work-based learning (WBL). *Development and Learning in Organisations*, 25 (5), 8–12.

Evison, R. (2006). Changing to learning cultures that foster life-long learners. In: Sutherland, P., and Crowther, J. (Eds.) *Life-long Learning: Concepts and Contexts*. Routledge, Abingdon.

Fenwick, T. (2008). Workplace learning: emerging trends and new perspectives. *New Directions for Adult and Continuing Education*, 118, 17–26.

Fenwick, T. (2014). Sociomateriality in medical practice and learning: attuning to what matters, *Medical Education*, 48, 44–52.

Fish, D., Twinn, S. (1997). *Quality Clinical Supervision*. Oxford, Butterworth-Heinemann.

Fraser, D., Murphy, R., Worth-Butler, M. (1997). *An Outcome Evaluation of the Effectiveness of Pre-registration Midwifery Programmes of Education*, London, The English National Board for Nursing, Midwifery and Health Visiting.

Gerrish, K. (2000). Still fumbling along? A comparative study of the newly qualified nurse's perception of the transition from student to qualified nurse. *Journal of Advanced Nursing*, 32 (2), 473–480.

Hager, P. (2004). Conceptions of learning and understanding learning at work. *Studies in Continuing Education*, 26 (1), 3–17.

Haigh, J. (2007). Expansive learning in the university setting: the case for simulated experience. *Nurse Education in Practice*, 7(2), 95–102.

Haslam, S.A., Platow, M.J. (2001). The link between leadership and followership: how affirming social identity translates vision into action. *Personality and Social Psychology Bulletin*, 27, 1469–1479.

Health Care Professions Council, (2012). *Standards of Continuing Professional Development*, London, HCPC.

Higgins, M.C., Kram, K.E. (2001). Reconceptualizing mentoring at work: a developmental network perspective. *The Academy of Management Review*, 26, 264–288.

Higgs, J. McAllister, L. Lincoln, M. McLeod, S. (1997). Learning to make clinical decisions. In: McAllister, L., Lincoln, M., McLeod, S. (Eds.). *Facilitating Learning in Clinical Settings*, Cheltenham, Stanley Thornes; p. 130–153.

Hodges, H.F. (2011). Preparing new nurses with complexity science and problem-based learning. *Journal of Nursing Education*, 50 (1), 7–13.

Hodkinson, P., Hodkinson H. (2004). The significance of individuals' dispositions in workplace learning: a case study of two teachers. *Journal of Education and Work*, 17(2), 167–182.

Hull, C., Quinn, F.M. (1998). Open learning and professional development: continuing professional development in nursing. In: Quinn, F.M. *Continuing Professional Development in Nursing*. Stanley Thornes, Cheltenham; 182–204.

Hunter, S., Arthur, A. (2016). Clinical reasoning of nursing students on clinical placement: clinical educators' perspectives. *Nurse Education in Practice*, 18, 73–79.

Illeris, K. (2007). *How we learn: Learning and Non-Learning in School and Beyond*. Abingdon, Routledge

Innes, R.B. (2004). *Reconstructing Undergraduate Education.* Lawrence Erlbaum, Mahwah.

Jensen, K., Lahn, L. (2005). The binding role of knowledge: an analysis of nursing students' knowledge ties. *Journal of Education and Work,* 18 (3), 305–320.

Knowles, M.S., Elwood, F.H., Swanson, R.A. (1998). *The Adult Learner* (fifth ed.) Houston, Gulf Publishing,

Kolb, D.A. (1984). *Experiential Learning: Experience as the Source of Learning.* Englewood Cliffs, New Jersey, Prentice-Hall.

Kram, K.E. (1983). Phases of the mentor relationship. *Academy of Management Journal,* 26 (4), 608–625.

Lave, J., Wenger, E. (1991). *Situated Learning: Legitimate Peripheral Participation.* Cambridge University Press, Cambridge.

Levett-Jones, T., Lathlean, J. (2009). 'Don't rock the boat': Nursing students' experiences of conformity and compliance. *Nurse Education Today,* 29, 342–349.

Lewin, D. (2007). Clinical learning environments for student nurses: key indices from two studies compared over a 25 year period. *Nurse Education in Practice,* 7, 238–246.

Lindeman, E.C. (1926). *The Meaning of Adult Education.* New York, New Republic.

MacLaren, J. (2018). Constellations of support for mentor development: exploring what is available to mentors in training. *Nurse Education in Practice,* 28, 66–75.

Manley, K., Titchen, A., Hardy, S. (2009). Work-based learning in the context of contemporary health care education and practice: a concept analysis. *Practice Development in Health Care,* 8 (2), 87–127.

McAllister, L., Lincoln, M., McLeod, S. (1997). An adult learning framework for clinical education: Facilitating Learning in Clinical Settings. In: McAllister, L., Lincoln, M., McLeod, S. (Eds.). *Facilitating Learning in Clinical Settings.* Cheltenham, Stanley Thornes, p. 1–26.

Marton, F. Säljö, R., Hounsell, D., Entwistle, N. (1984) Approaches to learning: the Experience of learning. In: Marton, F., Hounsell, D., Entwistle, N. (Eds.). *The Experience of Learning.* Edinburgh, Scottish Academic Press, p. 36–55.

May, N., Veitch, L., McIntosh, J. (1997). *Evaluation of Nurse and Midwife Education in Scotland: 1992 Programmes.* The National Board for Nursing, Midwifery and Health Visiting for Scotland, Edinburgh

Mezirow, J. (1981). A critical theory of adult learning in education. *Adult Education.* 32 (1), 3–24.

Moriaty, J., MacIntyre G., Manthorpe, J. (2010). My expectations remain the same. The student has to be competent to practise: practice assessor perspectives on the new social work degree qualification in England. *British Journal of Social Work,* 40, 583–601.

Morley, D. (2016). Applying Wenger's Communities of Practice to placement learning. *Nurse Education Today,* 39, 161–162.

Neary, M. (2000). *Teaching, Assessing and Evaluation for Clinical Competence.* Stanley Thornes, Cheltenham.

Newman, M. (2011). Reflection disempowered. In: Merriam, S. B., Grace, A. P. (eds). *The Jossey-Bass Reader on Contemporary Issues in Adult Education.* Jossey-Bass, San Francisco, pp. 315–339.

Newton, J.M., Billett, S., Ockerby, C.M. (2009). Journeying through clinical placements – an examination of six student cases. *Nurse Education Today,* 29, 630–634.

Newton, J.M., Henderson, A., Jolly, B., Greaves, J. (2015). A contemporary examination of workplace learning culture: an ethnomethodology study. *Nurse Education Today,* 35, 91–96.

NHS England (2016). *Leading Change: Adding Value.* London, NHS England.

Nordman, T., Kasen, A., Eriksson, K., Johns, C., Freshwater, D. (1998). Reflective practice – a way to the patient's world and caring. In: Johns, C., Freshwater, D. (Eds.). *Transforming Nursing Through Reflective Practice.* London, Blackwell Science, p. 161–176.

Nursing and Midwifery Council (2011). The *PREP Handbook.* Nursing and Midwifery Council, London.

Nursing and Midwifery Council (2018a). Standards for Student Supervision and Assessment, Available online at https://www.nmc.org.uk/globalassets/sitedocuments/education://www.nmc.org.uk/globalassets/sitedocuments/education-standards/student-supervision-assessment.pdf (Accessed 16 August 2019).

Nursing and Midwifery Council (2018b). Future nurse: Standards of Proficiency for Registered Nurses, available online at https://www.nmc.org.uk/standards/standards-for-nurses/standards-of-proficiency-for-registered-nurses/ (accessed 16 August 2019).

Nursing and Midwifery Council (2018c). The Code: Professional standards of practice and behaviour for nurses, midwives and nursing associates, London, Nursing and Midwifery Council

Nursing and Midwifery Council (2019). Revalidation: How to revalidate with the NMC, Available online at https://www.nmc.org.uk/globalassets/sitedocuments/revalidation/how-to-revalidate-booklet.pdf [Accessed 13 August 2019].

O'Driscoll, M.F., Allan. H.T., Smith, P.A. (2010). Still looking for leadership - who is responsible for student nurses' learning in practice. *Nurse Education Today,* 30, 212–217.

O'Lúanaigh, P.O. (2015). Becoming a professional: what is the influence of registered nurses on nursing students' learning in the clinical environment? *Nurse Education in Practice,* 15, 450–456.

Peters, E. (2018). Compassion fatigue in nursing: a concept analysis, *Nursing Forum,* 53, 466–480.

Phenix, P.H. (1964). *Realms of Meaning,* McGraw-Hill, New York.

Phillips, T., Schostak, J., Tyler, J. (2000). *Practice and Assessment in Nursing and Midwifery: Doing it for Real.* London, The English National Board for Nursing, Midwifery and Health Visiting.

Rogers, A. (1996). *Teaching Adults* (2nd edition). Buckingham, Open University Press.

Salami, S.O. Psychosocial factors as predictors of mentoring among nurses in Southwest Nigeria, *European Journal of Social Sciences,* 5 (2), 53–61.

Schön, D.A. (1987). *Educating the Reflective Practitioner.* San Francisco, Jossey-Bass.

Schön, D.A. (1983). *The Reflective Practitioner: How Practitioners Think in Action.* New York, Basic Books.

Solman, A., Wilson, V. (2016). Person-centredness in nursing strategy and policy. In: McCormack, B., McCance, T. (Eds). *Person-centred Practice in Nursing and Health Care: Theory and Practice* (2nd Edition). Wiley Blackwell, Chichester, p. 77–85.

Spouse, J. (1998). Scaffolding student learning in clinical practice. *Nurse Education Today* 18, 259–266.

Spouse, J. (2001). Bridging theory and practice in the supervisory relationship: a sociocultural perspective. *Journal of Advanced Nursing,* 33 (4), 512–522.

Stengelhofen, J. (1993) *Teaching Students in Clinical Settings,* London, Chapman & Hall.

Stuart, C.C. (2001). The reflective journeys of a midwifery tutor and her students. *Reflective Practice,* 2 (2), 171–184.

Stuart, C.C. (2000). A model for developing skills of reflection. *British Journal of Midwifery,* 8 (2), 111–117.

Thrysoe, L., Hounsgaard, L., Bonderup Dohn, N., Wagner, L. (2010). Participating in a community of practice as a prerequisite for becoming a nurse - trajectories as final year nursing students. *Nurse Education in Practice,* 30, 361–366.

Tilley, D.S., Allen, P., Collins, C. (2007). Promoting clinical competence: using scaffolded instruction for practice-based learning. *Journal of Professional Nursing,* 23 (5), 285–289.

Tolson, D., McAloon, M., Hotchkiss, R., Schofield, I. (2005). Progressing evidence-based practice: an effective nursing model? *Journal of Advanced Nursing,* 50 (2), 124–133.

Townsend, J. (1990) Teaching/learning strategies. *Nursing Times,* 86 (23), 66–68.

Usher, R., Boud, D., Cohen, R., Walker, D. (1993). Experiential learning or learning from experience: does it make a difference? In: Boud, D., Cohen, R., Walker, D. (Eds.), *Using Experience for Learning,* Buckingham, The Society for Research into Higher Education and Open University Press, p. 169–180.

Van Beek, A.P.A., Wagner, C., Spreeuwenberg, P.P.M., Frijters, D.H.M., Ribbe, M.W., (2011). Communication, advice exchange and job satisfaction of nursing staff: a social network analysis of 35 long term care units, available online at https://bmchealthservres.biomedcentral.com/track/pdf/10.1186/1472-6963-11-140 (accessed 09 March 2020)

Virktis, N.D., Herleth, A., Rewers, L. (2019). Closing nursing's experience-complexity gap, *Journal of Nursing Administration,* 49 (12), 580–582.

Wenger, E. (1998). *Communities of Practice,* Cambridge University Press, Cambridge.

White, R., Ewan, C. (1997). *Clinical Teaching in Nursing,* (2nd Ed.), Cheltenham, Nelson Thornes.

Windsor, A. (1987). Nursing students' perception of clinical experience. *Journal of Nursing Education,* 26 (4), 150–154.

Declaration of Good Health and Good Character in Support of an Application for Admission to a Part of the Nursing and Midwifery Council's Professional Register

(Reproduced with permission of the Nursing and Midwifery Council (NMC).)

I ……………………………………………… NMC PIN …………………………………

to the best of my knowledge of:

(full name of applicant) ………………………………………………………………….

whose NMC PIN is ……………………………………………………………………….

believe the above-named student's health and character are sufficiently good to enable safe and effective practice and that there is an intention to comply with the Code of Professional Conduct: NMC Standards for Conduct, Performance and Ethics. I also support their application to be entered in the professional register for nurses and midwives.

Signature* ……………………………………………………..……… Date ………………

Post held ……………………………………………………………………………………..

Stamp of education/training institution

*The individual signing this form must be registered with the NMC and should be the nursing registrant responsible for directing the educational programme. For midwifery programmes, this should be the lead midwife for education. In signing this supporting declaration of good health and good character, the individual should take account of the personal responsibilities and accountability that professional registration confers upon those practitioners registered with the NMC.

Sample Unit With Its Elements and One Element of Competence With Its Associated Performance Criteria

EXTRACT FROM NATIONAL VOCATIONAL QUALIFICATIONS (NVQS) IN HEALTH AND SOCIAL CARE LEVEL 3 – UNIT HSC35 AND ELEMENT HSC35A (SKILLS FOR HEALTH 2005)

Unit title: Promote choice, well-being and the protection of all individuals

About this unit

For this unit, you are expected to protect individuals whilst respecting their diversity, difference, preferences and choice.

Elements of competence

HSC35a Develop supportive relationships that promote choice and independence

HSC35b Respect the diversity and difference of individuals and key people

HSC35c Contribute to the protection of all individuals

Element HSC35a Develop supportive relationships that promote choice and independence

Performance criteria

You need to show that:

1. You respect the dignity and privacy of individuals and key people
2. You treat and value each person as an individual and ensure that the support you give takes account of their needs and preferences
3. You work with individuals and key people in ways that provide support that is consistent with individuals' beliefs, culture, values and preferences
4. You provide active support to enable individuals to participate in activities and maintain their independence
5. You support others with whom you work to work in ways that:
   • recognise and respect individuals' beliefs and preferences

   • take account of individuals' preferences in everything they do
   • acknowledge and respect diversity and difference
6. You reflect on, and challenge:
   • your own assumptions, behaviour and ways of working
   • the assumptions of others, their behaviour and ways of working
   • procedures, practices and information that are discriminatory
7. You seek advice when you are having difficulty promoting equality and diversity

SCOPE FOR ELEMENT HSC35A: DEVELOP SUPPORTIVE RELATIONSHIPS THAT PROMOTE CHOICE AND INDEPENDENCE. EXTRACT FROM NVQS IN HEALTH AND SOCIAL CARE LEVEL 3 – UNIT HSC35 AND ELEMENT HSC35A (SKILLS FOR HEALTH 2005)

Scope

Actions that could adversely affect the use of evidence in future investigations include: asking inappropriate and/or leading questions, not following organisation and legal procedures, putting undue pressure on individuals.

Communicate

Includes using: the individual's preferred spoken language; the use of signs, symbols, pictures, writing, objects of reference, communication passports, other nonverbal forms of communication, human and technological aids to communication.

Danger

Includes: imminent, in the short term, in the medium term, in the longer term.

Harm and abuse

Includes: neglect; physical, emotional and sexual abuse; bullying; self-harm; reckless behaviour.

Key people

Includes: family, friends, carers, others with whom the individual has a supportive relationship.

Risks

Include the possibility of: danger, damage and destruction to the environment and goods; injury and harm to people; self-harm; bullying; abuse; reckless behaviour.

Statements that could adversely affect the use of evidence in future investigations

Include: changing information, removing information, adding to information.

KNOWLEDGE AND UNDERSTANDING FOR UNIT HSC35: PROMOTE CHOICE, WELL-BEING AND THE PROTECTION OF ALL INDIVIDUALS. EXTRACT FROM NVQS IN HEALTH AND SOCIAL CARE LEVEL 3 – UNIT HSC35 (SKILLS FOR HEALTH 2005)

Knowledge specification for the whole of this unit

Competent practice is a combination of the application of skills and knowledge informed by values and ethics. This specification details the knowledge and understanding required to carry out competent practice in the performance described in this unit. When using this specification, it is important to read the knowledge requirements in relation to expectations and requirements of your job role.

You need to show that you know, understand and can apply in practice:

Values

1. Legal and organisational requirements on equality, diversity, discrimination, rights, confidentiality and sharing of information
2. How to provide active support and place the preferences and best interest of individuals at the centre of everything you do
3. Dilemmas between:
   - individuals' rights and their responsibilities for their own care and protection, the rights and responsibilities of key people and your role and responsibilities for their care and protection
   - individuals' views, preferences and expectations and how these can and are being met

- your own values and those of the individuals and key people
- your own professional values and those of others within and outside your organisations

4. How to work in partnership with individuals, key people and those within and outside your organisation to enable the individuals' needs, wishes and preferences to be met
5. Methods that are effective:
   - in promoting equality and diversity
   - when dealing with and challenging discrimination

Legislation and organisational policy and procedures

6. Codes of practice and conduct and standards and guidance relevant to your own and the roles, responsibilities, accountability and duties of others for valuing and respecting individuals and key people, taking account of their views and preferences and protecting them from danger, harm and abuse
7. Current local, national and European legislation and organisational requirements, procedures and practices for:
   - data protection, including recording, reporting, storage, security and sharing of information
   - health and safety
   - risk assessment and management
   - dealing with comments and complaints
   - the protection of yourself, individuals, key people and others from danger, harm and abuse
   - working with others to provide integrated services
8. Practice and service standards relevant to your work setting and relating to valuing and respecting individuals and key people, taking account of their views and preferences and protecting them from danger, harm and abuse
9. How to access records and information on the needs, views and preferences of individuals and key people
10. The purpose of, and arrangements for, your supervision and appraisal
    - **Theory and practice**
11. How and where to access information and support that **can inform your practice relating to valuing and respecting people, taking ac**count of their views and preferences and protecting them from danger, harm and abuse
12. Theories relevant to the individuals with whom you work, about:
    - human growth and development
    - identity and self-esteem

- loss and change
- power and how it can be used and abused

13. The effects of stress and distress
14. Role of relationships and support networks in promoting the well-being of individuals
15. Factors that affect the health, well-being, behaviour, skills, abilities and development of individuals and key people with whom you work
16. Methods of supporting individuals to:
    - express their needs and preferences
    - understand and take responsibility for promoting their own health and care
    - identify how their care needs should be met
    - assess and manage risks to their health and well-being
17. Factors that may lead to danger, harm and abuse
18. How to protect yourself, individuals, key people and others with whom you work from danger, harm and abuse
19. Signs and symptoms of danger, harm and abuse
20. Correct actions to take when you suspect danger, harm and abuse or where it has been disclosed
21. The types of evidence that is valid in investigations and court, actions and statements that could contaminate the use of evidence
22. Methods that are effective in forming, maintaining and ending relationships with individuals and key people
23. Different ways of communicating with individuals, families, carers, groups and communities about choice, well-being and protection

(Reproduced with permission of Skills for Health and Skills for Care and Development from Skills for Health website, http://www.skillsforhealth.org.uk. Accessed: December 2005. National Occupational Standards are reviewed and updated on a regular basis: see the National Occupational Standards Directory website, http://www.ukstandards.org.uk.)

Skills Checklist

GUIDELINES ON THE USE OF THIS RECORD OF ACHIEVEMENT

This record section is designed to help you direct your learning in relation to your clinical skills development and assist you in keeping a record of your progress. You may find it is useful in providing additional evidence for your professional portfolio.

It lists the core skills addressed within the main text. Clearly, the list of skills is not exhaustive; in recognition of this fact, spaces are included for you to add any skills unique to your personal learning experiences.

It is suggested that you initial and date the first column when you have been instructed in or studied the theoretical underpinnings of the skill and initial and date the other columns when:

Level 1 – you have observed the procedure in the practice setting

Level 2 – you have participated in the skill under direct supervision

Level 3 – you have performed the skill on a number of occasions and now require minimal supervision

Level 4 – you can perform the skill safely and competently, giving the rationale for your actions

Level 5 – you have taught the skill to others

It is recommended that initials denoting achievement of Levels 4 and 5 be those of a registered nurse assessor, although this will clearly require local negotiation, as this document is not intended to circumvent your locally determined summative assessment(s) of practice.

When performing each skill, remember it is important to not only exhibit the psychomotor element but also the affective and cognitive components (i.e., attitude and knowledge).

TABLE A3.1 Skills Related to the Activity of Breathing						
Skill	**Instructed/Studied**	**1**	**2**	**3**	**4**	**5**
Assess individual's ability to breathe normally						
Monitor and record respiratory rate						
Monitor and record peak flow						
Maintain airway of:						
infant						
child						
adult						
Monitor and record expectorant						
Disposal of sputum secretions						
Obtain sputum specimen						
Maintain safe administration of oxygen as prescribed via:						
mask						
nasal cannulae						
humidifier						
Perform rescue breathing (artificial respiration):						
infant/child/adult						

TABLE A3.2   Skills Related to the Activity of Mobility

Skill	Instructed/Studied	1	2	3	4	5
Assess individual's ability to mobilize safely						
Care of self						
Assess task, individual capacity, load and environment						
Move inanimate objects						
Moving and handling of a range of clients into the following positions:						
upright						
recumbent						
semirecumbent						
lateral						
semiprone (recovery)						
prone						
side to side						
Move a range of clients from:						
chair to chair						
bed to chair						
chair to bed						
up the bed						
up in the chair						
cot						
Care for an individual who is falling						
Care for the individual who has fallen						

TABLE A3.3   Skills Related to the Activity of Personal Cleansing and Dressing

Skill	Instructed/Studied	1	2	3	4	5
Make a bed/cot that is:						
unoccupied						
occupied						
Changing a sheet on an occupied bed:						
top to bottom						
side to side						
Dispose of linen that is:						
uncontaminated						
contaminated						
Assist individuals requiring a:						
shower						
general bath						
wash						
Assist individuals maintain their oral hygiene:						
cleansing of teeth/dentures/mucous membranes						
use of mouthwashes/dental floss/interdental sticks						
Administration of eye care						

Continued

TABLE A3.3	**Skills Related to the Activity of Personal Cleansing and Dressing—cont'd**						
Skill	**Instructed/Studied**	**1**	**2**	**3**	**4**	**5**
Facial shaving:						
with a safety razor						
with an electric shaver						
Care of hair:						
washing in bed						
dealing with infestation						
Assist a variety of individuals to dress:						
infant						
child						
adult						

TABLE A3.4	**Related to the Activity of Maintaining a Safe Environment**						
Skill	**Instructed/Studied**	**1**	**2**	**3**	**4**	**5**
Universal precautions—effective:						
handwashing						
use of gloves						
use of plastic aprons						
safe disposal of equipment						
Adheres to Health and Safety at Work						
Act in relation to:						
disinfection policies						
disposal of infected materials						
dealing with mercury spillage						
dealing with blood and body fluids						
Radiation:						
report untoward occurrences						
Perform a simple dressing using aseptic						
technique						
Obtain a wound swab						
Monitor pulse:						
radial						
carotid						
apex						
femoral						
Monitor and record blood pressure using:						
a mercury sphygmomanometer						
an aneroid sphygmomanometer						
an electronic device						
Administration of medicines (under direct						
supervision in keeping with trust policies)						
Storage of medicines						
Respond in the event of an actual or						
suspected fire						
Respond in the event of a cardiac arrest						
Respond in the event of other emergency						
(state type)						

TABLE A3.5 Skills Related to the Activity of Eating and Drinking

Skill	Instructed/Studied	1	2	3	4	5
Assess individual's nutritional status						
Assist clients in selecting appropriate meals/ fluids						
Monitor and record nutritional intake						
Monitor and record fluid balance						
Assist clients with feeding						
Assist clients with drinking						
Feed dependent clients						
Recognize and report changes in clients' condition						
Provide first aid to a client who is choking						

TABLE A3.6 Skills Related to the Activity of Communicating

Skill	Instructed/Studied	1	2	3	4	5
Respond appropriately to telephone calls						
Assess the communication needs of clients						
Communicate effectively with clients who have a:						
hearing difficulty						
speaking difficulty						
language difficulty						
comprehension difficulty						
Manage a client exhibiting an aggressive outburst						
Recognize and report changes in clients' condition						
Give and receive reports of clients' condition: orally						

TABLE A3.7 Skills Related to the Activity of Dying

Skill	Instructed/Studied	1	2	3	4	5
Communicate with dying patients						
Communicate with relatives of dying patients						
Communicate with the bereaved						
Perform last offices						

TABLE A3.8 Skills Related to the Activity of Eliminating						
Skill	Instructed/Studied	1	2	3	4	5
Assess individual's ability to eliminate effectively						
Assist clients to use:						
bedpan						
urinal						
toilet/commode						
Apply/change a nappy						
Empty a catheter bag						
Monitor and record urinary output						
Monitor and record bowel actions						
Monitor and record vomit/gastric aspirate						
Obtain specimen of urine/faeces/vomit for laboratory examination						
Identify and report changes in client's condition						

TABLE A3.9 Skills Related to the Activity of Maintaining Body Temperature						
Skill	Instructed/Studied	1	2	3	4	5
Assess an individual's ability to maintain a normal body temperature						
Assist individual's select suitable attire to maintain a normal body temperature						
Monitor and accurately record the temperature of a(n):						
infant						
child						
adult						
Orally						
Axillary						
Aurally						
Using fever strips						
Use appropriate strategies to raise body temperature						
Use appropriate strategies to lower body temperature						
Participate in the assessment of clients' ability to maintain body temperature						

TABLE A3.10 Skills Related to the Activity of Expressing Sexuality						
Skill	**Instructed/Studied**	**1**	**2**	**3**	**4**	**5**
Maintain privacy and dignity						
Assess individual's ability to express their sexuality:						
child						
adult						
Assist individuals express their sexuality:						
child						
adult						

TABLE A3.11 Skills Related to the Activity of Working and Playing						
Skill	**Instructed/Studied**	**1**	**2**	**3**	**4**	**5**
Assess individual's ability to work and play						
Assist individual's select appropriate work activities						
Assist individual's select appropriate recreational activities						

TABLE A3.12 Skills Related to the Activity of Sleep and Rest						
Skill	**Instructed/Studied**	**1**	**2**	**3**	**4**	**5**
Assess individual's needs related to sleep and rest						
Monitor and record individual's sleep and rest patterns						
Assist individuals to achieve a balance between activity and rest						

TABLE A3.13 Additional Skills						
Skill	**Instructed/Studied**	**1**	**2**	**3**	**4**	**5**

(Reproduced by permission of John Wiley & Sons Ltd, from
Hilton PA. Record of achievement. In: Hilton PA, Fundamental
Nursing Skills. Whurr Publishers Ltd., London:2004, pp. 306–313.)

Professional Behaviours Inventory

1. RELIABILITY IN CARE DELIVERY WITHIN EXPECTED CAPABILITY

Achieved

Exceptionally reliable at all times

Achieved

Very good level of reliability

Achieved

Satisfactory level of reliability

Not achieved

Unreliable

2. ATTENDING TO CLIENTS' NEEDS AND REQUESTS WITHIN EXPECTED CAPABILITY

Achieved

Exceptionally attentive and conscientious at all times

Achieved

Very attentive and conscientious

Achieved

Satisfactory level of attention and response paid to clients' needs and requests

Not achieved

Insufficient level of attention and response paid to clients' needs and requests

3. CONSISTENCY OF EFFORTS TO ACHIEVE THE REQUISITE STANDARD OF CARE

Achieved

Constantly and consistently makes best efforts in pursuit of excellence

Achieved

Constantly makes good effort to achieve high standards of care

Achieved

Makes satisfactory effort to achieve high standards of care

Not achieved

Perfunctory effort made to achieve required standard of care

4A. RELATING AND WORKING WITH COLLEAGUES AND OTHER TEAM MEMBERS

Achieved

Outstanding ability to work as a team member

Achieved

Good ability to work as a team member

Achieved

Functions satisfactorily as a team member

Not achieved

Uncooperative in the team

4B. RELATING AND WORKING WITH COLLEAGUES AND OTHER TEAM MEMBERS

Achieved

Contributes very actively

Achieved

Contributes well

Achieved

Makes occasional contributions

Not achieved

Does not contribute to the team

4C. RELATING AND WORKING WITH COLLEAGUES AND OTHER TEAM MEMBERS

Achieved	Achieved	Achieved	Not achieved
Has outstanding rapport	Has good rapport	Has satisfactory rapport	Unable to establish rapport

5A. ACKNOWLEDGEMENT OF COLLEAGUES' EXPERIENCE AND OPINIONS

Achieved	Achieved	Achieved	Not achieved
Polite, listens carefully and highly respectful of colleagues' experience and opinions at all times	Listens carefully and shows a good level of respect for colleagues' experience and opinions most of the time	Satisfactory level of respect for colleagues' experience and opinions most of the time	Poor respect for colleagues' experiences and opinions

5B. ACKNOWLEDGEMENT OF COLLEAGUES' EXPERIENCE AND OPINIONS

Achieved	Achieved	Achieved	Not achieved
Manages differences of opinion very well	Manages differences of opinion well	Manages differences of opinion fairly well	Unable to manage differences of opinions

6. MANAGEMENT OF PERSONAL OPINIONS

Achieved	Achieved	Achieved	Not achieved
Outstanding ability to contain and voice own opinions	Good ability to contain and voice own opinions	Some difficulty in containing and voicing own opinions	Voices own opinions inappropriately

7. RECOGNITION OF OWN LIMITATIONS WITHIN EXPECTED CAPABILITY

Achieved	Achieved	Achieved	Not achieved
Outstanding level of self-awareness and ability to recognize own limitations	Good self-awareness and recognition of own limitations	Satisfactory self-awareness and recognition of own limitations	Limited self-awareness; unaware of own limitations; potentially unsafe

8A. RESPONSE TO FEEDBACK

Achieved	Achieved	Achieved	Not achieved
Responds positively and in a mature manner to constructive feedback at all times; considers it carefully	Responds positively and in a mature manner to constructive feedback most of the time	Has some difficulty in responding appropriately to constructive feedback	Resents criticism; reluctant to accept feedback

8B. RESPONSE TO FEEDBACK

Achieved	Achieved	Achieved	Not achieved
Uses feedback to inform practice at all times	Uses feedback to inform practice most of the time	Uses feedback to inform practice some of the time	Does not change practice through feedback

9A. VERBAL AND NONVERBAL INTERPERSONAL SKILLS

Achieved	**Achieved**	**Achieved**	**Not achieved**
Verbal communication and interpersonal skills are congruent, clear, effective and appropriate at all times	Verbal communication and interpersonal skills are congruent, clear and appropriate most of the time	Verbal communication and interpersonal skills are satisfactory most of the time	Poor interpersonal skills; frequently gives mixed messages

9B. VERBAL AND NONVERBAL INTERPERSONAL SKILLS

Achieved	**Achieved**	**Achieved**	**Not achieved**
Nonverbal communication and interpersonal skills are congruent, clear, effective and appropriate at all times	Nonverbal communication and interpersonal skills are congruent, clear and appropriate most of the time	Nonverbal communication and interpersonal skills are satisfactory most of the time	Poor interpersonal skills; frequently gives mixed messages

10A. COMMUNICATION WITH WOMEN AND THEIR PARTNERS WITHIN EXPECTED CAPABILITY

Achieved	**Achieved**	**Achieved**	**Not achieved**
Exceptionally reassuring and supportive	Makes very good efforts to reassure and support	Satisfactory ability to reassure and support	Does not provide adequate reassurance and supporting care

10B. COMMUNICATION WITH WOMEN AND THEIR PARTNERS WITHIN EXPECTED CAPABILITY

Achieved	**Achieved**	**Achieved**	**Not achieved**
Very encouraging of their involvement as partners in care	Encouraging of their involvement as partners in care	Satisfactory ability to involve them as partners in care	Discourages their participation as partners

11. PROMOTION OF FAIR AND ANTIDISCRIMINATORY PRACTICE

Achieved	**Achieved**	**Achieved**	**Not achieved**
Actively promotes fair and antidiscriminatory practice at all times; always alert to discriminatory practice	Always maintains fair and antidiscriminatory practice; will recognize and act on evidence of discriminatory practice	Does not knowingly permit unfair or discriminatory practice; shows satisfactory awareness of the same	Shows poor awareness of fair and antidiscriminatory practice or promotes discriminatory practice

12. RESPECT FOR WOMEN AND THEIR FAMILIES

Achieved	**Achieved**	**Achieved**	**Not achieved**
Shows exceptional and consistent level of respect for women and their families	Very respectful of women and their families	Satisfactory level of respect for women and their families	Poor level of respect for women and their families

13. PROMOTION OF RIGHTS FOR WOMEN AND FAMILIES

Achieved	**Achieved**	**Achieved**	**Not achieved**
Always actively promotes rights for women and families; always alert to circumstances where rights may be overlooked	Always maintains rights for women and families; will recognise and act on evidence of rights being overlooked	Does not knowingly permit breach of rights for women and families; shows satisfactory awareness of the same	Shows poor awareness of, or disregards, rights for women and families

14. OBSERVATION OF ETHICAL PRACTICE

Achieved	**Achieved**	**Achieved**	**Not achieved**
Extremely effective in identifying ethical aspects of care and raising or handling ethical issues skilfully and collaboratively	Identifies ethical aspects of care well and always raises or handles ethical issues appropriately and collaboratively	Satisfactory awareness of ethical aspects of care, reflected in care given	Poor awareness of ethical aspects of care or handles ethical issues inappropriately

15. ATTENTION TO PROFESSIONAL APPEARANCE AND DRESS CODE

Achieved	**Achieved**	**Achieved**	**Not achieved**
Always maintains exemplary standard of professional appearance and dress code	Very good standard of professional appearance and dress code	Satisfactory standard of professional appearance and dress code	Careless or unprofessional standard of appearance and dress code

16. PUNCTUALITY AND TIMEKEEPING

Achieved	**Achieved**	**Achieved**	**Not achieved**
Completely dependable; always punctual	Very good level of reliability; usually punctual or communicates appropriately if unavoidably delayed	Satisfactory time-keeping; satisfactory communication if delayed	Unreliable; poor timekeeper and/or poor at communicating when delayed

INDEX

Page numbers followed by "*f*" indicate figures, "*t*" indicate tables, and "*b*" indicate boxes.